RENAL STONE DISEASE 2

RENAL STONE DISEASE 2

2nd International Urolithiasis Research Symposium

Indianapolis, Indiana 17 – 18 April 2008

EDITORS

Andrew P. Evan
Indiana University School of Medicine
Indianapolis, Indiana

James E. Lingeman
Methodist Hospital Institute for Kidney Stone Disease
Indianapolis, Indiana

James A. McAteer
Indiana University School of Medicine
Indianapolis, Indiana

James C. Williams, Jr.
Indiana University School of Medicine
Indianapolis, Indiana

All papers have been peer reviewed

SPONSORING ORGANIZATION
International Kidney Stone Institute

AMERICAN INSTITUTE OF PHYSICS

Melville, New York, 2008
AIP CONFERENCE PROCEEDINGS ■ VOLUME 1049

Editors:

Andrew P. Evan, Ph.D.
Department of Anatomy and Cell Biology
Indiana University School of Medicine
635 Barnhill Drive, MS 5035
Indianapolis, IN 46202-5120
United States

E-mail: evan@anatomy.iupui.edu

James A. McAteer, Ph.D.
Department of Anatomy and Cell Biology
Indiana University School of Medicine
635 Barnhill Drive, MS 5035
Indianapolis, IN 46202-5120
United States

E-mail: mcateer@anatomy.iupui.edu

James E. Lingeman, M.D.
Methodist Hospital Institute
for Kidney Stone Disease
1801 North Senate Boulevard
Suite 220
Indianapolis, IN 46202

E-mail: jlingeman@clarian.org

James C. Williams, Jr. Ph.D.
Department of Anatomy and Cell Biology
Indiana University School of Medicine
635 Barnhill Drive, MS 5035
Indianapolis, IN 46202-5120
United States

E-mail: williams@anatomy.iupui.edu

L.C. Catalog Card No. 2008935055
ISBN 978-0-7354-0577-6
ISSN 0094-243X
Printed in the United States of America

CONTENTS

III. URETERAL STENTS AND PHYSIOLOGY

IV. CLINICAL BIOLOGY OF STONE FORMERS

V. PROGRESS IN SHOCK WAVE LITHOTRIPSY

VI. OTHER TOPICS IN UROLITHIASIS RESEARCH

PREFACE

The 1st International Urolithiasis Research Symposium, held in Indianapolis, Indiana in November of 2006 was a remarkable success. Clearly the subject matter that dealt with the latest developments in the field of kidney stone disease and the unique format of the discussion periods allowed for an exciting atmosphere resulting in a robust interaction between the faculty and audience. There was an overwhelming response from the scientists, physicians and industrial representatives who attended this meeting that IKSI should continue organizing such symposiums in the future.

It was with great enthusiasm and anticipation that IKSI organized the 2nd International Urolithiasis Research Symposium in Indianapolis on April 17-18, 2008. The primary emphasis of the 2nd symposium was focused on several new concerns that have developed in this field. First, there have been several excellent studies showing a worrisome increase in the prevalence of calcium phosphate stones, a kidney stone that is much more difficult to treat than are calcium oxalate stones. What are the factors driving the conversion of calcium oxalate to calcium phosphate? Second, it is clear that a portion of the calcium oxalate stone formers develop bone disease, a condition that appears quite different from osteoporotic bone disease. How do these two bone disease differ? Lastly, substantial progress has been achieved recently to improve the safety of shock wave lithotripsy by manipulating the treatment protocols. What new protocols should the practicing urologist be implementing in his/her practice?

We would like to express our appreciation to the researchers/physicians who joined IKSI in Indianapolis to present and discuss their newest data. We also appreciate the outstanding effort and dedication of the International Kidney Stone Institute staff, Katy Cantor, and Hillary McCarley as well as professional skills of Cathy Sprunger. Finally, we are deeply appreciative for the support of the Methodist Health Foundation, of which the International Kidney Stone Institute is a component, as well as Clarian Health Partners and Indiana University School of Medicine for their support.

Andrew P. Evan, Ph.D.
James E. Lingeman, M.D.

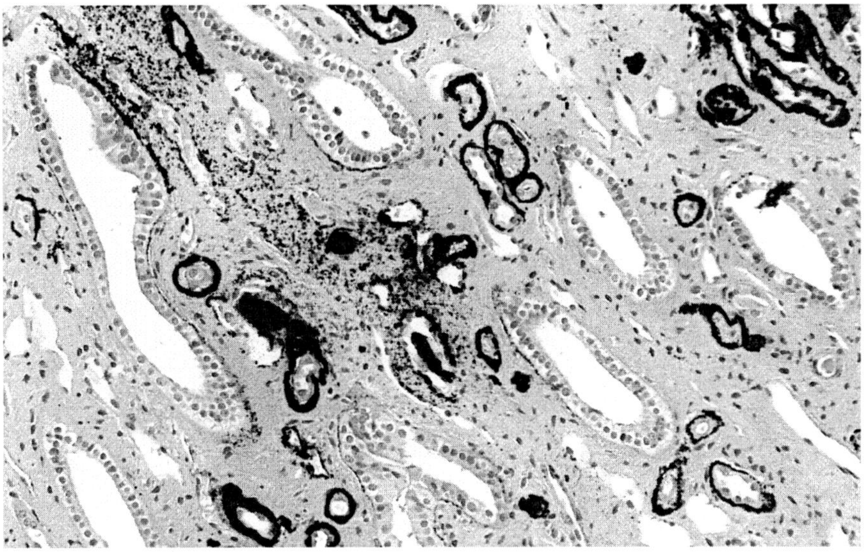

COVER IMAGE. Human papillary biopsy, stained with Yasue to show sites of calcium deposition (dark regions). It is these interstitial calcifications that coalesce to form Randall's plaque. Image courtesy of A.P. Evan.

THE INTERNATIONAL KIDNEY STONE INSTITUTE

The International Kidney Stone Institute (IKSI) is a charitable organization dedicated to supporting clinical and basic science research and education for the detection, management and prevention of kidney stone disease.

The Institute was established in 2004 by urologist James E. Lingeman, M.D. and kidney researcher Andrew P. Evan, Ph.D., to guide research in stone disease and to channel resources toward projects that deliver positive results in stone disease treatment and prevention. The International Kidney Stone Institute recognizes the accomplishments of kidney researchers and physicians who have:

- pioneered advances in minimally invasive treatments to clear stones from the body;
- dramatically refined the medical management of stone patients; and
- localized the site of stone formation in the kidney, a critical step toward developing strategies to prevent stones from forming.

Research initiatives of the International Kidney Stone Institute include:

- shock wave lithotripsy improvement
- studies in percutaneous kidney stone removal
- Randall's plaque and the prevention of stone disease
- dietary studies
- study of kidney stones in the bariatric population
- stone treatment and hypertension/bone disease

Education initiatives of the International Kidney Stone Institute include:

• Programs and conferences

IKSI will host its 3rd Urolithiasis Research Symposium on December 3-4, 2009, in Indianapolis. In addition, the Institute is developing educational programs and materials that will provide patients, medical care providers, school-age children and the general public with helpful information regarding kidney stone disease.

• Online atlas

A Web-based reference and resource of images and clinical scenarios from representative stone patients is now in development and will enable researchers and physicians worldwide to explore diagnoses, clinical decision-making, treatment options and outcomes.

• Fellowships

A two-year fellowship in stone disease and minimally invasive urology has been offered since 1990 by Methodist Hospital in affiliation with the Indiana University School of Medicine. The fellowship provides urologists who have completed their residency with an extensive clinical and basic science experience in all aspects of kidney stone disease. The fellowship is organized and approved by the Endourology Society.

SPONSORS FOR THE 2ND INTERNATIONAL UROLITHIASIS RESEARCH SYMPOSIUM

Platinum

Boston Scientific Corporation

Gold

Cook Urological, Inc.
Gyrus ACMI
National Institutes of Health (NIH)

Silver

Advanced Shockwave Technology, Inc.
Applied Medical
Cybersonics, Inc.
Direx
Litholink Corporation
Lumenis, Inc.
Mission Pharmacal
Olympus Surgical America
Quest Diagnostics, Inc.

Crystal

Bard Urological Division
Beck Analytical Services, LLC
Convergent Laser Technologies
Electro Medical Systems, (EMS)
Elsevier
FMD
Kosin Technologies
Laser Peripherals/Clarus Medical
PercSys

Corporate Donors

Clarian Health Partners, Inc.
Indiana University School of Medicine,
Department of Anatomy & Cell Biology
Methodist Health Foundation
Methodist Urology, LLC

Funding for this conference was made possible (in part) by grant R13 DK078503 from the National Institute of Diabetes and Digestive and Kidney Diseases (NIDDK). The views expressed in written conference materials or publications and by speakers and moderators do not necessarily reflect the official policies of the Department of Health and Human Services; nor does mention of trade names, commercial practices, or organizations imply endorsement by the U.S. Government.

2ND INTERNATIONAL UROLITHIASIS RESEARCH SYMPOSIUM

ORGANIZING COMMITTEE

Andrew P. Evan, PhD.
James E. Lingeman, M.D.
Fredric L. Coe, M.D.
Elaine M. Worcester, M.D.
James A. McAteer, Ph.D.
James C. Williams, Jr., Ph.D.
Philip M. Blomgren

With special thanks to:
Katy Cantor
Hillary McCarley
and
Cathy Sprunger

Sponsoring organization:
The International Kidney Stone Institute
P.O. Box 7168
Indianapolis, IN 46207-7168
(317) 962-9043
www.iksi.org

INTERNATIONAL KIDNEY STONE INSTITUTE ADVISORY BOARD

Mission Statement

The International Kidney Stone Institute (IKSI) is a charitable organization established to raise funds for clinical and basic science research, and education for the prevention, detection, and management of kidney stone disease. Further, it is the goal of the International Kidney Stone Institute to promote the highest standards of Urological clinical care.

Thursday, April 17, 2008

6:30-7:30 a.m.	Registration and Continental Breakfast	
7:30-7:35 a.m.	Introduction to the meeting	James E. Lingeman, M.D. Indianapolis, Indiana
7:35-7:55 a.m.	Pathogenesis of stone disease	Elaine M. Worcester, M.D. Chicago, Illinois
7:55-8:15 a.m.	Surgical treatment of stone disease	Glenn M. Preminger, M.D. Durham, North Carolina

Session 1 Factors that regulate normal and abnormal mineralization: Session I

Moderators: Sharon Moe, M.D., Indianapolis, Indiana
David A. Bushinsky, M.D., Rochester, New York

8:15-8:30 a.m.	Hypercalciuric bone disease	Murray J. Favus, M.D. Chicago, Illinois
8:40-8:55 a.m.	Bone genes and other determinants of pathologic calcification in blood vessels	Marc McKee, Ph.D. Montreal, Canada
9:05-9:20 a.m.	Bone genes in kidney of stone formers	Andrew P. Evan, Ph.D. Indianapolis, Indiana
9:30-9:45 a.m.	Cell biology of thiazide bone effects	Gerardo Gamba, M.D., Ph.D. Mexico City, Mexico
9:55-10:15 a.m.	Break	

Session 2 Factors that regulate normal and abnormal mineralization: Session II

Moderators: Murray J. Favus, M.D., Chicago, Illinois
Joseph Bidwell, Ph.D., Indianapolis, Indiana

10:15-10:30 a.m.	Bone proton receptor regulation of mineralization	David A. Bushinsky, M.D. Rochester, New York
10:40-10:55 a.m.	Pyrophosphate transport and stones	John Sayer, Ph.D. Newcastle Upon Tyne, United Kingdom
11:05-11:20 a.m.	FGF-23, Klotho and Leptin in regulation of mineral dynamics	Orson W. Moe, M.D. Dallas, Texas
11:55 a.m.-12:40 p.m.	Lunch	

Session 3 **Medullary and papillary cell biology**

Moderators: Lise Bankir, Ph.D., Paris, France
Andrew P. Evan, Ph.D., Indianapolis, Indiana

12:40-12:55 p.m.	IMCD cell biology—proton and urea transport	Susan Wall, Ph.D. Atlanta, Georgia
1:05-1:20 p.m.	New animal model of interstitial plaque, OPN/THP knockout	Xue-Ru Wu, M.D. New York, New York
1:30-1:45 p.m.	Papillary epithelial cells in stone disease — new cell line	Hari K. Koul, Ph.D. Denver, Colorado
1:55-2:10 p.m.	Production of hyaluronan by interstitial cells	Louise Rugheimer, Ph.D. Uppsala, Sweden
2:20-2:35 p.m.	Hyaluronan and stone disease	Marino Asselman, M.D. Rotterdam, The Netherlands
2:45-3:00 p.m.	Stones in idiopathic calcium oxalate stone disease are attached to sites of interstitial plaque	Nicole L. Miller, M.D. Nashville, Tennessee
3:10-3:30 p.m.	Break	

Session 4 **Ureteral stents and physiology**

Moderators: Stephen P. Dretler, M.D., Boston, Massachusetts
James E. Lingeman, M.D., Indianapolis, Indiana

3:30-3:45 p.m.	Implications of biofilm formation on urological devices	Peter Cadieux, Ph.D. London, Ontario
3:55-4:10 p.m.	Drug eluting stents: in vitro studies	Ben H. Chew, M.D. Vancouver, B.C.
4:20-4:35 p.m.	Drug eluting urological stents: fact or fiction	John D. Denstedt, M.D. London, Ontario
4:45-5:00 p.m.	Ureteral stents: new designs and materials	Manoj Monga, M.D. Minneapolis, Minnesota
5:10-5:25 p.m.	Dynamic and static models for the assessment of biofilm and encrustation formation on urological materials	Sean P. Gorman, Ph.D. Belfast, Ireland
5:35-5:50 p.m.	Ureteral stent coatings: what is here and what is coming?	Hassan Razvi, M.D. London, Ontario
6:30-8:30 p.m.	Reception/Poster Session	

Friday, April 18, 2008

6:30-7:30 a.m. Continental Breakfast

Session 5 **Clinical biology of stone formers**

Moderators: John R. Asplin, M.D., Chicago, Illinois
David S. Goldfarb, M.D., New York, New York

7:30-7:45 a.m.	Circadian variations of stone risk	Elaine M. Worcester, M.D. Chicago, Illinois
7:55-8:10 a.m.	Bariatric surgery and stone disease	John C. Lieske, M.D. Rochester, Minnesota
8:20-8:35 a.m.	Uric acid and diabetes	Naim M. Maalouf, M.D. Dallas, Texas
8:45-9:00 a.m.	Kidney stone morphology—implications for stone pathogenesis	Michel Daudon, Ph.D. Paris, France
9:10-9:25 a.m.	Very long follow-up of treated stone patients	Fredric L. Coe, M.D. Chicago, Illinois
9:35-9:55 a.m.	Break	

Session 6 **Progress in shock wave lithotripsy**

Moderators: Lawrence A. Crum, Ph.D., Seattle, Washington
Stephen Y. Nakada, M.D., Madison, Wisconsin

9:55-10:10 a.m.	The advantage of a broad focal zone in SWL	Robin O. Cleveland, Ph.D. Boston, Massachusetts
10:20-10:35 a.m.	Standards for lithotriptor performance	Reiner Schultheiss, Ph.D. Illighausen, Switzerland
10:45-11:00 a.m.	The characteristics of broad and narrow focal zone lithotriptors	Yuri Pishchalnikov, Ph.D. Indianapolis, Indiana
11:10-11:25 a.m.	Treatment protocols to reduce injury and improve stone breakage in SWL	James A. McAteer, Ph.D. Indianapolis, Indiana
11:35-11:50 a.m.	Renal hemodynamics during SWL	Rajash K. Handa, Ph.D. Indianapolis, Indiana
12:00-12:45 p.m.	Lunch	
12:45-1:00 p.m.	Outcomes assessment in SWL	David A. Tolley, M.D. Edinburgh, UK
1:10-1:25 p.m.	Determining the SW-treatment endpoint	Michael R. Bailey, Ph.D. Seattle, Washington
1:35-1:50 p.m.	Real-time monitoring of lithotriptor performance	Tim Leighton, Ph.D. Southampton, UK
2:00-2:15 p.m.	Perspective on lithotripsy adverse effects	Thomas Knoll, M.D. Mannheim, Germany

2:25-2:40 p.m.	Long-term effects of SWL and PNL	Amy E. Krambeck, M.D. Rochester, Minnesota
2:50-3:05 p.m.	Urolithiasis in space	Jeffrey A. Jones, M.D. Houston, Texas
3:15-3:45 p.m.	Meeting Summary: Pathogenesis of stone disease	Fredric L. Coe, M.D. Chicago, Illinois
3:45-4:15 p.m.	Meeting Summary: Urologic aspects	Margaret S. Pearle, M.D. Dallas, Texas
4:30 p.m.	Adjourn	

ACKNOWLEDGMENTS:
IKSI gratefully acknowledges the following for educational grants in support of this program:

Symposium Sponsor
Boston Scientific

Faculty Dinner Sponsor
Gyrus ACMI

Gold Level Sponsor
Cook Urological

Silver Level Sponsors
Applied Medical
AST Advanced Shockwave Technology GmBH
Direx Systems Corporation
Lumenis
Mission Pharmacal
Olympus America, Inc.
Quest Diagnostics

Bronze Level Sponsors
Convergent Laser Technologies
EMS Electro Medical Systems SA

OVERVIEW

Pathogenesis of Stone Disease

Elaine M. Worcester[a], Andrew P. Evan[b], and Fredric L. Coe[a]

[a] *Department of Medicine, Nephrology Section, MC 5100, University of Chicago, 5841 South Maryland Avenue, Chicago, Illinois, 60637, USA*
[b] *Department of Anatomy and Cell Biology, Indiana University School of Medicine, Indianapolis, IN 46202, USA*

Abstract. All stones share similar presenting symptoms, and urine supersaturation with respect to the mineral phase of the stone is essential for stone formation. However, recent studies using papillary biopsies of stone formers provide a view of the histology of renal crystal deposition which suggests that the early sequence of events leading to stone formation may differ depending on the type of stone and on the urine chemistry leading to supersaturation. Three general patterns of crystal deposition are seen: interstitial apatite plaque in idiopathic calcium oxalate stone formers, which is the site of stone attachment; tubule deposition of apatite, seen in all calcium phosphate stone formers; and mixtures of apatite and another crystal phase, such as cystine or calcium oxalate, seen in patients with cystinuria or enteric hyperoxaluria. The presence of apatite crystal in either the interstitial or tubule compartment (and sometimes both) of the renal medulla in stone formers is the rule, and has implications for the initial steps of stone formation and the potential for renal injury.

Keywords: Randall's plaque, nephrolithiasis, calcium oxalate, calcium phosphate
PACS: 87.15.nt; 87.19.X-

INTRODUCTION

All forms of nephrolithiasis share certain common features [1]. They all require that the urine of the stone former be supersaturated (at least temporarily) with respect to the components of the stone, so that crystals may form in the urinary tract. In the case of the most common types of stone, those composed primarily of calcium salts, there may also be a deficiency of biological inhibitors that hold crystal formation in check in the face of almost unrelenting supersaturation with respect to calcium oxalate in urine. The clinical outcomes of stone—renal colic and ureteral obstruction—are not dependent on the nature of the crystal.

However, in seeking to understand and treat patients with stone disease, we look beyond these common themes, to search for the factors that lead to formation of a specific stone type in a given individual.

CP1049, *Renal Stone Disease 2, 2nd International Urolithiasis Research Symposium,*
edited by A. P. Evan, J. E. Lingeman, J. A. McAteer, and J. C. Williams, Jr.

TAXONOMY OF STONE DISEASE

Mineral Composition

We are most familiar with categorizing stone disease by the type of mineral found in the stone. We distinguish among calcium (and further, between calcium phosphate or calcium oxalate; monohydrate or dihydrate), uric acid, cystine, struvite, and other rarer types of stone because we are aware that knowledge of the major mineral component of the stone provides useful information. The natural histories of these stone types differ, and stone type also has implications for pathophysiology and treatment (both medical and surgical). Determination of stone type rests ultimately on analysis of a passed stone, or of fragments passed after lithotripsy, using infrared spectroscopy or X-ray crystallography.

Pathophysiology of Supersaturation

Stone type is a faithful representation of the supersaturation present in urine when the stone formed [2], and the fact that stones are often recurrent testifies to the chronic nature of that supersaturation in many cases. Our treatments for stone prevention are largely based on methods to decrease supersaturation effectively, and so we are interested in the pathophysiology leading to specific types of supersaturation.

However, many pathways can lead to urinary supersaturation. As one example, increased calcium oxalate supersaturation may result from low urine volume or excessive excretion of calcium or oxalate, or combinations of these factors. Hypercalciuria and hyperoxaluria can each result from interaction of genetic susceptibility and environmental triggers, in varying proportions. For example, hyperoxaluria may result from rare autosomal recessive genetic disorders of oxalate synthesis (primary hyperoxaluria types 1 and 2 [3]), increased intestinal oxalate absorption secondary to malabsorptive disease (enteric hyperoxaluria [4]), dietary habits (high oxalate intake coupled with low calcium intake [5]), alteration in gut flora which may decrease oxalate degradation in the colon [6], and potentially abnormalities of anion transporters found in both gut and kidney [7].

Histopathology

Another way of looking at stone formation has recently emerged: studies of the renal papillary tissue of stone formers [8]. These studies have provided evidence that stone formers differ with respect to the sites of crystal deposition in renal tissue. Not only do patterns of crystal deposition and tissue injury differ between patients with different stone types, but differences have also emerged between stone formers with stones of similar composition, highlighting the various mechanisms by which stones may form.

INTERSTITIAL APATITE DEPOSITS: RANDALL'S PLAQUE

The characteristic histological finding in patients with calcium oxalate stones associated with idiopathic hypercalciuria is Randall's plaque [8], a mixture of calcium phosphate (as apatite) and macromolecules confined to the medullary interstitium except for its site of origin in the basement membrane of thin limbs of Henle. Individual plaque particles are composed of layers of apatite with interposed layers of macromolecular matrix; the nature and origin of this matrix is still undetermined, but osteopontin [9] and heavy chain 3 of inter-alpha-trypsin inhibitor [10] have been identified there. Within the interstitium, plaque forms a syncytium with islands of mineral in a sea of matrix. Of interest is the apparent lack of inflammatory reaction to the plaque material, or abnormalities in surrounding tubule cells or interstitium.

Plaque is seen on the surface of many papillae in stone formers, and more rarely in normal subjects; the amount of papillary surface covered by plaque correlates positively with urine calcium and inversely with urine volume and pH [11], factors that also increase urinary supersaturation with respect to calcium oxalate. However, despite the fact that the terminal collecting duct is exposed to elevated levels of supersaturation, no crystal deposition has been found in tubule lumens of idiopathic calcium stone formers [12], in striking contrast to the abundant interstitial mineral deposits. Renal calcium reabsorption is reduced in most patients with idiopathic hypercalciuria, but the nephron site of disordered reabsorption, and the mechanism by which the excess calcium gains access to the interstitium, is not yet known [13].

Calcium oxalate stones often grow attached to the renal papillae, and observation both at autopsy [14] and during percutaneous nephrolithotomy [15] confirms that apatite plaque is the site of attachment. Inspection of passed stones has shown that calcium oxalate stones often have a nidus of calcium phosphate, which may include calcified tubule profiles, suggesting that the stone formed as an overgrowth on interstitial plaque. Recent work has illuminated the process by which formation of a stone on plaque surface occurs.

Plaque Surface as the Initiating Site for Stone Formation

Plaque formation starts in the basement membrane of the thin limbs, but eventually moves into the interstitium and gradually extends downward in the papilla until it reaches the urothelial barrier. In order for stone overgrowth on plaque to occur, the papillary epithelium must be breached, and the way in which this occurs is still unknown. Exposure of plaque surface allows the supersaturated urine to come in contact with the plaque mineral and its organic matrix; urine, of course, contains many macromolecules that interact with mineral, as well. The process by which a stone forms in this milieu has been clarified by recent studies carried out during percutaneous nephrolithotomy, in which stones have been removed from papillae along with the underlying tissue **(Figure 1)**, and prepared in a manner that allows study of the plaque-stone interface [16]. The area of plaque underneath the stone, to which it is attached, can be seen as a white cuff beneath the stone **(Figure 1 panel a)**;

using micro-CT, the plaque is seen as the tail of mineral extending from the stone downward into the tissue **(Figure 1 panel b)**.

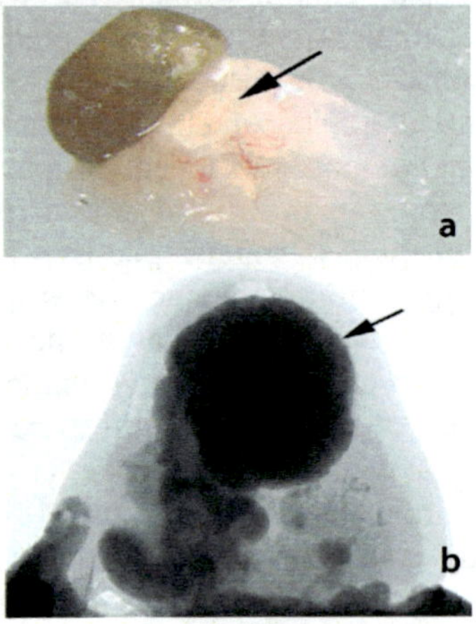

FIGURE 1. Attached stone with its tissue. **Panel a** shows *en bloc* biopsy of a calcium oxalate stone removed with its underlying papillary tissue. A white rim of plaque is below the stone (arrow). **Panel b** is a micro-CT shadow image of the stone (arrow) and displays a cuff of plaque extending downward from the base of the stone into the tissue.

Two stones were removed, one of which became detached from its plaque attachment site during demineralization; it is shown in the pre-detachment orientation **(Figure 2 panel a)**. The plaque in the tissue is stained black with Yasue stain, and a corresponding area of plaque is seen on the base of the stone. Papillary epithelial cells are absent from the plaque surface where stone was attached, but intact cells are seen at the periphery of the attachment site. The area enclosed by the box on the plaque surface facing the urinary space was studied further by transmission electron microscopy **(Figure 2, panels b and c)**. In panel b, the syncytium of mineral and matrix that makes up Randall's plaque is seen on the left, while the urinary space is on the right. At the boundary between the two is seen a multilayered ribbon, made up of alternating layers of light voids (where mineral has been dissolved) and dark organic matrix. Large crystals are seen anchored in the outermost matrix layer. The lamellated nature of the boundary suggests episodes of supersaturation during which mineral was laid down, followed by periods of time in which macromolecules bind to the mineral surface, entirely covering it. Succeeding layers of mineral then form on this organic surface. This may be seen in **Figure 2 panel c**, where spicules of mineral can be seen lined up along the outermost matrix layer, with newly forming matrix also visible. This matrix is presumably derived from urinary macromolecules. To the right, in the urinary space, are larger crystals, also embedded in matrix, continuous with the smaller crystals that are growing along the outermost layer of the macromolecular ribbon that covers the area of exposed plaque.

The nature of the mineral and matrix layers was investigated in the second stone, which remained attached to its plaque underpinnings, and was only partially decalcified [16]. This stone was sectioned, and alternating sections stained with either

Yasue stain, to highlight the mineral phase, or hematoxylin and eosin (H&E), for the tissue architecture. Using the H&E stained sections, the interface between plaque in the tissue and the stone mineral itself was determined, and then superimposed on the Yasue stained sections (**Figure 3, panel a, dotted lines**). Adjacent sections were used for determination of mineral phase by Fourier transform infrared spectroscopy (μ-FTIR) (**Figure 3, panel b**) and for immuno-histochemistry (**Figure 4, panels A and B**). The FTIR spectra of pure calcium oxalate and hydroxyapatite are seen at the top of **Figure 3, panel b**, with their characteristic bands. Samples of Randall's plaque show the band typical of biological apatite, while the area at the interface shows a broader band at the same location, characteristic of amorphous apatite. The area of the stone near the interface (Area 1 in Figure 3) again shows the apatite band, but farther into the stone (Area 2) both apatite and calcium oxalate were detected, and the spectra of Area 3, nearest to the urinary space, shows only calcium oxalate. This most likely represents the prevailing supersaturation in the urine.

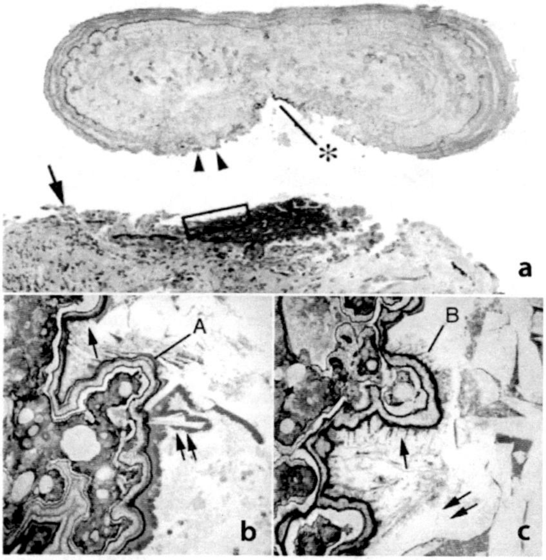

FIGURE 2. Light and TEM studies of an attached stone. **Panel a** shows the stone from Figure 1, detached and floating above the tissue site of its formation. The asterisk points to adherent plaque from the attachment site; arrowheads point to attached papillary epithelial cells. The arrow points to some papillary epithelial cells on the tissue. The small box highlights tissue plaque exposed to the original urine space, where the stone had been. **Panel b** shows a TEM of the plaque area enclosed by the small box. Plaque (left side of panel b) is covered by a multi-layered ribbon of matrix (black) and crystal (white) in a tree ring alternation. Innumerable small crystals (arrow) can be seen growing into the outermost ribbon layer and filling in the space above the mound of tissue labelled as 'A'. Double arrows point to a large crystal in matrix growing out of the ribbon layer. These attached crystals are contiguous with masses of crystals in the urine space to the right of the tissue. **Panel c** shows a higher magnification of the same area. Double arrows point to a large single crystal growing out of the tissue into a matrix within the urine space, and continuous with rafts of crystals filling that space. The single arrow points to innumerable small crystals growing in the outer lamina of the ribbon and anchoring the larger masses of crystal to the tissue.

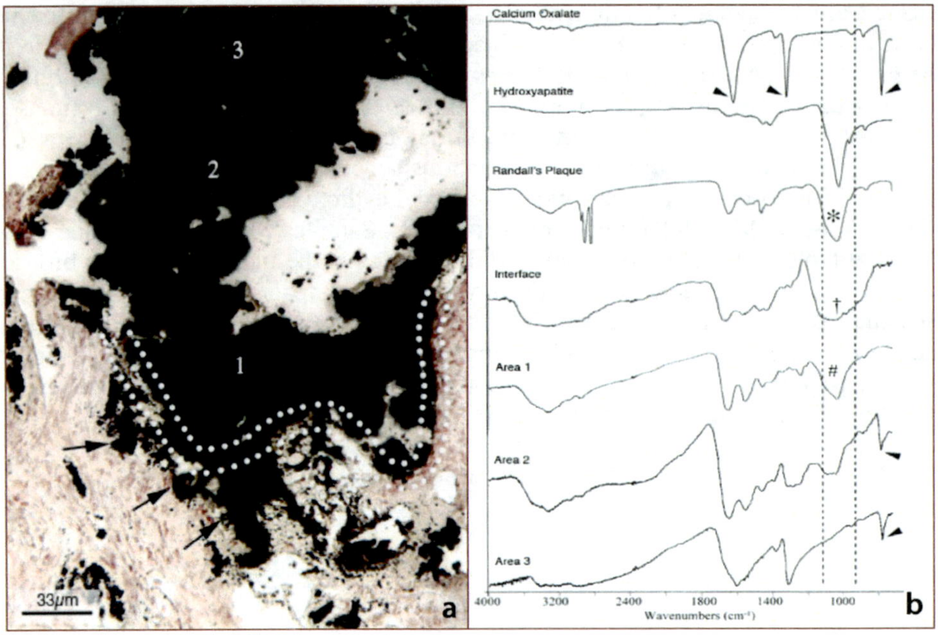

FIGURE 3. Light microscopic images of the stone-tissue interface. **Panel a** was generated from digital micrographs of identical regions on sequential serial sections, alternately stained with Yasue and H&E, and overlaid to make composites on which the interface (outlined by white dotted lines) could be readily seen and drawn. At the bottom of the panel, sites of Randall's plaque are seen near the stone interface (arrows), which cross the interface and merge into the mineral of the attached stone (area 1) just above the interface. Stone mineral extends continuously from region 1 into the stone interior (areas 2 and 3). White areas in the stone (adjacent to areas 1-3) are voids where mineral in the stone was lost during sectioning. The regions marked by area numbers and within the white dotted boundaries of the interface were studied using µFTIR. **Panel b**: The interface itself (between white dotted lines, panel a) revealed a broadened band (†) characteristic of amorphous apatite. Area 1 revealed a typical apatite band (#), and area 2 bands of apatite and calcium oxalate (CaOx, arrowhead) both were detected. Finally in area 3, toward the urinary space border of the stone, FTIR revealed only CaOx (arrowhead).

Immuno-histochemistry discloses the pattern of protein deposition within the mineral phase. Osteopontin **(Figure 4, panel A)** is found in both plaque and stone, whereas Tamm-Horsfall protein **(Figure 4, panel B)** is restricted to the area of the stone above the interface, clearly indicating that this protein was laid down on mineral bathed in urine.

These pictures suggest a sequence of stone formation for most common calcium oxalate stones. Plaque forms in the medullary interstitium in response to increased urine calcium excretion and reduced urine volume, but is covered by a layer of papillary epithelium. If this epithelial layer is breached, and plaque surface is exposed to the urine, macromolecules in the urine coat the exposed plaque surface. Subsequently, mineral phases can begin to form on the protein-coated surface of the exposed plaque, generated by supersaturation in the urine, which is then coated by another layer of protein. Eventually, urinary supersaturation overwhelms the available crystallization inhibitors, and increasing amounts of mineral are deposited at the plaque-urine interface. This deposited mineral is initially apatite, but more and more calcium oxalate is incorporated into the stone as it grows, eventually becoming the dominant mineral phase. As layers of mineral are laid down, they are coated by macromolecules in the urine, including osteopontin and Tamm-Horsfall protein, and probably many others.

The driving force for both plaque and stones is supersaturation, fostered by high urine calcium concentrations. Treatments that lower urinary supersaturation can prevent stone recurrence; whether plaque formation will also decrease is not yet known.

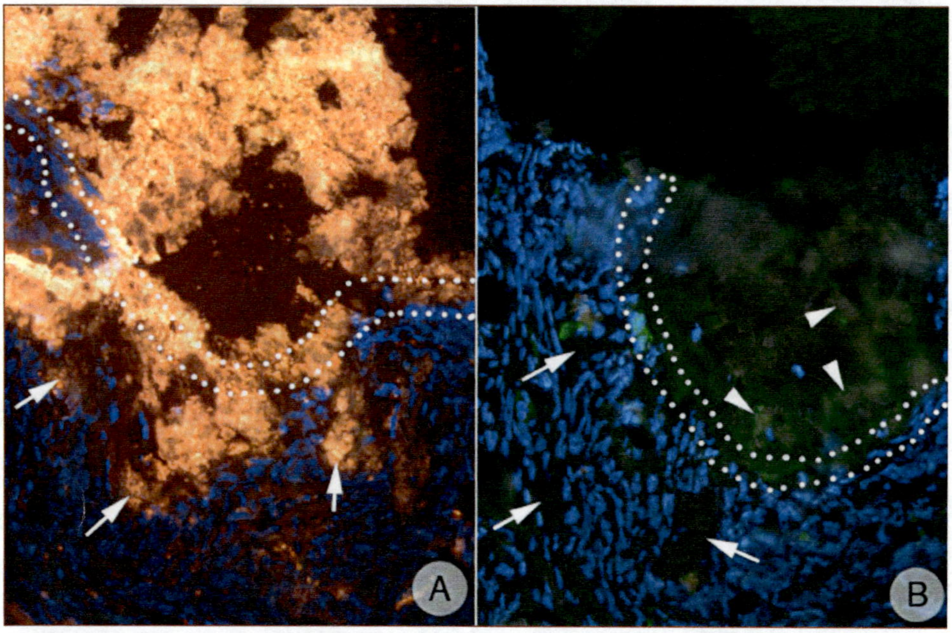

FIGURE 4. Immunocytochemistry of the stone-tissue interface. The interface region lies between the white dotted borders. **Panel A**: Osteopontin which is present in the urine and in renal tissue in Randall's plaque, spreads from the stone through the interface and into the tissue along the regions of plaque (arrows). **Panel B**: Tamm-Horsfall protein staining (arrowheads) spreads into the interface region but stops abruptly at the tissue border (arrows in panel B highlight the areas of plaque that are unstained for Tamm-Horsfall protein).

INTRATUBULAR CRYSTAL DEPOSITS

Apatite Deposits

In contrast to patients with idiopathic calcium oxalate stones, who deposit mineral only in the interstitium and not in the tubules, all other stone formers studied so far have prominent deposition of mineral in the inner medullary collecting duct (IMCD) lumens (**Figure 5**). This is true for all patients with stones composed mainly of calcium phosphate, in whom deposits of biological apatite are found filling the IMCD and often protruding from the mouths of Bellini ducts. These were named "type 2" deposits by Randall, in contrast with the interstitial apatite deposits, which he termed "type 1". Such tubular apatite crystal plugs have been identified in patients whose stones were composed mainly of brushite [17], and in patients with apatite-containing stones associated with distal renal tubular acidosis [18] and primary hyperparathyroidism [19]. Interstitial plaque may also be present in these patients, who are almost always hypercalciuric, although it was seldom seen in patients with distal RTA [18], who may be polyuric.

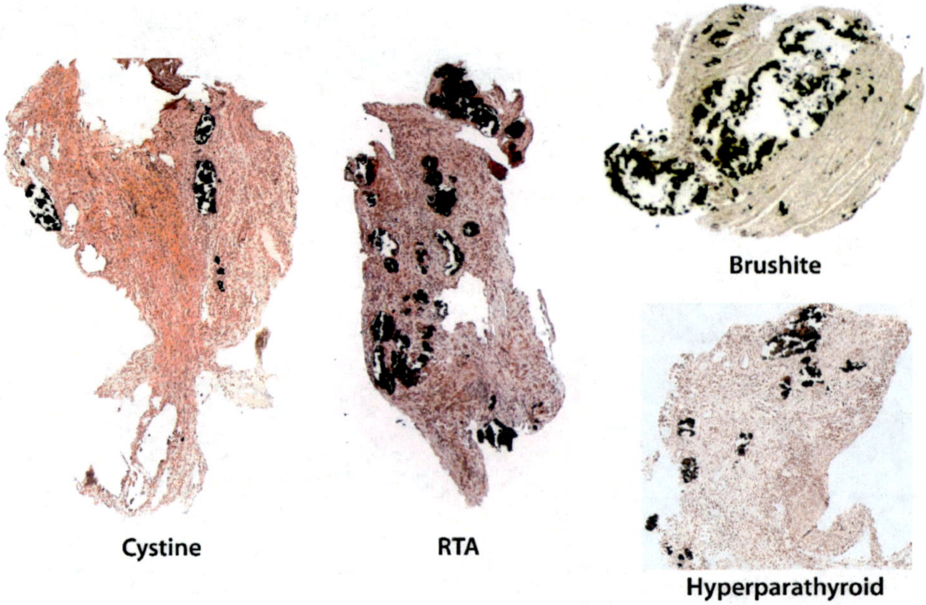

FIGURE 5. Composite of biopsies taken from four different types of stone formers, shown together to point out the major similarity, which is the presence of intratubular crystal deposits (Yasue stain). Lesions of this type were also described by Randall, and were designated type 2 plaque. In each case, the crystals fill the tubule lumen, which is dilated. Tubule lining cells are abnormal or absent, and there is interstitial fibrosis. In the cystine patients, the major crystal present is cystine, and apatite is present in smaller amounts. In the RTA and brushite patients, on the other hand, the crystal consists entirely of apatite. In some cases, crystal protrudes from the mouth of the duct of Bellini, and may be a point of attachment for stone. Patients with hyperparathyroidism are unique among all patients that have been biopsied and described thus far, because they combine both interstitial plaque and intratubular deposits.

Deposits are associated with injury or death of collecting duct cells in the affected tubules, which may be quite dilated. The surrounding interstitium is usually fibrotic, and inflammatory cells may be present. In addition, the papilla may be scarred or flattened, and there may also be cortical involvement with scarring.

Cystine and Apatite Deposits

A similar pattern is seen in patients with cystine stones, except that the crystal plugs contain mostly cystine, with an admixture of apatite (**Figure 5**). This may reflect the alkalinization that is carried out in the treatment of cystinuria, which can lead to formation of calcium phosphate crystals and stones in these patients. The magnitude and extent of crystal deposition

The pattern of intra-tubular crystal deposition appears to lead to a more destructive renal lesion. Stones may be attached to the deposits that protrude from the mouths of the ducts of Bellini.

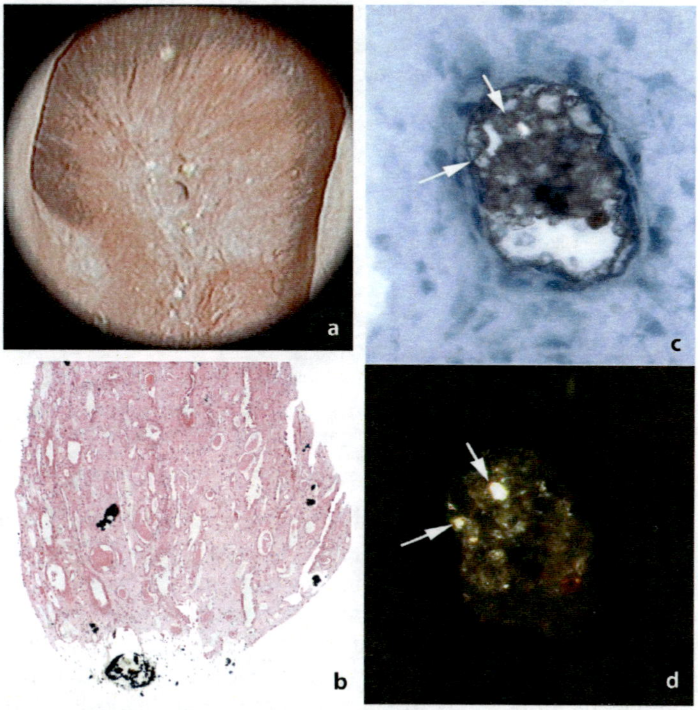

FIGURE 6. Panel a shows an intra-operative image of the papilla of a patient with enteric hyperoxaluria and calcium oxalate stones. These patients commonly show dilated ducts of Bellini with evident mineral plugs (**panel b**). No Randall's plaque is seen by endoscopic or histopathologic examination. The plugs contain largely apatite by FTIR. However, as shown in **panel c** (Yasue stain) and **d** (polarized optics), some plugs have been found to contain a mixture of both birefringent (arrows) and non-birefringent crystal, presumably a mixture of calcium oxalate and apatite.

Apatite Deposits in Hyperoxaluria

The medullary histopathology of patients with enteric hyperoxaluria (EH) presents a surprising contrast to the two pathologies already presented. Although the stones in these patients are invariably calcium oxalate, the medullary tissue is never found to contain islands of interstitial apatite plaque, as in idiopathic calcium oxalate stone formers. Rather these patients have intratubular crystal plugs (**Figure 6, panels a and b**). However, although the urine is supersaturated with calcium oxalate (**Figure 7**), the plugs contain largely calcium phosphate as apatite, this despite a urine pH consistently below 5.5, which would not support apatite as a stable mineral phase. This requires that local tubule fluid pH must differ from that of the bulk urine. The lack of calcium oxalate in these plugs was unexpected, however, and is difficult to explain. With exhaustive scrutiny of 1500 tissue sections taken from idiopathic calcium oxalate stone former biopsies and compared with tissue from patients with EH, the patients with EH were found to have rare sites of birefringent crystal deposited as a scrim on apical cell membranes and rarely intermixed with non-birefringent crystal plugs (**Figure 6, panels c and d**); these were never found in the idiopathic stone formers. We infer that the birefringent crystals are calcium oxalate.

Idiopathic CaOx SF		**Bypass CaOx SF**	
24 hr urine (mg/d):		24 hr urine (mg/d):	
Calcium	312 ± 89	Calcium	81 ± 29
Oxalate	40 ± 13	Oxalate	106 ± 11
Citrate	485 ± 278	Citrate	144 ± 107
UpH	5.89 ± 0.5	U pH	5.57 ± 0.25
CaOx SS	11 ± 4	CaOx SS	5 ± 2
CaP SS	1.4 ± 0.8	CaP SS	0.09 ± 0.05

$p < 0.01$ all values

FIGURE 7. Contrasting urine stone risk chemistries in idiopathic calcium oxalate stone formers and patients with calcium oxalate stones and enteric hyperoxaluria after jejunoileal bypass, studied with papillary biopsies.

In other words, two groups of calcium oxalate stone formers with differing pathophysiologies display radically different histopathologies. The hypercalciuric common stone formers produce stones as overgrowths on papillary surfaces over interstitial plaque. In contrast, the hyperoxaluric patients form intratubular apatite deposits, never form plaque, and never manifest attached calcium oxalate stones in their kidneys. The stones are invariably found free in the renal pelvis, and there appears to be no relationship between the intratubular deposits and the stones themselves.

ACKNOWLEDGMENTS

This work was supported by NIH grant P01 DK56788.

REFERENCES

1. Coe FL, Evan A and Worcester E. Kidney stone disease. *J Clin Invest* 115: 2598-2608, 2005.
2. Asplin JR, Parks JH, Lingeman JE, Kahnowski R, Mardis H, Goldfarb D, Grasso M, Lacey S and Coe F. Supersaturation and stone composition in a network of dispersed treatment sites. *J Urol* 159: 1821-1825, 1998.

3. Milliner DS. The primary hyperoxalurias: an algorithm for diagnosis. *Am J Nephrol* 25: 154-160, 2005.
4. Worcester EM. Stones from bowel disease. *Endocrinol Metab Clin North* Am 31: 979-999, 2002.
5. von Unruh GE, Voss S, Sauerbruch T and Hesse A. Dependence of oxalate absorption on the daily calcium intake. *J Am Soc Nephrol* 15: 1567-1573, 2004.
6. Kaufman DW, Kelly JP, Curhan GC, Anderson TE, Dretler SP, Preminger GM and Cave DR. Oxalobacter formigenes may reduce the risk of calcium oxalate kidney stones. *J Am Soc Nephrol* 19: 1197-1203, 2008.
7. Jiang Z, Asplin JR, Evan AP, Rajendran VM, Velazquez H, Nottoli TP, Binder HJ and Aronson PS. Calcium oxalate urolithiasis in mice lacking anion transporter Slc26a6. *Nat Genet* 38: 474-478, 2006.
8. Evan AP, Lingeman JE, Coe FL, Parks JH, Bledsoe SB, Shao Y, Sommer AJ, Paterson RF, Kuo RL and Grynpas M. Randall's plaque of patients with nephrolithiasis begins in basement membranes of thin loops of Henle. *J Clin Invest* 111: 607-616, 2003.
9. Evan AP, Coe FL, Rittling SR, Bledsoe SM, Shao Y, Lingeman JE and Worcester EM. Apatite plaque particles in inner medulla of kidneys of calcium oxalate stone formers: osteopontin localization. *Kidney Int* 68: 145-154, 2005.
10. Evan AP, Bledsoe S, Worcester EM, Coe FL, Lingeman JE and Bergsland KJ. Renal inter-alpha-trypsin inhibitor heavy chain 3 increases in calcium oxalate stone-forming patients. *Kidney Int* 72: 1503-1511, 2007.
11. Kuo RL, Lingeman JE, Evan AP, Paterson RF, Parks JH, Bledsoe SB, Munch LC and Coe FL. Urine calcium and volume predict coverage of renal papilla by Randall's plaque. *Kidney Int* 64: 2150-2154, 2003.
12. Evan AP, Coe FL, Gillen D, Lingeman JE, Bledsoe S and Worcester EM. Renal intratubular crystals and hyaluronan staining occur in stone formers with bypass surgery but not with idiopathic calcium oxalate stones. *Anat Rec (Hoboken)* 291: 325-334, 2008.
13. Worcester EM, Gillen DL, Evan AP, Parks JH, Wright K, Trumbore L, Nakagawa Y and Coe FL. Evidence that postprandial reduction of renal calcium reabsorption mediates hypercalciuria of patients with calcium nephrolithiasis. *Am J Physiol Renal Physiol* 292: F66-F75, 2007.
14. Randall A. The origin and growth of renal calculi. Annals of Surgery 105: 1009-1027, 1937.
15. Matlaga BR, Williams JC, Jr., Kim SC, Kuo RL, Evan AP, Bledsoe SB, Coe FL, Worcester EM, Munch LC and Lingeman JE. Endoscopic evidence of calculus attachment to Randall's plaque. *J Urol* 175: 1720-1724, 2006.
16. Evan AP, Coe FL, Lingeman JE, Shao Y, Sommer AJ, Bledsoe SB, Anderson JC and Worcester EM. Mechanism of formation of human calcium oxalate renal stones on Randall's plaque. *Anat Rec (Hoboken)* 290: 1315-1323, 2007.
17. Evan AP, Lingeman JE, Coe FL, Shao Y, Parks JH, Bledsoe SB, Phillips CL, Bonsib S, Worcester EM, Sommer AJ, Kim SC, Tinmouth WW and Grynpas M. Crystal-associated nephropathy in patients with brushite nephrolithiasis. *Kidney Int* 67: 576-591, 2005.
18. Evan AP, Lingeman J, Coe F, Shao Y, Miller N, Matlaga B, Phillips C, Sommer A and Worcester E. Renal histopathology of stone-forming patients with distal renal tubular acidosis. *Kidney Int* 71: 795-801, 2007.
19. Evan AP, Lingeman JE, Coe FL, Miller NL, Bledsoe SB, Sommer AJ, Williams Jr JC, Shao Y and Worcester EM. Histopathology and surgical anatomy of patients with primary hyperparathyroidism and calcium phosphate stones. *Kidney Int* 74: 223-229, 2008.

I. FACTORS THAT REGULATE NORMAL AND ABNORMAL MINERALIZATION

Hypercalciuric Bone Disease

Murray J. Favus

Section of Endocrinology, Diabetes, and Metabolism, Department of Medicine, University of Chicago Pritzker School of Medicine, 5841 S. Maryland Ave, MC 1027, Chicago, IL 60637, USA

Abstract. Hypercalciuria plays an important causal role in many patients with calcium oxalate (CaOx) stones. The source of the hypercalciuria includes increased intestinal Ca absorption and decreased renal tubule Ca reabsorption. In CaOx stone formers with idiopathic hypercalciuria (IH), Ca metabolic balance studies have revealed negative Ca balance and persistent hypercalciuria in the fasting state and during low dietary Ca intake. Bone resorption may also contribute to the high urine Ca excretion and increase the risk of bone loss. Indeed, low bone mass by DEXA scanning has been discovered in many IH patients. Thiazide diuretic agents reduce urine Ca excretion and may increase bone mineral density (BMD), thereby reducing fracture risk. Dietary Ca restriction that has been used unsuccessfully in the treatment of CaOx nephrolithiasis in the past may enhance negative Ca balance and accelerate bone loss. DEXA scans may demonstrate low BMD at the spine, hip, or forearm, with no predictable pattern. The unique pattern of bone histologic changes in IH differs from other causes of low DEXA bone density including postmenopausal osteoporosis, male hypogonadal osteoporosis, and glucocorticoid-induced osteoporosis. Hypercalciuria appears to play an important pathologic role in the development of low bone mass, and therefore correction of urine Ca losses should be a primary target for treatment of the bone disease accompanying IH.

Keywords: idiopathic hypercalciuria, bone mineral density, bone histomorphometry
PACS: 87.19.xv

INTRODUCTION

Idiopathic hypercalciuria (IH) is the single most common cause of calcium (Ca) oxalate (Ox) nephrolithiasis [1]. Since the initial description of IH [2] metabolic balance studies and radio-labeled Ca tracer studies demonstrated that the source of the high urine Ca is not only from intestinal Ca hyperabsorption and decreased renal tubule Ca reabsorption, but also from Ca released from bone [3,4,5]. Reduced bone mass was not appreciated at the time Albright and colleagues published their original description of IH stone disease [2]; however contemporary characterization of IH must now include low bone mass and increased fracture risk along with hypercalciuria and CaOx nephrolithiasis. This review will focus on the evidence for a bone disease accompanying IH, what is known about the pathogenesis of the low bone mass including the role of hypercalciuria, and consideration of therapeutic approaches.

CP1049, *Renal Stone Disease 2, 2nd International Urolithiasis Research Symposium,*
edited by A. P. Evan, J. E. Lingeman, J. A. McAteer, and J. C. Williams, Jr.

EVIDENCE FOR BONE DISEASE

Ca Balance Studies

The first suggestion that IH may be associated with low bone mass came from mineral balance studies which showed that some IH stone formers were in negative Ca balance, which is defined as urine Ca loss being greater than net Ca absorption [papers summarized in 5]. The negative Ca balance in IH stone formers was present over a range of Ca intake and was most pronounced when Ca intake was low. During equilibration on a low dietary Ca intake (2.0 mg Ca/Kg body weight and lower) non-stone formers conserve Ca by reducing urine Ca excretion, whereas 30 to 50% of IH patients fail to reduce urine Ca and so are in negative Ca balance [6]. As a portion of the excess urine Ca excreted by IH patients during low Ca intake must come from bone, the balance studies performed in the 1950's and 1960's predicted loss of bone mass during prolonged low Ca intake.

Bone Mineral Density

By the early 1980's the availability of non-invasive techniques to quantify bone mass permitted measurements of bone mineral density (BMD) in IH patients. Several clinical studies reported low BMDs of the lumbar spine, proximal femur, distal radius, and mid-radius in IH patients of all ages. A number of variables including age, menopausal state, and genetic background may be responsible for the variations of anatomic sites involved and the frequency of low BMD among patients. BMD of the lumbar spine was a primary site of low bone mass in some studies, whereas other studies revealed low hip BMD with or without low spine BMD. A summary of the results of over 11 published studies [7-17] in which bone density was measured in IH are summarized in Table 1. The studies in the aggregate indicate a general risk for low BMD in IH patients. Stone formation and/or passage are not a requisite for low bone mass. Where measured, the lowest BMD levels were associated with the highest rates of urine Ca excretion.

Table 1. Bone Mineral Density measurements in over 600 patients with IH from 15 published studies. SPA is single photon absorptiometry; DPA is dual photon absorptiometry; DXA is dual x-ray absorptiometry; and qCT is quantitative CT.

Obtained using either SPA, DPA, DXA, qCT
Lumbar spine BMD low in 11% to 92% of cases
Femoral neck BMD normal or low
Distal radius BMD normal

Femoral neck Z-score in IH stone formers and their first degree family members were inversely related to urine Ca and ammonium excretions [15]. In a subsequent three-year follow up of BMD, more severe hypercalciuria was associated with a greater decline in femoral neck Z score [16]. A weaker inverse relationship was observed between hypercalciuria and lumbar spine Z score.

Clinical Consequences of Low Bone Mass

There is limited data on the effects of low bone mass on fracture risk in IH; however, comparable reductions of BMD in patients with osteoporosis are associated with increased fracture rates. One retrospective analysis of kidney stone formers [18] revealed an increase in spine and hip fractures with increasing time from the onset of first stone event. At any interval, the fracture rates in stone formers were 3- to 4-fold greater than that predicted by fracture rates for the general population. As 50% of all stone formers have IH, it is possible that about 50% of the stone patients reporting fracture in the Mayo Clinic Study had IH. Clearly, there is a need for a prospective study of fractures in IH patients to assess the magnitude of the fracture risk. Other than RTA, no other common stone forming states has been associated with fracture.

PATHOGENESIS OF LOW BONE MASS

Role of Hypercalciuria

Hypercalciuria is life-long and can be detected during childhood at approximately the same frequency as found in the adult population. Low bone density has been documented in children and adolescents with IH [19]; however, skeletal growth and development proceed normally despite the persistent hypercalciuria. Indeed, children with IH have no gross skeletal deformity or reduction in peak height. Whether there is an increased frequency of fracture during childhood and adolescence is not known.

Calcium Intake

As noted above, Ca balance in IH becomes more negative during dietary Ca restriction, and often does not normalize urine Ca excretion. If sustained, negative Ca balance predicts the appearance of progressive bone loss. Ca restriction does not normalize urine Ca and does not reduce recurrence of Ca kidney stones [20,21]. Treatment of hypercalciuria should include sufficient but not excessive Ca intake and avoidance of calcium restriction.

1,25-Dihydroxyvitamin D (1,25D, Calcitriol)

Low bone mass is reported to be more common in patients with unremitting hypercalciuria such as those with morning fasting hypercalciuria and hypercalciuria during dietary Ca restriction compared to those with so-called absorptive hypercalciuria in which urine Ca excretion appears to arise solely from intestinal Ca hyperabsorption [11,12,17]. However, others have low BMD in IH patients with absorptive hypercalciuria [13,14] as well.

Increased intestinal Ca absorption is found in most all patients with IH. About one-half have elevated serum 1,25D levels due to renal over-production [5,22]. However, patients with normal serum 1,25D have comparable levels of intestinal Ca hyperabsorption and hypercalciuria [23]. A model of human IH has been developed by breeding male and female spontaneously hypercalciuric rats [24]. Hypercalciuria was more common among male and female offspring, and through successive generations the intensity and frequency of the hypercalciuria has increased [25]. The genetic hypercalciuric stone-forming (GHS) rats share many features with human IH in that the rats have high intestinal Ca absorption, reduced renal tubule Ca reabsorption, persistent hypercalciuria, negative Ca balance during low Ca intake, and low bone mass [24-34]. Serum 1,25D levels are normal in GHS rats as found in about 50% of IH patients. Elevated tissue vitamin D receptor (VDR) levels bind 1,25D and increase expression of VDR-dependent genes that produce proteins involved in Ca transport. Elevated peripheral blood monocyte VDR levels have been found in male IH stone formers, suggesting that like GHS rats, at least some with human IH could be caused by excess VDR [35].

Thiazide Diuretics

Thiazide diuretic agents inhibit NaCl but not Ca reabsorption along the loop of Henle [36]. Under steady state conditions with chronic thiazide administration distal Ca delivery declines and contributes to the reduction in urine Ca excretion. In addition, thiazide directly increases distal convoluted tubule Ca reabsorption in the rat and may also exert this action in humans [37]. In IH patients elevated urine Ca excretion can be reduced to normal by the chronic administration of thiazide diuretic agents [19,38-41]. Thiazide administration has been reported to decrease or have no effect on intestinal Ca absorption [38-41], but the effects appear to be small compared to the large decrease in urine Ca excretion. Therefore the increase in distal tubule Ca reabsorption changes negative Ca balance to neutral or positive balance [19]. Positive Ca balance can be sustained with chronic thiazide therapy and may increase lumbar spine and hip bone density [42,43]. No prospective randomized trials have been conducted to determine the impact of thiazide on fracture rate; however follow-up data from hypertensive patients treated with thiazide therapy show increased BMD [42] and reduction in hip fracture rate in those taking thiazide for six years and longer [44]. Quantitative analysis of bone biopsy specimens from IH patients before and after thiazide therapy shows reduction in bone turnover [45], which suggests a mechanism for the improvement in bone mass.

Models of Low Bone Mass

One model of low bone mass has the defect in renal tubule Ca reabsorption as the primary event. It proposes that urine Ca loss results in Ca mobilization from bone through osteoclastic mediated bone resorption. An alternative model suggests that hypercalciuria may result from a primary defect in Ca incorporation into the bone matrix. The defect in bone mineralization results in excess Ca absorption and urine excretion of the Ca normally destined for deposition in the bone matrix. Evidence for the primary renal tubular Ca transport defect model is largely derived from the effects of thiazide to normalize urine Ca and thereby increase bone density. The model does not incorporate the effect of thiazides to inhibit bone cell carbonic anhydrase (CA), which may inhibit bone resorption [46]. Whether the usual doses of thiazide can inhibit CA is not known.

Some IH patients have elevated serum parathyroid hormone (PTH) and 1,25D levels [5], which could stimulate osteoclast-mediated bone resorption and thereby cause bone loss. Thiazide administration reduces PTH and 1,25D levels in some IH patients [39-41], and so thiazide could also preserve bone mass through the reduction of these hormones.

All models of IH bone disease must take into account genetic contributions. IH is familial and follows a pattern consistent with an autosomal dominant mode of inheritance [5,47]. Hypercalciuria occurs in children and is life long. The role of inheritance in IH bone disease studied by Asplin and colleagues [16,17] revealed high urine Ca excretion among IH stone formers and some family members that predicted lower lumbar spine or femoral neck BMD Z-score. However, no inverse relationship between urine Ca and BMD Z-score was present in members with normal urine Ca excretion and there was no low BMD among first degree relatives who had normocalciuria.

Bone Histomorphometry

A limited number of bone biopsy specimens have been obtained from IH patients. Many of the patients who undergoing bone biopsy have not been well characterized with respect to Ca metabolism and calciotropic hormone levels [45,48]. Quantitative analysis of bone formation parameters on bone biopsy specimens requires administration of two doses (21 days apart) of oral tetracycline prior to taking the biopsy. Tetracycline accumulates along bone surfaces undergoing mineralization, and thereby identifies surfaces involved in new bone formation. The distance between the two lines of tetracycline accumulation permits calculation of the amount of bone (in microns/day) formed during the interval between the first and second dose of tetracycline. Bone resorption may be estimated from the percent of the bone surface disrupted by resorption pits, but activity level of these pits cannot be determined. Therefore, parameters of bone resorption are not as quantitative as that for osteoblastic new bone formation.

Bone biopsy specimens from IH patients (Table 2) show a delay in bone apposition rate and a mild defect in mineralization. The delay in mineralization is subtle and different from the florid defects in mineralization of osteomalacia. Bone resorption pits on trabecular surfaces are normal to slightly increased in number. Osteoclast number is not substantially increased. There is no abnormality of the multi-nucleated osteoclasts. Reduction in trabecular bone mass is reflected in greater spacing between trabeculae and more extensive disruption of trabecular connectivity [45,48]. Thus, histomorphometric analysis of bone biopsy specimens from IH patients reveals changes that are very different from the changes in bone formation and resorption and bone turnover that are characteristic of bone loss in postmenopausal women, men with hypogonadism, and men and women with steroid-induced bone loss.

TABLE 2. Histomorphometric changes of bone formation and resorption in bone biopsy specimens obtained from patients with IH and compared to postmenopausal osteoporosis (PMO), hypogonadal male osteoporosis (HMO), and glucocorticoid-induced osteoporosis (GIO) in men and women.

Parameter	IH	PMO	HMO	GIO
Bone formation	**Dec**	**Inc**	**Dec**	**Dec**
Mineral apposition rate	**Del**	**Inc**	**Dec**	**Dec**
Mineralization lag time	**Pro**	**Inc**	**Nl**	**Nl**
Osteoid volume	**Nl or Inc**	**Nl**	**Nl**	**Nl**
Osteoblastic activity	**Low**	**Inc**	**Dec**	**Dec**
Resorption	**Nl or mild Inc**	**Inc**	**Inc**	**Inc**

Parameters: Decreased (DEC), Delayed (Del), Prolonged (Pro), Normal (Nl), Increased (Inc), or Low (L)

Bone Cell Function

Bone biopsy analyses indicate subtle changes in both bone formation and resorption dynamics with decreased osteoblastic bone formation and either normal or mildly increased osteoclastic bone resorption. Bone turnover markers measured in blood or urine have been either mildly increased [17, 49, 50] or normal [15,16], indicating a modest decreases in bone formation (osteocalcin, bone specific alkaline phosphatase) and normal or slightly increased bone resorption (hydroxyproline, RANKL, IL-6, IL-1, GM-CSF, NTX). ^{47}Ca tracer kinetic studies in IH patients demonstrated increased bone resorption and formation [4]. Bone biopsy, tracer, and turnover marker data are consistent with a mild defect in bone formation and normal or mildly elevated bone resorption. The histomorphometric pattern of changes is very different from postmenopausal bone loss, hypogonadal osteoporosis in men, and steroid-induced osteoporosis in men and women.

CONCLUSIONS

Idiopathic hypercalciuria (IH) is associated with low bone density and increased fracture risk. The histologic changes characterize delayed mineralization, reduced osteoblast activity, and normal or slightly increased bone resorption. Therefore, the bone disease should be recognized as a separate entity from other causes of osteoporosis or low bone mass as occurs in males and pre- and post-menopausal women. Life-long hypercalciuria plays an important causal role in the development of low bone density, and reduction of urine Ca excretion with thiazides improves bone density. Long term use of thiazide reduces hip fracture risk. The awareness of asymptomatic low bone mass and increased fracture risk in men and women with IH should lead to an aggressive evaluation of bone density status and institution of appropriate treatment.

ACKNOWLEDGMENTS

The author wishes to express great appreciation for longstanding collaborations with Drs. Fredric L. Coe and David A. Bushinsky, and for the laboratory research contributions of Drs. Man-Sau Wong, Shaochun Bai, Alexander Karnauskas, and Hongwei Wang. A portion of the work was supported by the University of Chicago Osteoporosis Research Fund.

REFERENCES

1. F.L. Coe, *Ann Int Med* 87,404 (1977).
2. F. Albright et al., *N Engl J Med* 259,802 (1958)
3. A. Caniggia, C. Gennari, L. and Cesari, *Brit Med J* 1,247 (1965).
4. U.A. Liberman, et al., *J Clin Invest* 47,2580 (1968).
5. F.L. Coe, M.J. Favus, and J.R. Asplin, in *The Kidney*, Edited by B.M. Brenner (Saunders, Philadelphia, 2004), p1819.
6. F.L. Coe et al., *Am J Med* 72,25 (1982).
7. J. Barkin et al., *Miner Electrolyte Metab* 11,19 (1985).
8. E.M. Alhava, M. Juuti, and P. Karjalainen, *Scand J Urol Nephrol* 10, 154 (1976).
9. L. Borghi et al., *J Urol* 146,1334 (1991).
10. J.R. Zanchetta et al., *Nephron* 73,557 (1996).
11. S. Lawoyin et al., *Metabolism* 28,1250 (1979).
12. R. Pacifici et al., *J Clin Endocrinol Metab* 71, (1990)
13. P. Bataille et al., *Kidney Int* 39,1193 (1991)
14. F. Pietschmann, N.A. Breslau, and C.Y. Pak, *J Bone Miner* Res 7, 1783 (1991)
15. J.R. Asplin et al., *Kidney Int* 63, 662 (2003)
16. J.R. Asplin et al., *Kidney Int* 70,1463 (2006)
17. I.P. Heilberg, and J. R. Weisinger, *Curr Opin Nephrol Hypertens* 15, 394 (2006)
18. L.J. Melton et al., *Kidney Int* 53, 459 (1998)
19. F.L. Coe et al., *Kidney Int* 33,1140 (1988)
20. G.C. Curhan et al., *N Engl J Med* 328, 833 (1993)
21. G.C. Curhan et al., *Ann Int Med* 126,497 (1997)
22. A.E. Broadus et al., *N Engl J Med* 311, 73 (1984)
23. R.A. Kaplan et al., *J Clin Invest* 59, 71,56 (1977)
24. M.J. Favus, and F. L. Coe, *Mineral Electrolyte Metab* 2, 150 (1979)
25. D.A. Bushinsky, *Seminars in Nephrology* 16, 448 (1996)
26. M.J. Favus et al., *J Clin Invest* 82, 218 (1988)
27. D.A. Bushinsky and M.J. Favus *J Clin Invest* 82,1585 (1988)
28. N.S. Krieger et al., *Am J Physiol (Cell Physiol)* 271, C130 (1996)
29. S. Tsuruoka et al., *Kidney Int* 51, 1540 (1997)
30. J. Yao et al., *J Clin Invest* 101,2223 (1998)
31. A.J. Karnauskas et al., *J Bone Miner Res* 20, 447 (2005)
32. J. Yao et al., *J Am Soc Nephrol* 16, 1300 (2005)
33. X.-Q. Li et al., *J Clin Invest* 91, 661 (1993)
34. M. Kim et al., *Kidney Int* 43, 189 (1993)
35. M.J. Favus, et al., *J Clin Endocrinol Metab* 89,4937 (2004)
36. B.R. Edwards et al., *J Clin Invest* 52, 2418 (1973)
37. L.S. Costanzo et al., *Am J Physiol* 235, F492 (1978)
38. J.R. Hassim, and B.A. Higgins *Brit Med J* 1, 675 (1965)
39. U. Ehrig, J.E. Harrison, D.R. Wilson *Metabolism* 23, 139 (1974)
40. D.E. Barilla et al., *Metabolism* 27, 125 (1978)

41. J. E. Zerwekh, and C.Y. C. Pak *Metabolism* 29,13 (1980)
42. R.D. Wasnich et al., *N Engl J Med* 309, 344 (1983)
43. J.S. Adams, C.F. Song, and V. H. Kantorovich *Ann Int Med* 130, 658 (1999)
44. A.Z. LaCroix et al., *N Engl J Med* 322, 286 (1990)
45. T. Steinche et al., *APMIS* 97, 302 (1989)
46. A. Lalande et al., *J Bone Min Res* 16, 361 (2001)
47. F.L. Coe, J.H. Parks, and E.S. Moore *N Engl J Med* 300, 337 (1979)
48. H.H. Malluche et al. *J Clin Endocrinol Metab* 50, 654 (1980)
49. R.A.L. Sutton, V.R. Walker *Metabolism* 35,485 (1986)
50. M. Urivetzky, P.S Anna, and A.D. Smith *J. Urol.* 139, 12 (1988)

Extracellular Matrix Proteins, Alkaline Phosphatase and Pyrophosphate as Molecular Determinants of Bone, Tooth, Kidney and Vascular Calcification

Marc D. McKee

Division of Biomedical Sciences, Faculty of Dentistry, and Department of Anatomy and Cell Biology, Faculty of Medicine, McGill University, 3640 University Street, Montreal, Quebec, Canada H3A 2B2
marc.mckee@mcgill.ca

Abstract. Progress in biomineralization research in recent years has identified, characterized and described functions for key noncollagenous extracellular matrix proteins regulating crystal growth in the skeleton and dentition. Some of these same proteins expressed in soft tissues undergoing pathologic calcification also inhibit ectopic crystal growth. In addition to extracellular matrix proteins regulating matrix mineralization, the enzyme tissue-nonspecific alkaline phosphatase – which is highly expressed by cells in mineralized tissues – cleaves pyrophosphate, an anionic small-molecule inhibitor of mineralization. Together with the required mineral ion availability necessary for crystal growth, these molecular determinants appear to function in limiting the spread of pathologic calcification seen in soft tissues such as blood vessels and kidneys. Osteopontin, in particular, is a potent calcification inhibitor that accumulates in mineralized tissues and in calcified deposits during vascular calcification and nephrolithiasis/urolithiasis. Additional research is required to establish the exact temporal sequence in which the molecular determinants of pathologic calcification appear relative to mineral crystal growth in different tissues, and to establish their relationship (if any) to the activation of osteogenic differentiation programs.

Keywords: Bone, teeth, kidney, blood vessels, arteries, biomineralization, pathologic calcification, vascular calcification, kidney stones, urolithiasis, nephrolithiasis, Randall's plaques, calcium oxalate, hydroxyapatite, extracellular matrix, alkaline phosphatase, pyrophosphate, osteopontin, review.
PACS: 01.30.Cc; 87.14.ej

EXTRACELLULAR MATRICES, MATRIX PROTEINS AND PHYSIOLOGIC MINERALIZATION IN VERTEBRATES

Mineralization of cartilage, bone and teeth (includes dentin, cementum and enamel) occurs within extracellular matrices typically characterized by an abundance of fibrillar elements (*e.g.* type I collagen fibrils—except in enamel) which form a scaffold for cell adhesion and mineral deposition [1]. Within this matrix scaffolding, a myriad of other proteins, proteoglycans and enzymes contribute to its cell signaling properties and render the matrices competent for the deposition of nano-sized

CP1049, *Renal Stone Disease 2, 2nd International Urolithiasis Research Symposium*,
edited by A. P. Evan, J. E. Lingeman, J. A. McAteer, and J. C. Williams, Jr.

inorganic calcium-phosphate crystals having the chemistry and stoichiometry of a substituted hydroxyapatite. Another type of mineral, calcium carbonate, deposits within the inner ear in the form of small otoconia particles (otoliths / statoconia in fish and other species) residing on sensory cells as part of the vestibular system, and these likewise have an abundant organic matrix [2]. In the apatite-containing mineralized tissues, noncollagenous proteins—as part of the extracellular matrix—regulate cell adhesion and cell activity via outside-in (matrix-cell) signaling typically through integrin receptors. Indeed, cell differentiation of progenitor cells can be regulated by the stiffness of the surrounding extracellular matrix, with stiffer matrices leading to induction of the osteoblast phenotype, and less stiff matrices leading to fibroblast differentiation [3]. Extracellular matrix stability and rigidity are imparted in part by crosslinking enzymes, with the best characterized crosslinking enzymes being lysyl oxidase for collagen and elastin [4], and transglutaminase 2 for noncollagenous proteins [5]. Crosslinking of the noncollagenous proteins by transglutaminase 2 also modulates their assembly and activities, and creates noncollagenous protein networks interlacing with the collagen scaffolding [6]. Interactions between the noncollagenous protein networks, proteoglycans and the collagen scaffolding are less well characterized but are thought to occur to establish an integrated extracellular matrix whose properties regulate cell activity and mineralization. Both monomer and crosslinked multimer forms of the noncollagenous proteins likely contribute to matrix maturation and mineralization, although their respective contributions remain to be determined.

Physiologic mineralization of the skeleton and dentition proceeds as heterogeneous mineral deposition events at discrete locations within, at the surface of, and between, collagen fibrils (except enamel)[1]. Initial nucleation events are controlled locally by concentrations of mineral ions and by the presence, or absence, of mineral nucleators and inhibitors. Many noncollagenous proteins are acidic phosphoproteins that bind strongly to mineral, typically through their negatively charged phosphate groups, to regulate the induction and growth of the inorganic mineral phase such that the crystals are of the proper number, size, shape and alignment within their respective extracellular matrices [7,8]. Initially, critical nuclei of mineral ions reach a size and stability that subsequently mature to form crystals with a significant degree of long-range order with well-defined and characteristic crystallographic faces. For bones and teeth, these crystals are typically platelet-shaped crystallites with dimensions that vary depending on their physical location within the structure of the pre-established extracellular matrix [1,9]. Those crystals depositing within the collagen fibrils clearly form within a chemical environment entirely different from those depositing at the surface of, or between, the collagen fibrils. The arrangement of charge groups and the matrix interaction domain in type I collagen have recently been well characterized [10], but much less is known about the chemical environment contributing to mineral crystal nucleation and propagation outside the fibrils. However, evidence for the role of acidic, negatively charged mineral-binding proteins being important in regulating this interfibrillar mineralization process is accumulating, and this family of proteins (also having cell-signaling properties) is referred to as the SIBLING family (small integrin-binding ligand N-linked glycoproteins)[11]. While crystal deposition within the collagen fibril is thought to occur independently from that between the fibrils, Price and colleagues [12] have recently proposed a linked mineralization process whereby crystals formed at the surface of the fibrils might migrate to locations within the fibril. Alternatively, or as an additional mechanism, membrane-bound matrix vesicles released by chondrocytes, osteoblasts, odontoblasts and cementoblasts have also been proposed to initiate mineralization at specific sites within the extracellular matrix [13]. In this latter case, crystals form within the vesicle under the control of vesicular components including integral proteins of the limiting membrane. Following initial crystal growth within the matrix vesicle, and then rupture of the vesicle membrane by continued crystal growth, it is likely that the same extracellular matrix molecules that would otherwise regulate nonvesicle-mediated matrix mineralization would be similarly active in controlling crystal growth [14].

ALKALINE PHOSPHATASE AND PYROPHOSPHATE REGULATION OF MINERALIZATION

Tissue-nonspecific alkaline phosphatase (TNAP; also known as TNSALP, ALPL, AKP2 and liver/kidney/bone alkaline phosphatase) has long been known as an early osteoblast marker [15,16]. Its function in mineralized tissues was surmised many years ago by Fleisch and colleagues [17] where it was proposed that its enzymatic function might be related to cleavage of mineralization-inhibiting pyrophosphate produced as a metabolic byproduct of many intracellular processes [18]. TNAP also can remove phosphate groups from extracellular matrix phosphoproteins, thus modulating their mineral-binding capacity and potentially providing a source of phosphate for mineralization [19]. Other characterized alkaline phosphatases include the intestinal and placental forms. Alkaline phosphatases have recently been thoroughly reviewed by Millan [20].

Pyrophosphate is a potent inhibitor of many types of mineralization [17,21]. Industrially, it is commonly used as an anti-scaling agent to prevent mineral accumulation (of calcium carbonate and other minerals) in plumbing conduit systems. Biomedically, pyrophosphate is an active ingredient added to toothpastes to prevent calculus (tartar) formation at the surface of teeth which unchecked at gingival margins in the oral cavity can lead to gingivitis and periodontal disease. Bisphosphonates—commonly used drugs to treat osteoporosis, Paget's disease and osteogenesis imperfecta—are pyrophosphate analogues where the central oxygen is replaced by a nonhydrolyzable carbon atom, with variable side groups conferring different cytotoxic potencies [22]. These drugs were designed based on principles of pyrophosphate binding to mineral, and thus the core of the bisphosphonates is used to target these drugs to the apatitic mineral of bone where they subsequently act principally by being toxic to the bone-resorbing osteoclasts by inhibiting intracellular metabolic pathways in these cells [22].

In organismal biology, pyrophosphate is a metabolic byproduct of many intracellular pathways [18]. Its transport across the cell membrane into the extracellular environment is achieved by a membrane protein called ANK, or it can be produced outside the cell directly from extracellular nucleotides via the action of the membrane protein ENPP1 (ectonucleotide pyrophosphatase/phosphodiesterase 1; also known as NPP1, NPPS and PC1) [23]. Transgenic mice lacking these membrane proteins functioning to provide extracellular inhibitory pyrophosphate show increased extracellular calcification [24,25], whereas TNAP-deficient mice (*Akp2*-/-) conversely show decreased extracellular mineralization in the absence of TNAP required to remove this inhibitory pyrophosphate [26,27].

Pyrophosphate is a substrate for TNAP, whose enzymatic action cleaves this inhibitor to produce two phosphate ions; thus, not only is a small-molecule inhibitor of mineralization removed, but two phosphates are liberated for use in apatitic crystal growth. Of these two mineralization-regulating molecules, it is generally thought that the removal of pyrophosphate as an inhibitor is the more dominant change facilitating mineralization. Human hypophosphatasia results from loss-of-function mutations in the *TNAP* (*ALPL*) gene [20]. In the skeleton and dentition, elevated pyrophosphate in these patients leads to hypomineralized bone and tooth extracellular matrices. *Tnap*-deficient mice (*Akp2*-/- mice) have been developed as a mouse model for this disease, and likewise show an osteomalacic skeleton and hypomineralized teeth [26,27]. Of clinical note, systemic administration of a bone-targeted form of TNAP in these mice prevents hypophosphatasia [28].

COMMON DETERMINANTS REGULATING PHYSIOLOGIC AND PATHOLOGIC (KIDNEY AND VASCULAR) CALCIFICATION

In recent years, it has gradually become more apparent that the molecular determinants regulating physiologic mineralization in the skeleton and dentition can also become active in soft tissues that do not normally mineralize—but do so pathologically [29]. This latter pathologic mineralization, where soft tissues calcify ectopically, most commonly occurs within a collagenous extracellular matrix (like for bones and teeth), although several examples exist where elastin is the predominant extracellular matrix component (*e.g.*, in vascular medial arterial calcification [Mönckeberg's Sclerosis] and in calcification of the dermis of the skin in pseudoxanthoma elasticum).

Pathologic calcification of soft tissues has been studied most extensively in blood vessels, kidney and articular cartilage. All these tissues have extensive exposure to circulating fluids that include plasma, urine and synovial fluid, respectively, and thus may be particularly sensitive to changes in freely diffusible small molecules that might influence mineralization—such as pyrophosphate and citrate. Systemically circulating proteins, like fetuin A, have been shown to be widely inhibitory of soft tissue calcification; indeed, mice lacking fetuin A (α_2HS glycoprotein)(*Ahsg*-/-) show extensive ectopic calcification of many of their soft tissues [30]. Collagens type I and III, and elastin, are usually abundant proteins present where calcification occurs (including in Randall's plaques in the kidney), except when it occurs directly in a tissue fluid such as in urine in urolithiasis, in synovial fluid in pseudogout, and in some other joint pathologies.

Noncollagenous proteins and macromolecules produced locally have a significant effect on ectopic calcification, where they seem to be mostly inhibitory. In particular, osteopontin (OPN) has been documented to accumulate abundantly at essentially all sites of pathologic calcification, where its expression is usually upregulated in tissue-resident cells [31,32]. OPN, a heavily phosphorylated glycoprotein of the SIBLING family, potently inhibits both *de novo* crystal growth and seeded crystal growth, with its inhibitory potency being orders of magnitude greater than other well-characterized noncollagenous proteins [33,34]. Consistently, OPN expression and accumulation has been documented at essentially all mineralization sites (both physiologic and pathologic), whereas expression and accumulation of other SIBLING and noncollagenous proteins typical of mineralizing tissues is less obvious and often contradictory amongst various studies. Because of its consistent association with ectopic calcification sites, OPN has been proposed to be secondary "reactive" inhibitor used by body defenses to limit the spread of crystal growth once initiated in soft tissues [29,32]. In normal mineralized tissues, OPN is considered to be part of the physiologic regulatory pathway by which crystals attain their tissue-specific size, shape and orientation appropriate to meeting the tissue-specific biomechanical demands placed upon skeletal and dental tissues [1]. In addition to pyrophosphate and systemically circulating proteins, primary, proteinaceous tissue-resident inhibitors of calcification are thought to reside in most soft tissues, perhaps best illustrated by the extensive calcification of arteries in mice lacking inhibitory matrix Gla protein (MGP)[35].

During vascular calcification and kidney calcification (both for calcium oxalate and for the apatite of Randall's plaques), OPN is particularly prominent and its expression by local cells consistently correlates with an abundance of this protein in nearby calcified deposits [32,36-38]. More specifically, high-resolution electron microscopic studies have revealed concentric or sequentially deposited planar accumulations of OPN that appear to correspond to cyclic growth patterns in calcified masses where periodic crystal growth spurts are followed by inhibition by a layer of protein containing abundant OPN; this is particularly evident in calcium oxalate kidney stones and in induced crystalluria particles in a rat model of urolithiasis [38]. OPN also accumulates with the calcium-phosphate mineral deposited in the interstitium of the kidney in Randall's plaques [37], and in the case of a knockout mouse lacking the sodium phosphate co-transporter 2 (*Npt2*-/-) whose renal phosphate wasting leads to elevated urinary phosphate and precipitation of spherulitic apatite deposits in the renal tubules [39]. Sequentially deposited layers of OPN also appear with vascular calcification of elastic lamellae and interlamellar collagen fibrils of the extracellular matrix in the arterial media of mice lacking matrix Gla protein (*Mgp*-/-)[35]. In these knockout mice, waves of calcification proceed along elastic lamellae, inducing OPN expression by neighboring vascular smooth muscle cells. Secreted OPN coats the surfaces of the calcified elastic lamellae to form a layer of protein referred to as a lamina limitans [32]. The *Mgp*-/- calcification phenotype is 100% penetrant; thus in the absence of MGP, and without any vascular redundancy to prevent the arterial calcification, OPN is called upon as a "second line of defense" to limit as best as possible this detrimental calcification event.

While our understanding of crystal growth inhibition is far more advanced than our understanding of how, where and under what conditions crystals nucleate in extracellular matrices, progress in recent years has decidedly pointed to the induction of a bone (osteoblast) or cartilage (chondrocyte) cell-type differentiation program in arteries (and potentially other soft tissues) that calcify pathologically [40-42]. While bone ossicles may form in the vascular wall [43], these clearly represent a very late-stage event. Calcification of extracellular matrix occurs long before the formation of a bone ossicle, and very likely even before *bona fide* osteogenesis. Isolated membrane-bounded vesicles within the vascular wall [44,45] have long been implicated as initiators of calcification, and osteogenic sequelae may result only as a consequence of this.

Cultured kidney cells have recently been shown to have an upregulation of TNAP and intracellular organellar calcification when provided with an exogenous source of phosphate [46], and expression of the pyrophosphate transporter ANK [47] has been shown in another kidney cell line. Other recent evidence points to an important role for TNAP and pyrophosphate in regulating the phosphate/pyrophosphate balance in soft tissues having an abundant extracellular matrix—like the dermis of skin and the media of blood vessels [48]. While less matrix is present in the kidney, there is nevertheless abundant basement membranes and some collagen in the interstitium of the renal medulla and papillae, and these sites calcify pathologically with apatite to form Randall's plaques [49]. It is possible that perturbation of the phosphate/pyrophosphate balance in the kidney interstitium might lead to the first mineralization events appearing just before the more obvious formation of larger Randall's plaques, which may then be associated with osteogenic events.

A discussion of a potential role for TNAP in various soft tissues pathologies has been presented previously [50]. In transgenic mice where tissue-specific gene promoters were used to selectively drive a high level of TNAP expression by cells within an abundant extracellular matrix, skin dermal collagen and arterial medial collagen (and elastic fibers) were heavily mineralized by the expression of this enzyme and the subsequent removal of inhibitory pyrophosphate at these sites [48]. Once calcification is initiated, it is likely that subsequent responsive signaling processes are locally activated which might lead to chondroblastic and/or osteoblastic programming. Thus, while likely connected, there remains the need to dissociate early mineralization events with those signaling events that trigger and develop the cartilage and bone program in soft tissues. More attention needs to be given to both the very earliest events of this pathologic calcification, and to transcription factor expression and regulation once calcification has begun. Encouraging progress in this area has recently been forthcoming in both the fields of vascular, kidney and joint biology, but much remains to be determined about how pathologic calcification is triggered, and how this might lead to the expression of genes associated with normal mineralized tissues.

ACKNOWLEDGMENTS

The author wishes to thank William N. Addison, Monzur Murshed, Jose Luis Millan, Philippe Crine and Lydia Malynowsky for their input and contributions to much of the work summarized here. Most of the work described from the author's own laboratory has been funded by the Canadian Institutes of Health Research.

REFERENCES

1. M. D. McKee, W. N. Addison and M. T. Kaartinen, *Cells Tissues Organs* **181**, 176-188 (2005).
2. C. D. Fermin, D. Lychakov, A. Campos, H. Hara, E. Sondag, T. Jones, S. Jones, M. Taylor, G. Meza-Ruiz and D. S. Martin, *Histol. Histopathol.* **13**, 1103-1154 (1998).
3. A. J. Engler, S. Sen, H. L. Sweeney and D. E. Discher, *Cell* **126**, 677-689 (2006).
4. S. P. Robins, *Biochem. Soc. Trans.* **35**, 849-852 (2007).
5. M. Nurminskaya and M. T. Kaartinen, *Front. Biosci.* **11**, 1591-1606 (2006).
6. H. F. Al-Jallad, Y. Nakano, J. L. Chen, E. McMillan, C. Lefebvre and M. T. Kaartinen, *Matrix Biol.* **25**, 135-148 (2006).
7. A. L. Boskey, *Ann. N.Y. Acad. Sci.* **760**, 249-256 (1995).
8. D. A. Pampena, K. A. Robertson, O. Litvinova, G. Lajoie, H. A. Goldberg and G. K. Hunter, *Biochem. J.* **378**, 1083-1087 (2004).
9. X. Su, K. Sun, F. Z. Cui and W. J. Landis, *Bone* **32**, 150-162 (2003).
10. S. M. Sweeney, J. P. Orgel, A. Fertala, J. D. McAuliffe, K. R. Turner, G. A. Di Lullo, S. Chen, O. Antipova, S. Perumal, L. Ala-Kokko, A. Forlino, W. A. Cabral, A. M. Barnes, J. C. Marini and J. D. San Antonio, *J. Biol. Chem.* (2008).
11. L. W. Fisher and N. S. Fedarko, *Connect. Tissue Res.* **44 Suppl 1**, 33-40 (2003).
12. D. Toroian, J. E. Lim and P. A. Price, *J. Biol. Chem.* **282**, 22437-22447 (2007).
13. H. C. Anderson, *Curr. Rheumatol. Rep.* **5**, 222-226 (2003).
14. T. Kirsch, *Crit. Rev. Eukaryot. Gene Expr.* **18**, 1-9 (2008).
15. J. L. Millan, *Purinergic Signal* **2**, 335-341 (2006).
16. M. Hui, M. Hu and H. C. Tenenbaum, *Cell Tissue Res* **274**, 429-437 (1993).
17. R. G. Russell, S. Bisaz, A. Donath, D. B. Morgan and H. Fleisch, *J. Clin. Invest.* **50**, 961-969 (1971).
18. A. Kornberg, *Horizons on Biochemistry*, Academic Press Inc., New York, 1962.
19. W. N. Addison, F. Azari, E. S. Sørensen, M. T. Kaartinen and M. D. McKee, *J. Biol. Chem.* **282**, 15872-15883 (2007).
20. J. L. Millan, *Mammalian Alkaline Phosphatases*, Wiley-VCH, Weinheim, 2006.
21. E. C. Moreno, T. Aoba and H. C. Margolis. *Compend Contin Educ Dent Suppl* **8**, S256-S266 (1987).
22. M. J. Rogers, S. Gordon, H. L. Benford, F. P. Coxon, S. P. Luckman, J. Monkkonen and J. C. Frith, *Cancer* **88**, 2961-2978 (2000).
23. R. A. Terkeltaub, *Am. J. Physiol. Cell Physiol.* **281**, C1-C11 (2001).
24. A. M. Ho, M. D. Johnson and D. M. Kingsley, *Science* **289**, 265-270 (2000).
25. L. Hessle, K. A. Johnson, H. C. Anderson, S. Narisawa, A. Sali, J. W. Goding, R. Terkeltaub and J. L. Millan, *Proc. Natl. Acad. Sci. U.S.A* **99**, 9445-9449 (2002).
26. K. N. Fedde, L. Blair, J. Silverstein, S. P. Coburn, L. M. Ryan, R. S. Weinstein, K. Waymire, S. Narisawa, J. L. Millan, G. R. MacGregor and M. P. Whyte, *J. Bone Miner. Res.* **14**, 2015-2026 (1999).
27. K. G. Waymire, J. D. Mahuren, J. M. Jaje, T. R. Guilarte, S. P. Coburn and G. R. MacGregor, *Nat. Genet.* **11**, 45-51 (1995).
28. J. L. Millan, S. Narisawa, I. Lemire, T. P. Loisel, G. Boileau, P. Leonard, S. Gramatikova, R. Terkeltaub, N. Pleshko Camacho, M. D. McKee, P. Crine and M. P. Whyte, *J. Bone Miner. Res.* (2007).
29. C. M. Giachelli, *Orthod. Craniofac. Res.* **8**, 229-231 (2005).
30. C. Schafer, A. Heiss, A. Schwarz, R. Westenfeld, M. Ketteler, J. Floege, W. Muller-Esterl, T. Schinke and W. Jahnen-Dechent, *J. Clin. Invest.* **112**, 357-366 (2003).
31. C. M. Giachelli, M. Y. Speer, X. Li, R. M. Rajachar and H. Yang, *Circ. Res.* **96**, 717-722 (2005).
32. M. T. Kaartinen, M. Murshed, G. Karsenty and M. D. McKee, *J. Histochem. Cytochem.* **55**, 375-386 (2007).
33. J. Sodek, B. Ganss and M. D. McKee, *Crit. Rev. Oral Biol. Med.* **11**, 279-303 (2000).

34. G. K. Hunter, P. V. Hauschka, A. R. Poole, L. C. Rosenberg and H. A. Goldberg, *Biochem. J.* **317 (Pt 1)**, 59-64 (1996).
35. G. Luo, P. Ducy, M. D. McKee, G. J. Pinero, E. Loyer, R. R. Behringer and G. Karsenty, *Nature* **386**, 78-81 (1997).
36. E. R. O'Brien, M. R. Garvin, D. K. Stewart, T. Hinohara, J. B. Simpson, S. M. Schwartz and C. M. Giachelli, *Arterioscler. Thromb.* **14**, 1648-1656 (1994).
37. A. P. Evan, F. L. Coe, S. R. Rittling, S. M. Bledsoe, Y. Shao, J. E. Lingeman and E. M. Worcester, *Kidney Int.* **68**, 145-154 (2005).
38. M. D. McKee, A. Nanci and S. R. Khan, *J. Bone Miner. Res.* **10**, 1913-1929 (1995).
39. H. Chau, S. El-Maadawy, M. D. McKee and H. S. Tenenhouse, *J. Bone Miner. Res.* **18**, 644-657 (2003).
40. S. L. Cheng, J. S. Shao, N. Charlton-Kachigian, A. P. Loewy and D. A. Towler, *J. Biol. Chem.* **278**, 45969-45977 (2003).
41. Y. Tintut, Z. Alfonso, T. Saini, K. Radcliff, K. Watson, K. Bostrom and L. L. Demer, *Circulation* **108**, 2505-2510 (2003).
42. C. Farrington-Rock, N. J. Crofts, M. J. Doherty, B. A. Ashton, C. Griffin-Jones and A. E. Canfield, *Circulation* **110**, 2226-2232 (2004).
43. M. Jeziorska, C. McCollum and D. E. Wooley, *Virchows Arch.* **433**, 559-565 (1998).
44. Y. V. Bobryshev, M. C. Killingsworth, T. G. Huynh, R. S. Lord, A. J. Grabs and S. M. Valenzuela, *Basic Res. Cardiol.* **102**, 133-143 (2007).
45. J. S. Shao, J. Cai and D. A. Towler, *Arterioscler. Thromb. Vasc. Biol.* **26**, 1423-1430 (2006).
46. F. Azari, H. Vali, J. L. Guerquin-Kern, T. D. Wu, A. Croisy, S. K. Sears, M. Tabrizian and M. D. McKee, *J. Struct. Biol.* In Press, (2008)
47. G. Carr, J. A. Sayer and N. L. Simmons, *Cell Physiol. Biochem.* **20**, 507-516 (2007).
48. M. Murshed, D. Harmey, J. L. Millan, M. D. McKee and G. Karsenty, *Genes Dev.* **19**, 1093-1104 (2005).
49. A. P. Evan, J. E. Lingeman, F. L. Coe, J. H. Parks, S. Bledsoe, Y. Shao, A. J. Sommer, R. F. Paterson, R. L. Kuo and M. Grynpas, *J. Clin. Invest.* **111**, 607-616 (2003).
50. M. Hui and H. C. Tenenbaum, *Anat Rec* **253**, 91-94 (1998).

Bone Genes in the Kidney of Stone Formers

Andrew P. Evan and Sharon B. Bledsoe

Department of Anatomy and Cell Biology, Indiana University, School of Medicine, 635 Barnhill Drive, Indianapolis, Indiana, 46223

Abstract. Intraoperative papillary biopsies from kidneys of idiopathic-calcium oxalate stone formers (ICSF) have revealed a distinct pattern of mineral deposition in the interstitium of the renal papilla. The earliest sites of these deposits, termed Randall's plaque, are found in the basement membrane of thin loops of Henle and appear to spread into the surrounding interstitium down to the papillary epithelium. Recent studies show kidney stones of ICSF patients grow attached to the renal papilla and at sites of Randall's plaque. Together these observations suggest that plaque formation may be the critical step in stone formation. In order to control plaque formation and thereby reduce future kidney stone development, the mechanism of plaque deposition must be understood. Because the renal papilla has unique anatomical features similar to bone and the fact that the interstitial deposits of ICSF patients are formed of biological apatite, this paper tests the hypothesis that sites of interstitial plaque form as a result of cell-mediated osteoblast-like activity.

Keywords: plaque; osteoblast-like activity; protein matrix; biopsy tissue; human stone formers
PACS: 87.18.–h

Randall's Discovery of Interstitial Plaque in the 1940's

Papillary Lesion Type I. The early studies of Randall on 1,154 kidneys examined after autopsy with just a hand lens, revealed a cream colored area near the tip of the renal papilla, which was subepithelial in location [1]. A total of 227 kidneys or 19.6% showed such a feature on one or more papillae. On microscopic examination and staining, the cream colored areas were found to be plaques of calcium salts deposited in the interstitial tissue of the renal papilla and definitely not in tubular lumens. These sites of calcium plaque were termed papillary lesion type I. In addition, Randall found evidence of cellular destruction and round-cell infiltration in only 4% of the papilla. He reasoned that such changes are inevitable findings at the autopsy table and believed that it represented a secondary factor from pre-existing pathological conditions.

Randall's next critical observation was the discovery of a secondary deposit of some black material about 1 mm in diameter on a site of subepithelial plaque. Microscopic examination of that material and the plaque associated with it revealed a site of interstitial plaque denuded of an epithelial covering and deposited on the surface of the plaque was the black colored material. This black material was later determined to be the earliest evidence of a renal stone.

The third important finding was the discovery of visible calcium plaque supporting a stone, which projected into the lumen of the minor calyx. A total of sixty-five

CP1049, *Renal Stone Disease 2, 2nd International Urolithiasis Research Symposium*,
edited by A. P. Evan, J. E. Lingeman, J. A. McAteer, and J. C. Williams, Jr.

kidneys were found to have one or more stones attached to the renal papilla at sites of calcium plaque. Further chemical analysis of the sites of calcium plaque and associated stone found the calcium plaque to be composed of calcium carbonate and phosphate while the stones varied from calcium phosphate for the smallest stones to calcium oxalate in the larger stones.

There are obvious problems with Randall's studies. First, he did not have detailed medical records or metabolic data to determine the type of stone disease these patients had. So he had to generalize his observations. Second, he had autopsy-quality material to examine, which limits the level of cellular change one can link to a disease process vs. autolysis. Despite these issues Randall concluded from his observations: "*Here, for the first time, we find a lesion of not infrequent occurrence (19.6%) and of rather constant character and chemical composition. This lesion, innocent enough while buried in the wall of a renal papilla, can lose its epithelial covering and from then on be bathed in calycine urine, and then, acting as a foreign body, it becomes the nidus upon which a different urinary salt crystallizes. Here, likewise, we can picture the reason that renal calculi can remain stationary while increasing in size. Here we can account for a common origin of stone formation, which also allows of the known variation of salts so deposited to form stone, and we can assume that the salt which crystallizes to form a calculus is the one which, at that epoch, is most readily precipitated from solution [1].*"

Randall's Description of Intratubular Calcification or Nephrocalcinosis

Papillary Lesion Type II. In twenty-three of the one thousand-one hundred and fifty-four total cases, Randall observed a second pattern of mineral deposition in the renal papilla [1]. On gross inspection of each papilla Randall noted yellowish lines converging toward the papillary tip with the cribriform membrane heavily impregnated with visible salt deposits. Microscopic examination of these papilla revealed varying degrees of tubular plugging, from where every collecting duct was involved to just a solitary tubule. In four kidneys, the intraluminal mineral deposits were uric acid while the remaining nineteen kidneys the collecting ducts were plugged with calcium phosphate. Evidence of infection was seen in eight of nineteen kidneys. Marked fibrosis with cellular injury of the nearby plugged collecting ducts was seen in all specimens. Frequently the tip of the papilla was necrotic and in three cases a stone was found growing at the papilla tip as part of the calcium deposits. Randall concluded that the lower incidence of the type II lesion suggests that its cause is based upon some infectious, dietary, metabolic, or glandular disturbances, which were more rare then the conditions causing type I lesions.

New Studies Revealing Interstitial Plaque (Randall's Plaque) in Idiopathic Calcium Oxalate Stone Formers

While there have been significant advances in treatment modalities for kidney stones, as well as in the metabolic evaluation of kidney stone disease, little progress has been made in our understanding of the pathogenesis of kidney stone formation. However, with the advent of the digital endoscope and now the digital ureteroscope, our group designed a series of studies to test the hypothesis that sites of Randall's plaque develop in unique anatomical sites of the kidney and that its formation is conditioned by specific stone-forming pathophysiologies [2]. To test this hypothesis, we studied a series of well characterized idiopathic calcium oxalate stone formers (ICSF), intestinal bypass patients for obesity, brushite, renal tubular acidosis, cystine, primary hyperparathyroidism and ileostomy patients with stones [2,3]. Our protocol incorporated thorough metabolic analyses of those patients we studied surgically with the new digital, surgical instruments, which permitted us to carefully map all renal papilla of a particular kidney at very high image resolutions followed by biopsy of selected papilla for histopathologic examination.

In this paper, only our findings in idiopathic calcium oxalate stone formers, the most common type of stone former, are described. During the endoscopic examination of the renal papilla, irregular, whitish subepithelial sites of plaque were easily seen just as described by Randall (the type 1 calcium plaque). Histological examination of such sites revealed deposits of plaque first in the basement membrane of the thin loops of Henle (Figure 1a). These initial sites of plaque appear to spread from the loops into the surrounding interstitial space and become very dense around thin loops/collecting ducts (Figure 1b) migrating down the papillary tip where it is directly beneath this epithelial layer. Within the basement membranes, plaque consists of individual laminated particles in which zones of crystal and organic matrix overlay each other in a tree-ring pattern (Figures 1c and d). The mineral type is biological apatite. In the matrix, both osteopontin and heavy chain 3 of inter-alpha-trypsin were immuno-loacalized [3]. In the interstitium, these particles fuse to form a syncytium of crystal islands in an organic sea. Plaque is never found in the lumens of tubules or vessels, or within epithelial cells; it is uniquely located in the basement membranes and the interstitium. There is no evidence of inflammation. Therefore as expected, the renal epithelial cells invariably appear normal, as does the cellular interstitium.

Great significance is placed on interstitial plaque because of our observation in ICSF patients that their stones grow attached to renal papillae at sites of exposed interstitial plaque, a finding Randall also noted for stones attached to the renal papilla (Figures 2a and b). Several investigators have described a depression at the attachment region or "umbilication" on the concave (tissue side) of an attached stone [4,5,6] that is thought to represent the interface area between the interstitial plaque and the developing stone, the stone-tissue attachment region. This region is generally small and is whitish in color (Figure 2b). By scanning electron microscopy, tubular profiles are easily seen within this region [4,5] and the mineral content is primarily carbapatite

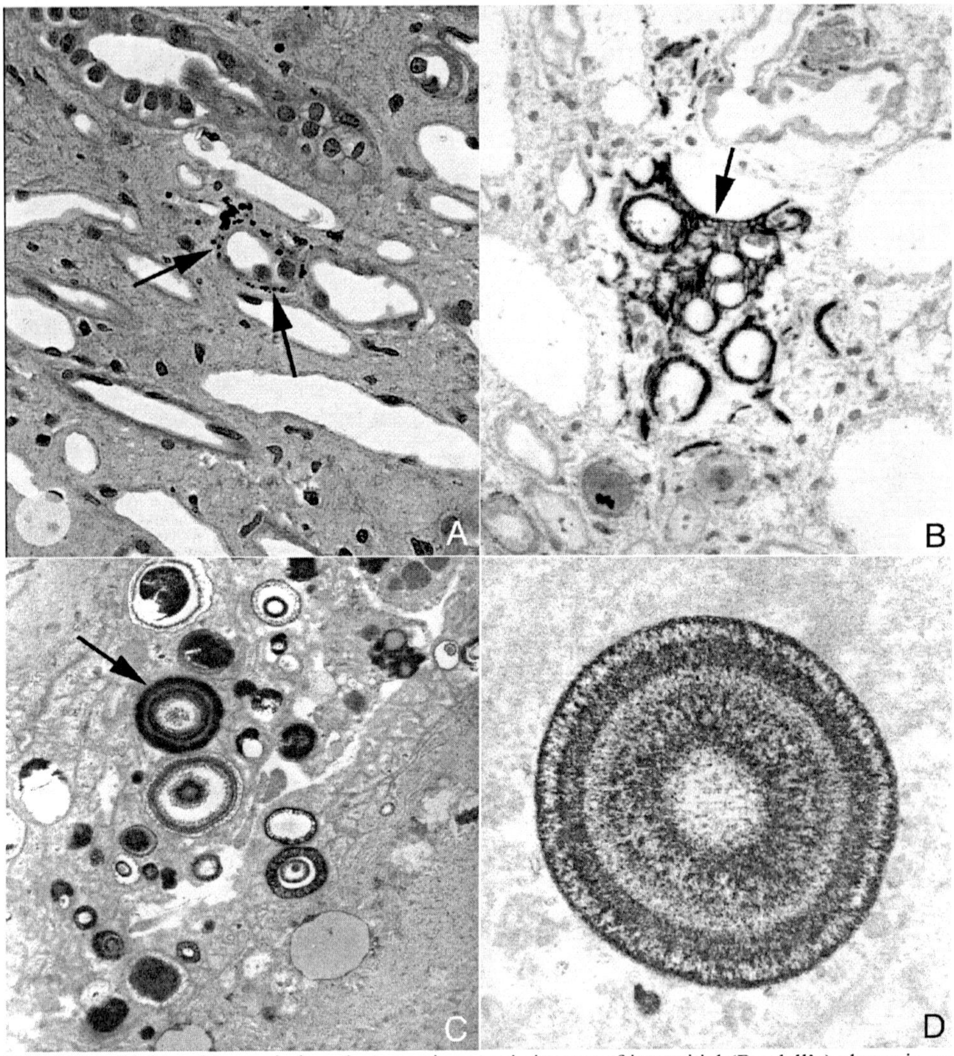

FIGURE 1. Light and transmission electron microscopic images of interstitial (Randall's) plaque in an ICSF patient. Panel A is a light microscopic image showing the initial sites of interstitial plaque deposits (arrows) in the basement membranes of thin loops of Henle. Panel B shows a region of the interstitium filled with plaque (arrow) that surrounds thin loops of Henle but also accumulates in interstitial space. Panel C is a transmission electron micrograph showing a similar site of mineralization seen in panel A. Individual deposits (arrow) vary in size but are generally spherical in shape with a multilayered, tree ring-like internal structure. The electron dense (dark) layers are formed of matrix material while the electron lucent (light) layers are composed of hydroxyapatite mineral.

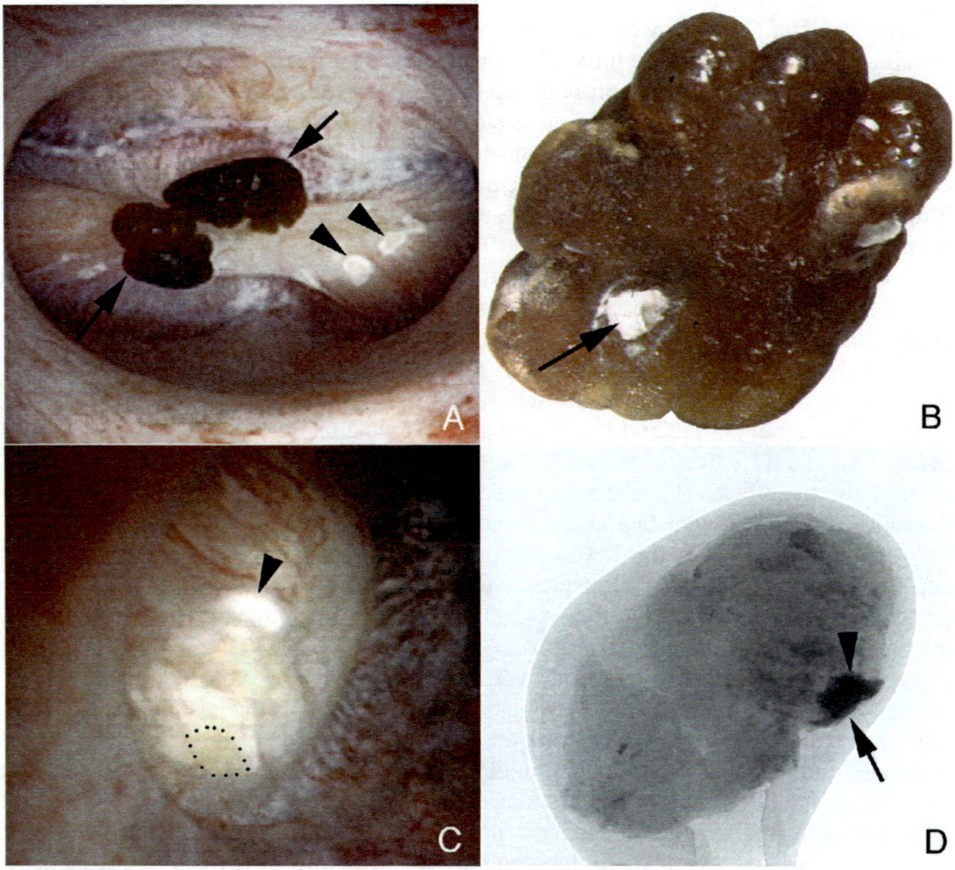

FIGURE 2. Endoscopic, light microscopy and μ-CT images of attached stones prior to and after removal. Panel A is an endoscopic view of two stones (arrows) attached to a compound papilla. Off to the right of the stones are several regions of Randall's plaque (arrowheads). Inspection of attached stones (panel B) such as illustrated in panel A after removal always reveals a whitish area (arrow) on the tissue (concave) side of the stone that lines up with a site of Randall's plaque. Panel C shows a 0.5 millimeter attached stone (outlined in dotted line) that was removed *en bloc* with biopsy forceps. Panel D shows the same stone by μ-CT. The stone (arrow) is clearly seen at the surface of the sample and resting on a region of interstitial plaque (arrowhead) deep to it.

with some uric acid [6]. To more carefully analyze the ultrastructural features of the stone-tissue attachment region to determine the potential steps to stone formation, we biopsied a 0.5 millimeter stone *en bloc* (Figure 2c and d) [7]. After this stone was demineralized and sectioned, the transition area between the interstitial plaque and the developing stone was examined and was found to be lacking papillary epithelial cells. The outer surface of the interstitial plaque was covered with a ribbon-like layer made up of numerous alternating layers of mineral and matrix presumably formed from urinary ions and proteins. Abruptly, this mineralization pattern changed such that rafts of large and small crystals were seen embedded into the outer most layer of the ribbon, which is matrix material. The mineral of the interface region is amorphous apatite. The process of deposition of amorphous apatite on the ribbon-like barrier represents mineral overgrowth and is what initiates stone formation. The overgrowth process also allows the developing stone to be fixed to the papilla and thereby, permitting slow and, we think, progressive growth of the stone for many months or years. Progressing further into the developing stone, the mineral changes to biological apatite and eventually to calcium oxalate.

In order to establish if stone formation and growth in ICSF patients is growth on Randall's plaque, Miller and colleagues [8] formally tested the hypothesis that "in a population of ICSF, the majority of stones grew attached to interstitial plaque" and reported the results in this proceedings. A total of 115 stone were observed at the time of percutaneous nephrolithotomy or ureteroscopy. It was determined if each stone was attached to a renal papilla and if attached was the attachment to a region of interstitial plaque? Of the 115 stones studied 81 were attached and to plaque. These data fully support the hypothesis that the mechanism of stone formation is ICSF is growth on Randall's plaque (Figures 2a and b). These findings strongly suggest a critical role for the interstitial plaque in the development of kidney stones. Stated another way, it appears that sites of interstitial plaque are a requirement for the development of kidney stones in ICSF patients. If one could eliminate the interstitial plaque, one would prevent all if not most stone formation.

Lastly, it is important to point out that interstitial plaque is a characteristic finding of ICSF patients and not the other groups of stone formers we have studied [3]. These other stone forming groups have unique histopathologic characteristics centered on common findings of intraluminal plugging of inner medullar collecting ducts and adjacent interstitial fibrosis. The distinct histopathologic findings between ICSF and other stone formers suggest separate pathogenetic pathways for stone formation between groups and therefore, each potentially requiring different treatment strategies.

Mechanisms for Interstitial Plaque Formation

Current hypotheses:

This present paper has clearly established the critical role interstitial plaque plays in the initiation of stone formation. If we are to develop therapeutic approaches to alter the course of plaque development, we must understand the mechanism for plaque formation. Two potential models appear reasonable to explain plaque formation. The first model states that the interstitial cells of the renal medulla transdifferentiate into osteoblast-like cells and initiate a cell-mediated process of bone formation much like what has been described in coronary and renal arteries and heart valves. The second idea suggests that there is an increased calcium and phosphate levels in the papillary interstitium, which leads to an increased calcium/phosphate ion product resulting in the deposition and growth of apatite crystals on regions of collagen matrix.

We have decided to test the idea of a cell-mediated osteoblast-like activity for three reasons. First, as early as 1942, Vermooten [9] suggested that the sites of interstitial crystal deposition were similar to the first stages of "bony ossification." Second, the structural organization and specialization of the interstitial compartment of the inner medulla would appear to be able to support bone formation. Lastly, there is ectopic calcification in a variety of organs [10] resulting from mineral (usually biological apatite) precipitating in soft tissues through a cell-mediated process [11].

Structural similarities of inner medulla to developing bone

Central to the formation of embryonic bone is a source of multipotential mesenchymal stem cells (MSC) that can form osteogenic cells (osteoblasts). These cells under the appropriate stimuli secrete osteoid, which contains hyaline ground substance composed of type I collagen, osteopontin, bone sialoprotein, osteocalcin and other bone matrix proteins. It is on this osteoid (particularly on the type 1 collagen) that hydroxyapatite mineral crystallizes in a controlled fashion.

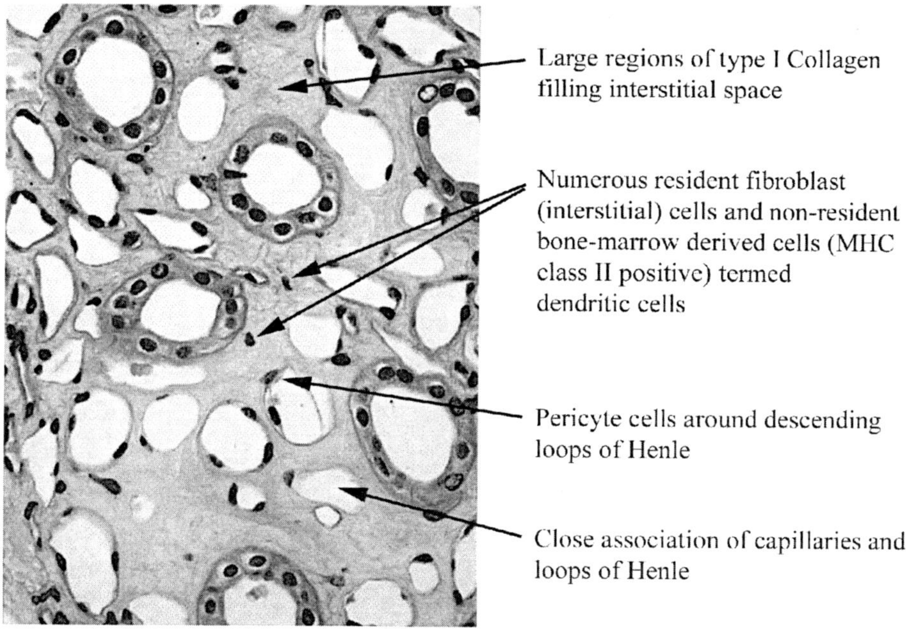

FIGURE 3. Light micrograph of the inner medulla of a human kidney near the tip of the papilla. Each of the unique features of the papilla at this level of the renal medulla is pointed out.

The inner medulla of the kidney also has an internal source of stromal fibroblasts termed interstitial cells, type 1 (Figure 3). These cells are physically connected to nearby basement membranes of tubules and vessels by cellular attachments and to each other by intermediate-like junctions. They are in contact with nerve terminals and migrating nonresident bone marrow-derived cells. The ultrastructure of the medullary interstitial cell is much like other fibroblasts in other parenchymal organs and possess extensive cell processes with prominent a cytoskeleton (actin filaments) and lipid inclusions. There are numerous reports documenting the phenotypic modulation of these cells in vivo under conditions of environmental factors, such as extracellular matrix composition, cytokines and growth factors. In other words, these cells can transform to myofibroblasts under conditions of interstitial inflammation [12]. Renal medullary interstitial cells display lipid droplets in their cytoplasm that can be changed by specific environmental conditions established by the inner medullary collecting ducts. These interstitial cells are thought to help regulate urinary osmolarity, produce prostaglandin E_2 and glycosaminoglycans and contain aminopeptidase A. In healthy kidneys, there is also a bone marrow-derived interstitial cell termed dendritic cells are major histocompatibility complex (MHC) class II positive. They have spot-like cell contacts with the stromal fibroblasts. In addition, the descending loops of Henle are lined with numerous pericyte cells. These cells have been shown to also have the potential for transdifferentiation into osteogenic cells [13].

Another unique feature of the renal medulla is that the medullary interstitial volume at the papillary tip greatly increases from that of the outer medulla (from 30-40% to 3-5%, respectively) especially in kidneys that have a simple medulla like in man [14]. The extracellular matrix is composed of interstitial reticulum (types 1, 3 & 6 collagen), proteoglycans, glycosaminoglycans, glycoproteins (like fibronectin, laminin) and interstitial fluid. Most important to this hypothesis is that the amount of type 1 collagen greatly increases at the papillary tip as the extracellular volume increases.

Induction of Osteogenic Cells During Normal Bone Formation

Osteogenic cells like the osteoblast arise from what is termed multipotential mesenchymal stem cells (MSC). These stem cells have the capacity to not only form osteoblast cells but also other lineages that include chondroblasts, fibroblasts, adipocytes and myoblasts. The development of these MSC into mature osteoblasts is through a sequence of cellular transitions demonstrated by morphological and molecular criteria [12]. Two key genes for osteoblast differentiation are Cbfa1 (recently named Runx2), a member of the runt homology domain transcription factor family and osterix, a Kruppel-like Sp-1 binding factor with three zinc-finger motifs. Runx2 is thought to be the master gene for osteoblast differentiation while osterix may complete the differentiation process. Both genes drive the osteoblastic cells to produce alkaline phosphatase, osteopontin, osteocalcin, type 1 collagen and bone sialoprotein. These proteins/enzymes are well known to be bone extracellular matrix molecules and markers of osteoblast differentiation expressed during active mineralization.

Induction of Osteogenic Cells During Ectopic Calcification

Cells from a variety of tissues may be induced to differentiate into osteoblast-like cells, which can then actively mineralize the surrounding tissue. In particular, pericytes, smooth muscle cells and adventitial myofibroblasts have been shown to participate in ossification of blood vessels [10, 11]. These cells have been shown to have the capacity to undergo osteogenic/chondrogenic differentiation resulting in the production of bone morphogenetic protein, osteopontin, osteocalcin, type 1 collagen and matrix γ-carboxylated glutamate, all components of osteoid. Thus, calcification may proceed in a vessel wall in the same way as occurs in bone formation.

Induction of osteoblast-like cells in the medulla of kidney stone formers

The hypothesis this study tests is that resident or non-resident fibroblasts in the renal medulla of idiopathic calcium oxalate stone formers transdifferentiate into osteoblast-like cells resulting in a cell-mediated formation of interstitial (Randall's) plaque in the basement membranes of thin loops of Henle and the type 1 collage of the interstitium. To test this hypothesis, we used immunohistochemistry to run a set of pilot studies to determine the presence of Runx2 and osterix, the two key genes in osteoblast differentiation, in primary murine osteoblastogenic cells stimulated with ascorbic acid for 10 days, decalcified normal rat ribs, and in normal human renal papillary biopsies and renal papillary biopsied for idiopathic calcium oxalate kidney stone formers. To our knowledge, these two antibodies have not been previously localized in human renal papillary tissue. Both antibodies were purchased from Santa Cruz Biotechnologies (Santa Cruz, CA). Standard immunohistochemical techniques were used to identify the location of these proteins [15].

Our preliminary observations on the immuno-staining pattern of Runx2 in the non-confluent primary osteoblastogenic cells was to the nuclear region of these cells (Figure 4a). This is an expected finding in that Runx2 is a transcriptional factor. Osterix was immuno-positive in the cytoplasm of the non-confluent primary osteoblastogenic cells (Figure 4b), an unexpected finding in that osterix is also a transcriptional factor. This immuno-staining pattern may relate to the "shuttling" ability of this protein. We will test both of these antibodies on confluent primary osteoblastogenic cells to test the possibility that the stage of the cell cycle a cell is in may influence their gene expression of these proteins. We will also obtain monoclonal antibodies to both Runx2 and osterix to determine if there was any cross-reactivity related to the polyclonal nature of these antibodies.

Next we determined the immuno-staining pattern of Runx2 and osterix on renal papillary sections from a idiopathic calcium oxalate stone former. The polyclonal antibody to Runx2 was immuno-positive to the apical cell membrane of primarily inner medullary collecting ducts (Figure 4c) while osterix stained the entire cytoplasm of these same cells. The immuno-staining pattern for both Runx2 and osterix was unexpected in that they are transcriptional factors. This may be due to an unknown function of these proteins or more likely to the polyclonal nature of the antibodies. We have ongoing studies using monoclonal antibodies to Runx2, osterix, osteocalcin and bone sialoprotein.

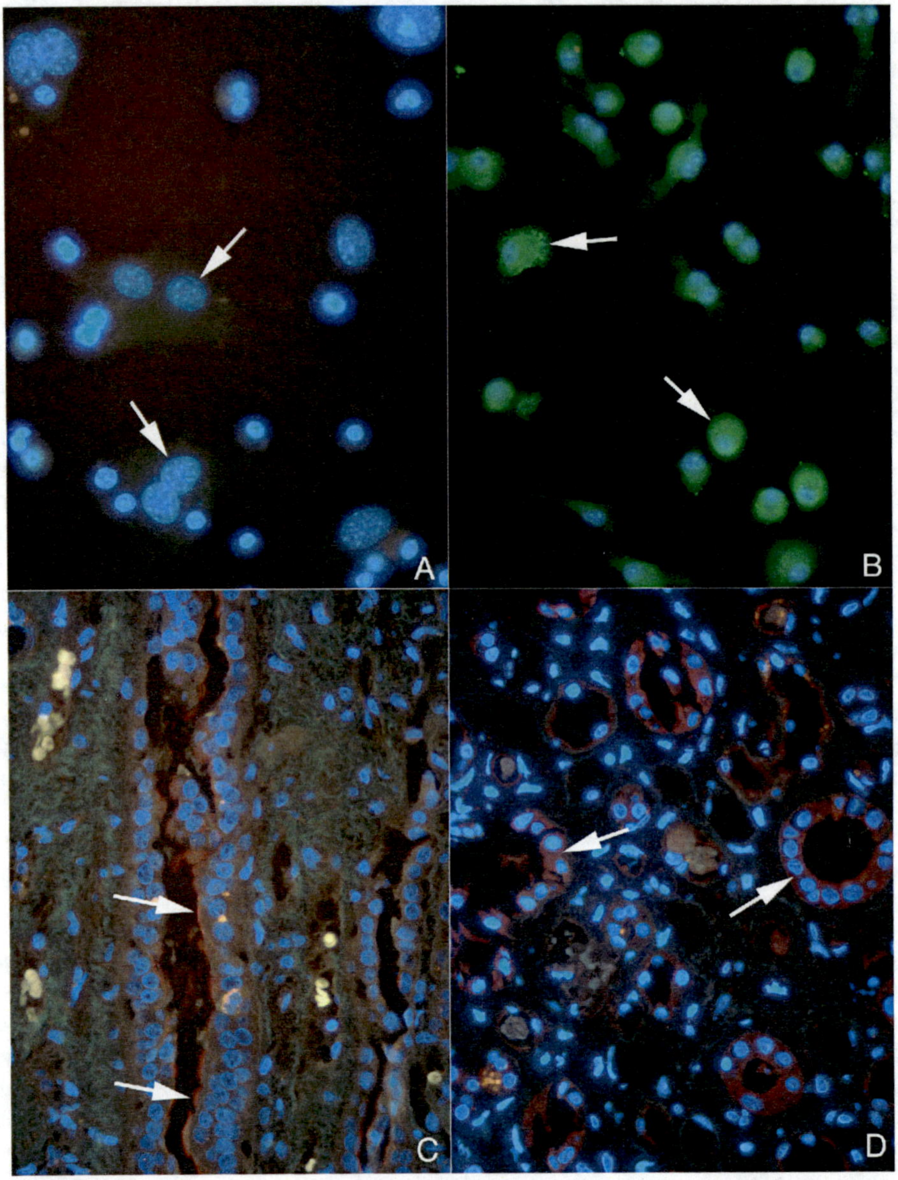

FIGURE 4. Immunohistochemical localization of two transcriptional factors, Runx2 and osterix, for osteoblast activity. Panel A shows immuno-positive staining of primary osteoblastogenic cells for Runx2 using a polyclonal antibody. The staining is localized to the nuclear region of the cells (arrows) as expected. Panel B shows immuno-positive staining for osterix in the same cells. Staining is seen in the cytoplasm (arrows), an unexpected pattern. Panel C shows Runx2 immuno-positive staining in inner medullary collecting ducts of tissue from ICSF patients. Staining was seen at the apical end of these cells (arrows), but not in the nucleus. Osterix stained the entire cytoplasm of the inner medullary collecting duct cells (arrows), but again not the nucleus.

CONCLUSION

This paper has attempted to outline the rationale that supports the hypothesis that interstitial plaque develops as a cell-mediated osteoblastic process of bone formation. The preliminary data generated in this study do not allow us to say that this hypothesis is correct or incorrect. Clearly, we have to obtain additional monoclonal antibodies to sort out our pilot data on the immuno-staining patterns of Runx2 and osterix on the non-confluent primary osteoblastogenic cells and the renal papillary sections for known kidney stone formers. Our current observations of the immuno-localization of Runx2 and osterix may be simply representing a non-specific staining pattern.

ACKNOWLEDGEMENTS

This work was supported by NIH grant P01 DK56788. We want to thank Dr. Joseph Bidwell for the primary osteoblastogenic cell culture cells and his scholarly input into the experimental design of this pilot study and Dr. James Williams for supplying Figure 2b.

REFERENCES

1. Randall A: The etiology of primary renal calculus. *Intl Abst Surgery,* 71, 209-240 (1940).
2. Evan AP, Lingeman JE, Coe Fl, Parks JH, *et al*: Randall's plaque of patients with nephrolithiasis begins in basement membranes of thin loops of Henle. *J Clin Invest*, 111, 607-616 (2003).
3. Evan AP, Lingeman JE, Coe FL, Worcester E: Randall's Plaque: pathogenesis and role in calcium oxalate nephrolithiasis. *Kidney Intl*, 69, 1313-1318 (2006).
4. Cifuentes Delatte L, Minon-Cifuents, JL, Medina JA: Papillary stones: calcified renal tubules in Randall's plaques. *J Urol*, 133, 490-494 (1985).
5. Pieras E, Costa-Bauza A, Ramis M, Grases F: Papillary and nonpapillary calcium oxalate monohydrate renal calculi: comparative study of etiologic factors. *TSW Urol*, 1, 116-124 (2006).
6. Daudon M, Traxer O, Jungers P, Bazin D: Stone morphology suggestive of Randall's plaque. In *1st Annual International Urolithiasis Research Symposium* (vol 900), edited by Evan AP, Lingeman JE, and Williams JC, Jr., Indianapolis, Indiana, American Institute of Physics, 2007, pp 26-34.
7. Evan AP, Coe FL, Lingeman JE, Shao Y, *et al*: Mechanism of formation of human calcium oxalate renal stones on Randall's plaque. *Anat Rec*, 290, 1315-1323 (2007).
8. Miller NL, Gillen DL, Williams JC, Evan AP, *et al*: Stones in idiopathic calcium oxalate stone disease are attached to sites of interstitial plaque. In: Evan, A.P., J.E. Lingeman, J.A. McAteer, and J.C. Williams, eds. *Renal Stone Disease 2: Proceedings of the Second International Urolithiasis Research Symposium.* American Institute of Physics, Melville, NY, 2008.
9. Vermooten V: The origin and development in the renal papilla of Randall's calcium plaques. *J Urol*, 48, 27-37 (1942).
10. Giachelli CM: Vascular calcification mechanisms. *J Am Soc Nephrol,* 15, 2959-2964 (2004).
11. Giachelli CM: Inducers and inhibitors of biomineralization: lessons from pathological calcification. *Orthod. Craniofac Res,* 8, 229-231 (2005).
12. Desmouliere A, Gabbiana G: Myofibroblast differentiation during fibrosis. *Exp Nephrol*, 3, 134-139 (1995).
13. Tintut Y, Alfonso Z, Saini T, Radcliff K, *et al*: Multilineage potential of cells from the artery wall. *Circulation*, 108, 2505-2510 (2003).
14. Kriz W, Kaissling B: Structural organization of the mammalian kidney. In: Kidney: Physiology and Pathophysiology, W Seldin and G Giebisch eds, Lippincott Williams & Wilkins, Philadelphia, pp 587-654 (2000).
15. Evan AP, Coe FL, Rittling SR, Bledsoe SM, *et al*: Apatite plaque particles in inner medulla of kidneys of calcium oxalate stone formers: Osteopontin localization. *Kidney Intl*, 68, 145-154 (2005).

Cell Biology of Thiazide Bone Effects

Gerardo Gamba[a] and Daniela Riccardi[b]

[a]Molecular Physiology Unit, Instituto Nacional de Ciencias Médicas y Nutrición Salvador Zubirán and Instituto de Investigaciones Biomédicas, Universidad Nacional Autónoma de México, Tlalpan 14000 Mexico City, Mexico
[b]Cardiff University School of Biosciences and Cardiff Institute of Tissue Engineering and Repair, Cardiff, United Kingdom

Abstract. The thiazide-sensitive Na^{+}:Cl^{-} cotransporter (NCC) is the major pathway for salt reabsorption in the mammalian kidney. The activity of NCC is not only related to salt metabolism, but also to calcium and magnesium homeostasis due to the inverse relationship between NCC activity and calcium reabsorption. Hence, the thiazide-type diuretics that specifically block NCC have been used for years, not only for treatment of hypertension and edematous disease, but also for the management of renal stone disease. Epidemiological studies have shown that chronic thiazide treatment is associated with higher bone mineral density and reduced risk of bone fractures, which can only partly be explained in terms of their effects on the kidney. In this regard, we have recently shown that NCC is expressed in bone cells and that inhibition of NCC in bone, either by thiazides or by reduction of NCC protein with specific siRNA, is associated with increased mineralization *in vitro*. These observations open a field of study to begin to understand the cell biology of the beneficial effects of thiazides in bone.

Keywords: Diuretics, distal convoluted tubule, calcium, mineralization.
PACS: 01.30.Cc

INTRODUCTION

The thiazide-sensitive Na^{+}:Cl^{-} cotransporter (NCC) is the main pathway for salt reabsorption in the distal convolute tubule (DCT) in mammalian kidney and also plays an important role in bone mineralization [1]. Following our molecular identification of NCC cDNA from fish urinary bladder [2] and mammalian kidney [3] more than a decade ago significant progress has been made in understanding the physiology of NCC. This cotransporter is the pharmacological target of thiazide-type diuretics that are recommended as the first line treatment of arterial hypertension, either alone or in combination with other antihypertensive agents [4]. In addition, elderly patients under thiazide treatment exhibit decreased prevalence of osteoporosis-related bone fractures [5]. It has been clearly established that NCC plays an essential role in preserving the extracellular fluid volume, blood pressure and bone density, as demonstrated by the identification of NCC inactivating mutations as the cause of Gitelman's disease, an inherited disorder that features arterial hypotension, hypokalemia, metabolic alkalosis, hypocalciuria, hypomagnesaemia, and increased bone mineral density [6]. Additionally, a defect in NCC regulation by serine/threonine kinases WNK1 and WNK4 is implicated in the pathogenesis of a salt-dependent form of human

CP1049, *Renal Stone Disease 2, 2nd International Urolithiasis Research Symposium,*
edited by A. P. Evan, J. E. Lingeman, J. A. McAteer, and J. C. Williams, Jr.

hypertension, known as pseudohypoaldosteronism type II (PHAII), that is a mirror image of Gitelman's patients (hyperkalemia, metabolic acidosis, hypercalciuria), which also features decreased bone density and enhanced sensitivity to thiazides [7]. Thus, at the clinical level there is a clear inverse relationship between renal NCC activity and bone mineral density, where a reduction in the NCC activity is mirrored by a higher bone mineral density and vice versa. In the present chapter we review the current knowledge around the molecular physiology of NCC in the kidney and bone and our view of the mechanisms for the inverse relationship between NCC activity and bone mineralization.

NCC belongs to the super family of electroneutral cation-coupled chloride cotransporters (SLC12) from which nine members have been identified, two out of which remains orphan at the functional level [1]. Functional and structural analysis revealed that the SLC12 family can be divided in two major branches. NCC, together with two isoforms of the Na^+:K^+:$2Cl^-$ cotransporter, NKCC1 and NKCC2, compose the Na-driven branch (NKCCs). These membrane transporters translocate chloride ions together with sodium (with or without potassium). Thus, following the driving force generated by the Na^+:K^+:ATPase, these cotransporters move ions from outside to inside the cell. The other is the K^+-driven branch and is made by four genes encoding four isoforms of K^+:Cl^- cotransporters, known as KCC1 to KCC4. These transporters use potassium as the only cation coupled to chloride. Thus, they move ions from inside to outside the cells. SLC12 cotransporters are involved in many different physiological processes at the level of cellular physiology, such as regulation of cell volume and/or intracellular chloride concentration ($[Cl^-]_i$), at the level of specific organ physiology, such as modulation of neuronal excitability, and at the level of systemic physiology involving different organs, such as regulation of arterial blood pressure.

Most of the SLC12 family members are expressed in many organs or tissues, with the exception of three of them [1]. The Na^+:K^+:$2Cl^-$ cotransporter NKCC2 is expressed only in the apical membrane of the thick ascending limb of Henle's loop where it serves as an important salt reabsorption pathway and as a receptor for loop diuretics, like furosemide or bumetanide. The K^+:Cl^- cotransporter KCC2 is expressed only in the central nervous system, specifically in neurons. The third is NCC. For many years it was believed that NCC was expressed exclusively in the apical membrane of the distal convoluted tubule in the kidney. As is shown below, it has recently been shown that NCC is also expressed in bone [8] and probably in the intestine [9].

RENAL PHYSIOLOGY OF THE NA^+:CL^- COTRANSPORTER

The mammalian distal convoluted tubule (DCT) begins just a few cells after the macula densa, hence it is located in a region of the nephron in which any change in salt reabsorption can no longer be compensated for by tubuloglomerular feedback. [10-14]. 5-10% of glomerular filtrate is reabsorbed in DCT. The molecular mechanism of salt reabsorption in DCT is shown in Figure 1. Most of the studies in mammalian kidneys agree that NCC is the only sodium reabsorption pathway along the early DCT and shares this work with the sodium channel ENaC in late DCT [13;15-19]. The sodium gradient that drives transport from the lumen to the interstitium is due to the intense expression and activity of the Na^+:K^+:ATPase, which is polarized to the basolateral membrane [20]. Potassium that enters the cell through the Na^+:K^+:ATPase is secreted by the luminal membrane via ROMK K^+ channels [21] and by an apical K^+:Cl^- cotransporter [22]. Thus, the rates of Na^+:Cl^- reabsorption and K^+ secretion are positively correlated. The chloride entering in the apical membrane through NCC leaves the cell at the basolateral membrane by the way of the chloride channels CLC-KB and CLC-KA. NCC is highly regulated by the mineralocorticoid hormone aldosterone secreted by the adrenal glands [23-25]. As shown in Figure 1, the apical Na^+:Cl^- cotransporter in DCT is the receptor for thiazide-type diuretics, like chlorthalidone, hydrochlorothiazide, bendroflumethiazide, and metolazone [3;13;26], which are among the most commonly prescribed drugs in the world due to their beneficial effects in the treatment of arterial hypertension, edematous states, and renal stone disease [27].

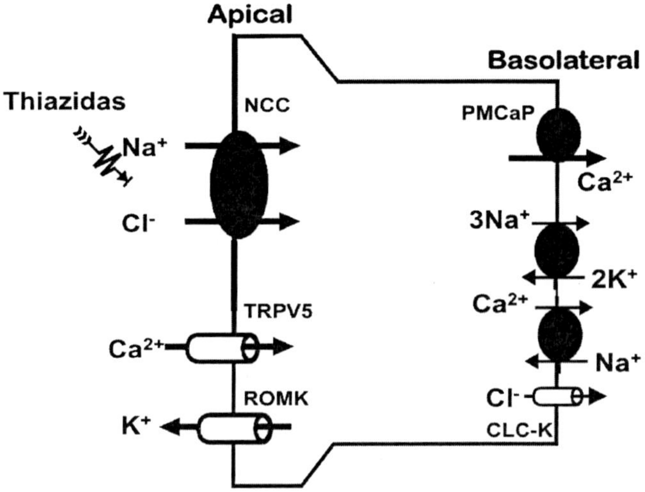

FIGURE 1. Molecular physiology or ion transport in DCT.

NCC also modulates calcium reabsorption, but this occurs in an inversely related fashion. The higher the NCC activity and hence, the sodium reabsorption, the lower the calcium reabsorption and vice versa [12]. DCT is the region of the nephron in which most of the calcium reabsorption takes place and it is specifically modulated by calcium sparing hormones, such as parathyroid hormone. The mechanism involved in calcium absorption in DCT is also depicted in Figure 1. Calcium ions enter the cell through the apical calcium channel known as TRPV5. Inside the cell, free calcium is trapped by calbindin D28K, also known as parvalbumin, and transported through the cell preventing an unwanted increase of this divalent cation in the cytoplasm. At the basolateral membrane, calcium ions leave the cell via the Na^+:Ca^{2+} exchanger or the plasma membrane Ca^{2+} ATPase [28].

Two different mechanisms for the inverse relation between NCC activity and calcium reabsorption in DCT have been proposed. Gesek and Friedman [29] studied the relationship between NCC activity, thiazide effect, and calcium reabsorption in a DCT cell line obtained and immortalized from mouse kidney. Based on their observations they proposed that when the NCC activity is reduced by thiazides, the entry of salt is diminished, but the efflux of chloride ions through the chloride channels at the basolateral membrane continues. This decrease in intracellular chloride hyperpolarizes the cell that in turn stimulates the opening of calcium channels (presumably TRPV5) in the apical membrane, allowing calcium ions to move into the cell. The other proposed mechanism was based on observations performed in TRPV5 null mice by Nijenhuls *et al.* [30]. Since in the absence of TRPV5 in this model the hypocalciuric response to thiazide was still present, the authors proposed that increased calcium reabsorption is due to a compensatory increase in fluid volume reabsorption in the proximal tubule, due to the slight dehydration that follows the diuretic treatment.

NCC AS A POTENTIAL LINK BETWEEN HYPERTENSION AND OSTEOPOROSIS

Studies carried out in both humans and in relevant rodent models have established a link between systemic hypertension and osteoporosis [31-34]. Indeed, high sodium intake can lead to urinary calcium loss compatible with bone demineralization over time, which is significantly ameliorated by a modest reduction in sodium intake [35-37]. The molecular mechanism responsible for the inverse relation between urinary calcium excretion and plasma sodium is not completely understood, but it is believed that the volume expansion caused by the sodium retention might cause the increased urinary calcium excretion. This, in turn, would evoke a homeostatic response by the parathyroid-kidney-bone axis to compensate the resulting a negative calcium balance. Such an explanation could account for the link between high blood pressure and skeletal demineralization, as demonstrated both in rodent models [33;38] as well as in human subjects [39] with systemic hypertension. In contrast, impairment of sodium reabsorption due to either pharmacological therapy (i.e., thiazide diuretics) or genetic defects (i.e., Gitelman's syndrome and type II pseudohypoaldosteronism) results in hypotension and a subsequent reduction in urinary calcium loss, with a potential increase in bone mass. Evidence gathered over the last 30 years has suggested that, at usual anti-hypertensive doses, thiazide diuretics increase bone mineral density at the hip and the spine [5], decrease the rate of bone mineral loss at the wrist, elbow and heel [40;41] and reduce the prevalence of hip fractures. Their beneficial effect has been related to their action on the kidney tubule to promote calcium reabsorption [29].

As described above, thiazides act by inhibiting NCC expressed at the luminal surface of the kidney distal convoluted tubule [1], decreasing the Na^+-Cl^- absorption and enhancing renal calcium retention, resulting in a more positive calcium balance [42]. Inactivating mutations in NCC in humans cause Gitelman's syndrome [43] and are associated with an increased bone mineral density in subjects with normal calciotropic hormone levels and bone resorption markers [44]. This phenotype is mirrored by the murine model of Gitelman's syndrome, which also shows an increased bone mineral density. On the other hand, patients with type II pseudohypoaldosteronism, who present with an increased NCC activity, exhibit reduced bone mineral density when compared to non-affected members of the family [7]. Taken together, these observations suggest a direct link between NCC function and bone metabolism. The bone-sparing effect of thiazides remains, however, ill-defined. Low-dose thiazides increase bone density in normotensive men and women [45]. Such dynamics would be expected to be associated with a small increase in serum free ionized calcium concentration, resulting in depression of parathyroid hormone (PTH) secretion and reduced bone turnover rate, but alterations in the concentrations of circulating calciotropic hormones in response to thiazides [46] have not been consistently reported. On the other hand, direct actions on osteoblast proliferation [47;48] and differentiation have yielded conflicting findings. Similarly, evidence that thiazides might also slow down osteoclastic bone resorption [49], possibly through inhibition of the carbonic anhydrase and attendant alkalinization, is also present. Given the potential therapeutic importance of chronic thiazide treatment in the prevention of age-related osteoporosis, we hypothesized that, at the cellular and molecular levels, the anabolic effects of thiazides could be ascribed to the presence of a Na:Cl cotransporter in bone. Indeed, NCC mRNA had been previously reported in bone-derived cell lines [50]. We therefore tested the hypothesis that thiazides increase bone mineral density by interacting directly with an osteoblast NCC using *in vitro* models of primary osteoblasts, namely fetal rat calvarial (FRC) cells, and in human, murine and rat osteoblast-derived cell lines, *i.e.*, MG63, 2T3, UMR106, respectively.

Using both paraffin-embedded and freshly frozen human and rat specimens, we found that NCC protein expression in skeletal tissue, specifically within the reversal lines of the bone matrix of frozen rat femur (not shown) and human mandible (Figure 2A and 2B).

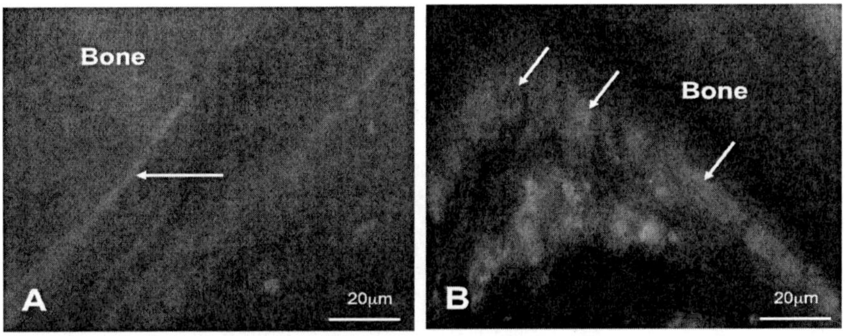

FIGURE 2. NCC is expressed in human bone.

NCC-specific immunoreactivity was found in the cells of the osteoblastic lineage, particularly in osteoblasts and some osteocytes, while NCC is absent from human osteoclasts and femoral cartilage (not shown). These results suggest that the osteoblast NCC, like the kidney NCC, may also be a target for thiazide diuretics. New bone formation could be the result of: a) an increased proliferation of the osteoblast progenitors; b) stimulation of osteoblast differentiation, or; c) a combination of both. Previously it has been shown that hydrochlorothiazide increases ^{3}H-thymidine incorporation in human [51] and mouse primary osteoblasts [52], whereas others report no such effect in human [53;54] and rat osteosarcoma cells [50]. Our experiments demonstrate that, in both human- (MG63) and rat-derived (FRC) models of osteoblasts, the thiazide-like metolazone and chlorothiazide did not increase cell proliferation [8]. Consistent with these findings is the absence of NCC in pre-confluent, proliferating cells. Indeed, NCC protein expression could only be detected in post-confluent cells, and it increased progressively with time in culture. These results point at an important role for NCC in osteoblast differentiation.

Having ruled out an effect of thiazides in the regulation of osteoblast proliferation, and given that NCC expression was confined to a differentiation-specific stage, we investigated the effects of the metolazone on osteoblast differentiation markers. Our data show that metolazone increased the expression of the osteoblast master transcription factor, Runx2, and the production of one of its downstream targets, osteopontin, in both MG63 and FRC cells [8]. Figure 3 shows that post-transcriptional gene silencing of NCC using siRNA prevented thiazide-dependent upregulation of Runx2, but not on the housekeeping gene actin or on the mitogen-activated protein kinase (MAPK, positive control) or that of AF-488 (negative control), indicating that changes in NCC gene expression are upstream of Runx2.

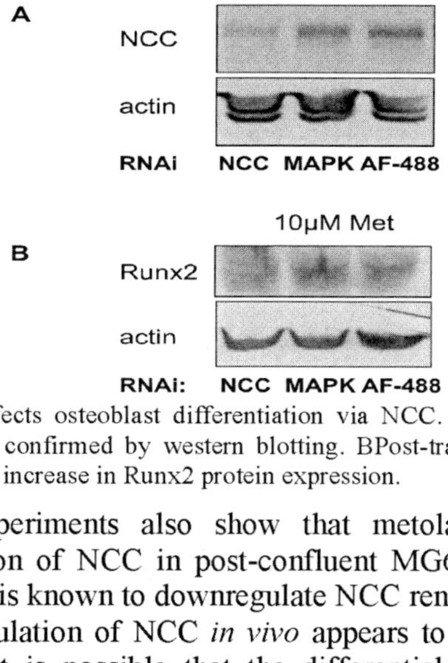

FIGURE 3. Metolazone affects osteoblast differentiation via NCC. A NCC knockdown by gene silencing in MG63 cells was confirmed by western blotting. BPost-transcriptional gene suppression abrogates metolazone-induced increase in Runx2 protein expression.

Interestingly, our experiments also show that metolazone treatment directly upregulates the expression of NCC in post-confluent MG63 cells (Figure 4) while chronic thiazide infusion is known to downregulate NCC renal expression *in vivo* [55]. Since the renal downregulation of NCC *in vivo* appears to be the consequence of a hypovolemic response, it is possible that the differential osteoblastic response to thiazides could be ascribed to the absence of extracellular volume contraction.

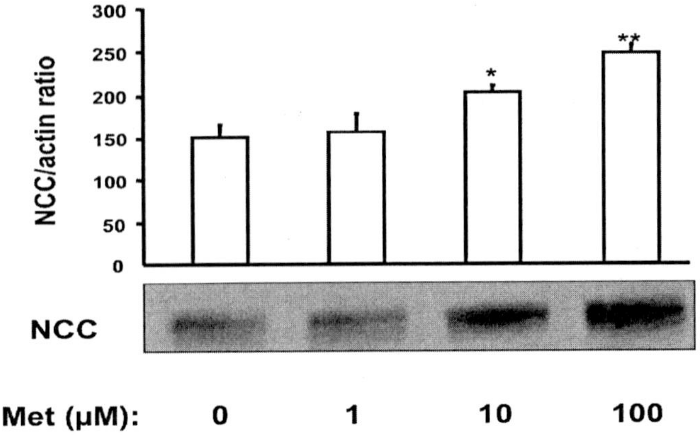

FIGURE 4. Metolazone treatment increases NCC protein expression by MG-63 cells.

The ultimate differentiation marker is formation of new bone and, consistently with the observed effects of thiazides on osteoblast differentiation, FRC cells grown in the presence of chronic metolazone treatment show a dose-dependent increase in the number of mineralized nodules (Figure 5). This effect is specific for thiazide diuretics as it could be mimicked by chrolothiazide, but not by the loop diuretic bumetanide [8].

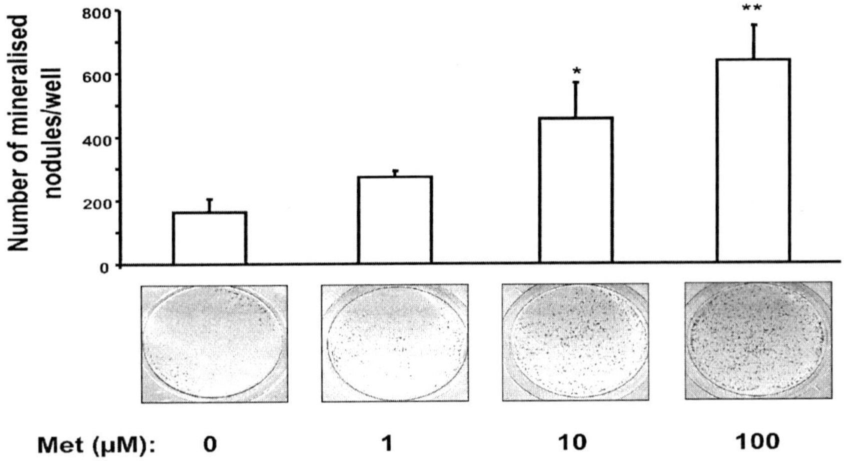

FIGURE 5. Metolazone treatment stimulates mineralized nodule formation in FRC cells.

In conclusion, our studies lend support to the hypothesis that NCC acts as the thiazide receptor in bone-forming cells, and that thiazides *directly* stimulate osteoblast differentiation and the formation of new bone *in vitro*. Together with the observations that inherited mutations of NCC affect bone mineral density, our findings indicate the involvement of the osteoblast NCC in the process of bone formation, and suggest that NCC provides a molecular link between high blood pressure, urinary calcium excretion and osteoporosis. In an aging population, osteoporosis is a highly debilitating disease associated with significant morbidity and mortality. The use of thiazides in osteoporosis prevention and therapeutic programs should be highly beneficial.

ACKNOWLEDGMENTS

GG would like to thank the NIDDK for the R01 grant DK64635 to study the Molecular Physiology of NCC and to all past and present members of the Molecular Physiology Unit involved in NCC studies, particularly to Norma Vázquez for her technical assistance. DR would like to thank the Arthritis Research Campaign (grant R0626) for supporting this work, Dr. Melita M. Dvorak and Dr. Cyrille De Joussineau for their involvement in the project. We both would like to express our eternal gratitude to the memory of our beloved mentor Steven C. Hebert.

REFERENCES

1. Gamba, G. (2005) *Physiol Rev.* **85**, 423-493
2. Gamba G, Saltzberg S N, Lombardi M, Miyanoshita A, Lytton J, Hediger M A, Brenner B M, and Hebert S C (1993) *Proc.Natl.Acad.Sci.USA* **90**, 2749-2753
3. Gamba G, Miyanoshita A, Lombardi M, Lytton J, Lee WS, Hediger MA, and Hebert SC (1994) *J.Biol.Chem.* **269**, 17713-17722
4. Chobanian, A. V., Bakris, G. L., Black, H. R., Cushman, W. C., Green, L. A., Izzo, J. L., Jr., Jones, D. W., Materson, B. J., Oparil, S., Wright, J. T., Jr., and Roccella, E. J. (2003) *JAMA* **289**, 2560-2571
5. LaCroix A Z, Wienpahl J, White L R, Wallace R B, Scherr P A, George L K, Cornoni-Huntley J, and Ostfeld A M (1990) *N Engl J Med* **322**, 286-290
6. Cruz, D. N., Simon, D. B., Nelson-Williams, C., Farhi, A., Finberg, K., Burleson, L., Gill, J. R., and Lifton, R. P. (2001) *Hypertension* **37**, 1458-1464
7. Mayan, H., Vered, I., Mouallem, M., Tzadok-Witkon, M., Pauzner, R., and Farfel, Z. (2002) *J.Clin.Endocrinol.Metab* **87**, 3248-3254
8. Dvorak, M. M., De Joussineau, C., Carter, D. H., Pisitkun, T., Knepper, M. A., Gamba, G., Kemp, P. J., and Riccardi, D. (2007) *J Am Soc Nephrol* **18**, 2509-2516
9. Bazzini, C., Vezzoli, V., Sironi, C., Dossena, S., Ravasio, A., Debiasi, S., Garavaglia, M., Rodighiero, S., Meyer, G., Fascio, U., Furst, J., Ritter, M., Botta, G., and Paulmichl, M. (2005) *J.Biol.Chem.* **280**, 19902-19910
10. Kunau R T, Weller D R, and Webb H L (1975) *J.Clin.invest.* **56**, 401-407
11. Velazquez H, Good D W, and Wright F S (1984) *Am.J.Physiol.(Renal Fluid Electrolyte Physiol.)* **247**, F904-F911
12. Costanzo L S (1985) *Am.J.Physiol.(Renal Fluid Electrolyte Physiol.)* **248**, F527-F535
13. Ellison D H, Velazquez H, and Wright F S (1987) *Am.J.Physiol.(Renal Fluid Electrolyte Physiol.)* **253**, F546-F554
14. Plotkin M D, Kaplan M R, Verlander J M, Lee W-S, Brown D, Poch E, Gullans S R, and Hebert S C (1996) *Kidney Int.* **50**, 174-183
15. Loffing, J. and Kaissling, B. (2003) *Am.J.Physiol Renal Physiol* **284**, F628-F643
16. Loffing, J., Loffing-Cueni, D., Valderrabano, V., Klausli, L., Hebert, S. C., Rossier, B. C., Hoenderop, J. G., Bindels, R. J., and Kaissling, B. (2001) *Am J Physiol Renal Physiol* **281**, F1021-F1027
17. Obermuller N, Bernstein P, Velázquez H, Reilly R, Moser D, Ellison D H, and Bachman S (1995) *Am.J.Physiol.(Renal Fluid Electrolyte Physiol.)* **269**, F900-F910
18. Campean, V., Kricke, J., Ellison, D., Luft, F. C., and Bachmann, S. (2001) *Am J Physiol Renal Physiol* **281**, F1028-F1035
19. Reilly, R. F. and Ellison, D. H. (2000) *Physiol Rev.* **80**, 277-313
20. Doucet A (1988) *Kidney Int.* **34**, 749-760
21. Xu, J. Z., Hall, A. E., Peterson, L. N., Bienkowski, M. J., Eessalu, T. E., and Hebert, S. C. (1997) *Am.J.Physiol Renal Physiol* **273**, F739-F749
22. Amorim, J. B., Bailey, M. A., Musa-Aziz, R., Giebisch, G., and Malnic, G. (2003) *Am.J.Physiol Renal Physiol* **284**, F381-F388
23. Masilamani, S., Kim, G. H., Mitchell, C., Wade, J. B., and Knepper, M. A. (1999) *J.Clin.Invest* **104**, R19-R23

24. Kim G-H, Masilamani S, Turner R, Mitchell C, Wade J B, and Knepper M A (1998) *Proc.Natl.Acad.Sci.USA* **95,** 14552-14557
25. Nielsen J, Kwon, T. H., Masilamani, S., Beutler, K., Hager H, Nielsen, S., and Knepper, M. A. Sodium transporter abundance profiling in the kidney: effect of spironolactone. Am J Physiol Renal Physiol 283, F923-F933. 2002.
26. Stokes J B, Lee I, and D'Amico M (1984) *J.Clin.invest.* **74,** 7-16
27. Rose B D (1991) *Kidney Int.* **39,** 336-352
28. de Groot, T., Bindels, R. J., and Hoenderop, J. G. (2008) *Kidney Int.*
29. Gesek F A and Friedman P A (1992) *J.Clin.invest.* **90,** 429-438
30. Nijenhuis, T., Vallon, V., van der Kemp, A. W., Loffing, J., Hoenderop, J. G., and Bindels, R. J. (2005) *J.Clin.Invest*
31. McCarron, D. A., Pingree, P. A., Rubin, R. J., Gaucher, S. M., Molitch, M., and Krutzik, S. (1980) *Hypertension* **2,** 162-168
32. Cirillo, M., Galletti, F., Strazzullo, P., Torielli, L., and Melloni, M. C. (1989) *Am.J.Hypertens.* **2,** 741-746
33. Brickman, A. S., Nyby, M. D., von Hungen, K., Eggena, P., and Tuck, M. L. (1990) *Hypertension* **16,** 515-522
34. Cruz, D. N. (2001) *Nephrol.Dial.Transplant.* **16,** 691-694
35. LaCroix, A. Z., Ott, S. M., Ichikawa, L., Scholes, D., and Barlow, W. E. (2000) *Ann.Intern.Med.* **133,** 516-526
36. Nordin, B. E. and Polley, K. J. (1987) *Calcif.Tissue Int.* **41 Suppl 1,** S1-59
37. Cappuccio, F. P. (2001) *JAMA* **285,** 2323-2324
38. Izawa, Y., Sagara, K., Kadota, T., and Makita, T. (1985) *Calcif.Tissue Int.* **37,** 605-607
39. Cappuccio, F. P., Meilahn, E., Zmuda, J. M., and Cauley, J. A. (1999) *Lancet* **354,** 971-975
40. Wasnich, R. D., Benfante, R. J., Yano, K., Heilbrun, L., and Vogel, J. M. (1983) *N.Engl.J.Med.* **309,** 344-347
41. Jones G, Nguyen T, Sambrook P N, and Eisman J A (1995) *J.Bone Miner.Res.* **10,** 106-111
42. Brickman, A. S., Massry, S. G., and Coburn, J. W. (1972) *J.Clin.Invest* **51,** 945-954
43. Simon D B, Nelson-Williams C, Johnson-Bia M, Ellison D, Karet F E, Morey-Molina A, Vaara I, Iwata F, Cushner H M, Koolen M, Gainza F J, Gitelman H J, and Lifton R P (1996) *Nature Genetics* **12,** 24-30
44. Nicolet-Barousse, L., Blanchard, A., Roux, C., Pietri, L., Bloch-Faure, M., Kolta, S., Chappard, C., Geoffroy, V., Morieux, C., Jeunemaitre, X., Shull, G. E., Meneton, P., Paillard, M., Houillier, P., and De Vernejoul, M. C. (2005) *J.Bone Miner.Res.* **20,** 799-808
45. Kamel, H. K. (2002) *Ann.Intern.Med.* **136,** 252-253
46. Van Den Berg, C. J., Tucker, R. M., and Dousa, T. P. (1982) *J.Clin.Endocrinol.Metab* **55,** 23-26
47. Lalande, A., Roux, S., Denne, M. A., Stanley, E. R., Schiavi, P., Guez, D., and De Vernejoul, M. C. (2001) *J.Bone Miner.Res.* **16,** 361-370
48. Aubin R, Ménard P, and Lajeunesse D (1996) *Kidney Int.* **50,** 1476-1482
49. Hall, T. J. and Schaueblin, M. (1994) *Calcif.Tissue Int.* **55,** 266-268
50. Barry E L R, Gesek F A, Kaplan M R, Hebert S C, and Friedman P A (1997) *Am.J.Physiol (Cell Physiol)* **272,** C109-C116
51. Lau, K. H., Song, X. D., Ochi, M., and Wergedal, J. E. (1996) *Calcif.Tissue Int.* **59,** 505-510
52. Aronow, M. A., Gerstenfeld, L. C., Owen, T. A., Tassinari, M. S., Stein, G. S., and Lian, J. B. (1990) *J.Cell Physiol* **143,** 213-221
53. Dallas, S. L., Park-Snyder, S., Miyazono, K., Twardzik, D., Mundy, G. R., and Bonewald, L. F. (1994) *J.Biol.Chem.* **269,** 6815-6821
54. Dvorak, M. M., Siddiqua, A., Ward, D. T., Carter, D. H., Dallas, S. L., Nemeth, E. F., and Riccardi, D. (2004) *Proc.Natl.Acad.Sci.U.S A* **101,** 5140-5145
55. Nijenhuis, T., Hoenderop, J. G., Loffing, J., van der Kemp, A. W., van Os, C. H., and Bindels, R. J. (2003) *Kidney Int.* **64,** 555-564

Acid-Base and the Skeleton

David A. Bushinsky

University of Rochester School of Medicine and Dentistry, Nephrology Division, University of Rochester Medical Center, 601 Elmwood Avenue, Box 675, Rochester, NY 14642

Abstract. Chronic metabolic acidosis increases urine calcium (Ca) excretion in the absence of a concomitant increase in intestinal Ca absorption resulting in a net loss of total body. The source of this additional urine Ca is almost certainly the skeleton, the primary reservoir of body Ca. *In vitro* metabolic acidosis, modeled as a primary reduction in medium bicarbonate concentration, acutely (<24h) stimulates Ca efflux primarily through physicochemical mineral dissolution while at later time periods (>24h) cell-mediated mechanisms predominate. In cultured neonatal mouse calvariae, acidosis-induced, cell-mediated Ca efflux is mediated by effects on both osteoblasts and osteoclasts. Metabolic acidosis inhibits extracellular matrix production by osteoblasts, as determined by measurement of collagen levels and levels for the non-collagenous matrix proteins osteopontin and matrix gla protein. Metabolic acidosis upregulates osteoblastic expression of RANKL (Receptor Activator of NFκB Ligand), an important osteoclastogenic and osteoclast-activating factor. Acidosis also increases osteoclastic activity as measured by release of β-glucuronidase, an enzyme whose secretion correlates with osteoclast-mediated bone resorption.

Keywords: bone; calcium; metabolic acidosis
PACS: 01.30.Cc

METABOLIC ACIDOSIS

Daily cellular metabolism of dietary amino acids in humans leads to production of ~1 mmole/kg of acid (protons, H^+) [34;122;135]. Additional endogenous H^+ production occurs during pathophysiological states such as diarrhea, diabetic ketoacidosis and lactic acidosis [22;25;27]. The subsequent reduction of systemic pH results in metabolic acidosis (MA). The mammalian physiologic response to MA is to rapidly increase extracellular fluid pH toward the physiologic neutral of 7.40 to maintain normal cellular function [22;24;25;27;29-31;33;34;42;47;54;121;122;135]. This homeostatic response to an acid challenge involves first buffering of the acid, then increasing respiratory rate to lower the partial pressure of carbon dioxide (Pco_2) and finally renal excretion of the additional H^+. The initial step, buffering of the additional H^+, is the most critical step in the immediate restoration of a neutral pH. The final step, renal excretion of H^+, begins hours after the acid challenge and is complete only days later. Renal acid excretion relies upon normal kidney function; as we age our ability to excrete acid declines and humans become slightly, but significantly, more acidemic [86;87].

CP1049, *Renal Stone Disease 2, 2nd International Urolithiasis Research Symposium*, edited by A. P. Evan, J. E. Lingeman, J. A. McAteer, and J. C. Williams, Jr.

Chronic MA, found in patients with renal insufficiency [25;27;146] and with renal tubular acidosis (RTA) [11;25], increases urinary Ca excretion [41;56;72;130;133;135] secondary to a direct reduction in renal tubular Ca reabsorption [193]. There is no [1;213] or an inadequate increase in intestinal Ca absorption [116;117] resulting in negative Ca balance (a net loss of body Ca) [7;41;130;132;135]. The source of much of this additional urinary Ca appears to be H^+-mediated dissolution and resorption of bone mineral [10;25;27;48;72;101;135]. Chronic MA appears to decrease bone mineral content [10;41;132;133] and has been shown to significantly decrease bone density, formation and growth [75;76;148;149]. Patients with proximal RTA, a defect in renal acid excretion, are shorter in height and have decreased radial bone densities and thinner iliac cortices than unaffected relatives [134]. In one study, patients with distal RTA, who also have a defect in renal acid excretion, had a lower bone mineral density in most areas when compared with normal controls and also had a decreased bone formation rate [75]. After treating these patients with the base $KHCO_3$ for 1 year, bone mineral density significantly improved in the trochanter and total femur and bone formation rate normalized [76].

During the ongoing MA of chronic renal failure, blood pH remains stable, although substantially reduced, in spite of progressive acid retention, suggesting the availability of large stores of proton buffers [182]. During renal failure there is ample clinical evidence that acidosis adversely affects bone [99;129;140;152] which may be corrected by HCO_3^- treatment [16;71;128]. Bone carbonate is decreased in acidic, uremic patients [115;164;165], which may represent dissolution of bone carbonate or replacement by phosphate, resulting in the incorporation of H^+ into the mineral [13;50;51]. In view of the deleterious effect of MA on bone, the National Kidney Foundation has recently published evidenced-based guidelines that recommend vigorous treatment of MA to help prevent renal osteodystrophy [156].

In addition to its effects on existing bone, MA also affects *de novo* bone formation. The independent effect of acidosis to suppress bone formation was elegantly demonstrated in children with RTA [67;148;149]. McSherry *et al.* found that 6 of 10 children with RTA were stunted (height < 2.5 S.D.), 2 were too young to be short (< 2 weeks old) and 2 were previously not acidemic [148;149]. With alkali therapy each patient attained and maintained normal stature, the mean height increased from 1.4 to 37th percentile and the rate of growth increased 2-3 fold.

The common high protein diet of North Americans, coupled with the known effects of bone to buffer an acid load [35;122], has led to the suggestion that excess dietary acid may play a role in the etiology of osteoporosis [8-10;35;85;135;136] especially coupled to the age-related decline in renal function [86;87]. Several studies have demonstrated that adequate dietary protein intake is necessary for optimal bone health [175]. Treatment of post-menopausal women with the base $KHCO_3$, which neutralizes endogenous H^+ production, leads to improved Ca retention, reduced bone resorption and increased bone formation [85;131;176;183]. Severe, life-threatening metabolic acidosis must be treated [25]; however, the mild metabolic acidosis present in the initial stages of renal insufficiency [135;181;182] and in aging [86;87], worsened in the latter case by a high protein diet [85;126;135], is rarely treated [25;35;135].

ANIMAL STUDIES

During *in vivo* acute MA (primary decrease in [HCO_3^-]), ~60% of the administered H^+ are buffered outside of the extracellular fluid [194] by soft tissues [2;138;168] and by bone [20-22;24;27;47-51;54]. The *in vivo* evidence that bone acutely buffers H^+, and in the process releases Ca, derives principally from the loss of bone Na and/or K [12;14;19;43;44;52;61;63;66] and carbonate [13;19;37;49-51;57;61] and the increase in serum Ca [120] observed during acute acidosis. Bone Na (or K) loss implies H^+ for Na (or K) exchange and carbonate loss suggests consumption of this buffer by the administered H^+. As at least 98% of body Ca is contained within bone [214;215], the increase in serum Ca is likely to derive from mineral stores.

We have studied the response of bone in vitro and in vivo to physiologically relevant acidosis [20;21;23;26;28;43;44;46;49-53;57-59;63;66;89;92;125;187] (reviewed in [22;24;27;31;33;34;37;42;45;47;48;54;55;60;61;90;91;93;121;122;124;135]). Initially, over the first few hours, there is buffering of the acidic medium pH [20;21;49;61] through physicochemical dissolution of bone mineral [51;63], releasing Ca as well as the H^+ buffers, carbonate and phosphate [4;49;50;57;61]), and exchange of bone Na and K for H^+ [43;44;52;61;63;66]. Hours later, cellular mechanisms increase bone resorption and decrease bone formation, both of which help normalize systemic pH [23;26;28;44;46;53;125]. Increased bone resorption further liberates carbonate and phosphate from the mineral [37;60], and decreased bone formation lessens the amount of acid produced during bone mineralization. We have shown that acidosis alters expression of a number of genes in osteoblasts [89-92] and increases osteoblastic prostaglandin E_2 (PGE_2) synthesis [55;124] leading to an increase in receptor activator of NFκB-ligand (RANKL) expression [91] and osteoclastic bone resorption.

The final step in osteoclastic bone resorption involves secretion of a H^+ into the microenvironment between the osteoclast and the mineral [17]. Carbonic anhydrase catalyzes the intracellular hydration of CO_2, producing equimolar H^+ and HCO_3^-. Thus, the osteoclast itself cannot contribute net acid or base to the body, as it secretes equimolar amounts of acid (H^+) and base (HCO_3^-). Only the bone mineral can provide a sink for H^+ in exchange for Na and K and contribute phosphates and carbonates, both of which will buffer the additional H^+ [122]. However, H^+ stimulation of osteoclastic bone resorption results in net consumption of bone carbonates and phosphates resulting in a mitigation of the acidosis at the expense of bone mineral stores. When cultured calvariae are exposed to an acid medium there is an influx of H^+ into the mineral [20;21;49;51;61], exchange for bone Na and K [43;52;63] and a reduction in bone carbonate and phosphate [37;60;61], implying that the mineral is involved in the H^+ buffering.

PROTON SENSING RECEPTOR

Bone must respond to MA through a coordinated homeostatic response aimed at normalizing systemic pH, often at the cost of decreased mineral content; however, the mechanism by which extracellular pH is sensed was previously not clear. While the existence of acid-sensitive ion channels, including ASICs, TRPV1, and TASK in nociceptor [209], skeletal muscle [97] and taste cells [139;208], has been extensively studied, until recently, the physiological mechanism whereby osteoblasts respond to environmental H^+ was not known. A novel class of G-protein coupled receptors that respond to both protons and lysosphingolipids has been recently characterized [205]. This family includes the ovarian G-protein coupled receptor 1 (OGR1, also termed GPR68) [143], GPR4 [143], T-cell death-associated gene 8 (TDAG8, also termed GPR65) [108;212] and G2A (also termed GPR132) [108;153], which share 40-50% homology. Activation of OGR1 [143] and G2A [153] by decreased pH leads to inositol phosphate (IP) accumulation, while GPR4 [143] and TDAG8 [108;212] are coupled to cAMP formation. However, the activation of G2A shows little pH dependence and H^+ sensing may be a minor role for this receptor [170].

Expression profiling by reverse transcriptase-mediated polymerase chain reaction (RT-PCR) revealed mRNA for OGR1 in MG63 human osteosarcoma cells [143]. The cells responded to physiological acidic pH with increased IP formation. Half-maximal activation was found at pH 7.46, very close to physiologic neutral pH of 7.40. Using an affinity-purified rabbit polyclonal antibody, OGR1 protein was observed in active osteoblasts, lining cells on the bone surface and matrix-embedded osteocytes in rat bones. OGR1 in human aortic smooth muscle cells [206] or expressed in CHO or COS7 cells [151] also activates cAMP formation, but with a different pH dependency than activation of IP accumulation; while IP accumulation is half-maximal at pH ~7.1, the cAMP effect is half-maximal at pH ~6.6. At pH >7.0, at the very acidic region of the normal physiological range [22;25;47], OGR1 signaling is primarily through IP. OGR1 is present in osteosarcoma cells, rat osteoblasts [143], and osteoclasts from rabbit and rat [119]. In addition the activity of osteoclasts is increased by a physiologic reduction of pH [150]. Differentiation of RAW264.7 mouse monocytes to osteoclasts with RANKL led to increased accumulation of OGR1 RNA and greater Ca_i responses to acid stimulation [119], consistent with a direct role for OGR1 activation in osteoclast stimulation.

Although *in vivo* evidence strongly suggests that bone is involved in the systemic response to acid-base disorders, until our studies there was little direct *in vitro* confirmation [22]. Neuman et al. found that a reduction of medium pH produced a marked increase in hydroxyapatite solubility [161]. Dominguez and Raisz [74] determined that an acid medium induced movement of prelabeled ^{45}Ca from bone.

We undertook a series of studies to test the hypothesis that cultured bone exposed to a physiologically acidic medium would release Ca into the medium and buffer the increased medium $[H^+]$ (decreased pH) [20;21;23;26;28;43;44;46;49-53;57-59;63; 66;89;92;125;187] (reviewed in [22;24;27;31;33;34;37;42;45;47;48;54;55;60;61;90; 91;93;121;122;124;135]. We utilized the model of cultured neonatal mouse calvariae, as the calvariae (frontal and parietal bones of the skull) have functioning osteoclasts and osteoblasts [82;123;179], respond to hormones and synthesize DNA and proteins as does bone *in vivo* [190]. We found that calvariae can be cultured in the physiologic CO_2/HCO_3^- buffer system [49] where medium pH can be regulated precisely by independently altering [HCO_3^-] or Pco_2 to model clinical "metabolic" or "respiratory" (respectively) acid-base disorders [25;49].

ACUTE ACIDOSIS – CALCIUM RELEASE

We found that cultured calvariae exhibit H^+-dependent net Ca efflux (J_{Ca}) during both acute (3h [49]) and more chronic (>24-99h) incubations [20;21;23;26;28;43;44; 46;49-53;55;57;59-61;63;66;89-92;124;125;187]). We found that the mechanism of H^+-mediated Ca efflux from bone during acute incubations was direct physicochemical Ca release and not cell-mediated [46]. We confirmed this finding by demonstrating Ca efflux from synthetic carbonated apatite (CAP) disks, a cell-free model of bone mineral [78-81;158-160], cultured in physiologically acid medium [58].

The type of bone mineral in equilibrium with the medium and thus altered by physicochemical forces might be carbonate or phosphate in association with Ca. We found that bone carbonate is solubilized during an acute reduction in pH leading to a release of Ca [50;51]. Further support for the role of carbonate in H^+-mediated bone mineral dissolution comes from our observation that at a constant pH, whether physiologically neutral or acid, Ca flux from bone is dependent on the medium [HCO_3^-]; the lower the [HCO_3^-], the greater the Ca efflux [57]. Bone carbonate appears to be in the form of carbonated apatite [18;102;159].

ACUTE ACIDOSIS – HYDROGEN ION BUFFERING

The *in vitro* evidence for H^+ buffering by bone is derived from studies of acidosis-induced H^+ flux into bone [20;21;49;51;61], ion microprobe evidence for a depletion of bone Na and K during acidosis [43;44;52;61;63;66] and from a depletion of bone carbonate and phosphate during acidosis [61]. When calvariae are cultured in medium acidified by a decrease in [HCO_3^-] (Met), there is a net influx of H^+ into bone, decreasing medium [H^+] and indicating that the additional H^+ are being buffered by bone, ultimately leading to an increase in medium pH [20;21;49;51;61]. During acute acidosis there appear to be two principal mechanisms by which the acid is buffered: H^+ for Na/K exchange [12;14;19;43;44;52;61;63;66] and consumption of the buffers carbonate and phosphate [13;19;37;49-51;57;61].

Proton for Na/K exchange. Bone is a reservoir for Na and K and its surface has fixed negative sites which normally complex with Na, K and H^+ [214;215]. We utilized a high resolution scanning ion microprobe [103;137;144] to determine how H^+ alter the ion composition of bone mineral [37-40;43-45;52;60-63;66]. We found that the calvarial surface is rich in Na and K relative to Ca [37-40;43-45;52;60-63;66]. The excess mineral K is maintained through cell-mediated processes [39].

Met causes release of bone Ca and leads to a decrease in the surface ratio of Na/Ca and K/Ca, indicating a greater relative release of mineral Na and K than Ca [52]. To better understand the effects of acidosis on K relative to Ca, we labeled the mineral *in vivo* with the stable isotope ^{41}K and found that mineral is indeed rich in K relative to Ca and that acidosis induces a fall in the ratio of $^{41}K/Ca$, indicating loss of this stable isotope from the bone mineral [43]. We also utilized the microprobe to study the acute physiochemical bone mineral dissolution caused by acidosis and found that physicochemical bone mineral dissolution causes relatively equal Ca and Na release [63].

Fall in bone carbonate and phosphate. Bone contains ~80% of the total carbon dioxide in the body [163]. Acute MA decreases bone total carbon dioxide [13]. Bone also contains a substantial amount of the total body phosphate, estimated to be ~90% [36], largely in the form of hydroxyapatite ($Ca_{10}(PO_4)_6(OH)_2$) and other forms of apatite [161]. During MA, protonation of the phosphate in apatite will consume H^+ and help restore the pH toward normal [34;42;122;135]. Using chemical analysis we demonstrated that Met induces the release of Ca and carbonate from bone [51] leading to a progressive loss of bone carbonate [50].

We utilized the microprobe to study the bone content of carbonate and phosphate in response to a model of acute MA [61]. We found a marked preferential loss of surface HCO_3^- and of cross-sectional phosphate. When both the *in vitro* and *in vivo* studies are considered together, there is clear evidence that bone is a H^+ buffer capable of maintaining the extracellular fluid pH near the physiologic normal. The loss of bone Na, K, carbonate and phosphate suggests that in addition to Na and K for H^+ exchange, bone carbonate and phosphate are lost from the mineral in response to acidosis, each of which helps to restore the pH toward normal.

CHRONIC ACIDOSIS – INCREASED BONE RESORPTION

Chronic MA induces the release of bone Ca, predominantly by enhanced cell-mediated bone resorption and decreased bone formation [20;23;26;28;37;44; 53;55;60;89-91;124;125;187], although there continues to be a component of direct physicochemical H^+-induced dissolution [21;43;46;49-52;57-59;61;63;66;187]. Osteoblastic collagen synthesis and alkaline phosphatase activity both were decreased after 48h incubation in Met compared to Ntl [125] *while RANKL synthesis was increased* [91;93]. Release of osteoclastic β-glucuronidase, a lysosomal enzyme whose secretion correlates with osteoclast-mediated bone resorption, was increased during culture in Met. Conversely, we observed that an increase in $[HCO_3^-]$, modeling metabolic alkalosis, decreases Ca efflux from bone through an increase in osteoblastic bone formation and a decrease in osteoclastic bone resorption [28].

Further support for a direct effect of MA to *regulate* osteoblastic function was obtained using primary cells isolated from the calvariae. These isolated osteoblasts synthesize collagen and form nodules of apatitic bone [15;77;186;192]. Compared to cell incubated in neutral medium, cells incubated in Met produced fewer nodules and had decreased Ca influx into the nodules [187].

In addition to the acidosis that occurs during clinical renal failure, there is also often an increase in parathyroid hormone (PTH) secretion [27;29;29;30;32;42; 100;184]. We found that acidosis and PTH independently stimulated Ca efflux from bone, inhibited osteoblastic collagen synthesis and stimulated osteoclastic β-glucuronidase secretion. In the presence of acidosis + PTH there was a greater effect on each of these parameters than either alone [53] suggesting an additive deleterious effect of PTH and acidosis on bone.

CHRONIC ACIDOSIS – ROLE OF PGE_2

Acidosis increases the level of prostaglandins in a variety of model systems. In both toad bladder [84;88] and rat kidney [109], PGE_2 levels increase in response to chronic MA, leading to enhanced H^+ excretion. In the rat, acute MA increases urinary prostaglandin excretion, which may regulate renal ammonia synthesis and acid excretion. Prostaglandins, especially PGE_2, are potent multifunctional regulators with complex effects on both bone resorption and formation [171;172]. Prostaglandins have been shown to promote new bone formation in vivo [113;211] and in isolated osteoblasts [110;217]. However in bone organ culture PGE_2, the most abundant eicosanoid in bone, has been shown to directly stimulate bone resorption [95;118;124;172;202;210]) and to stimulate RANKL expression in calvarial osteoblasts [141]. PGE_2 has also been shown to mediate bone resorption stimulated by a variety of cytokines and growth factors [95;172;189;198-201]. The relative effects of prostaglandins on bone may be dependent on timing or magnitude of dose [173], as has been found for PTH [169;195], or dependent on stage of osteoblast differentiation [65;104;197]. Thus, on the cellular and molecular level, regulation of PGE_2 remains important to understand the intracellular mechanisms of action of acidosis in the osteoblast.

In support of an earlier finding [98], we demonstrated that incubation of neonatal mouse calvariae in acidic medium increases medium PGE_2 in parallel with an increase in net Ca efflux [124]. Inhibition of PGE_2 production by indomethacin strongly limited this acidosis-induced bone Ca release *as well* as acid stimulation of RANKL [91]. Culture of calvariae in neutral pH medium with an amount of exogenous PGE_2 similar to that found in medium of calvariae incubated in Met induces net Ca efflux from bone [124]. Incubation of primary mouse calvarial bone cells, which consist mostly of osteoblasts [123], in Met led to a marked increase in medium PGE_2 levels which was again completely suppressed by indomethacin [124]. The magnitude of this H^+-induced increase in medium PGE_2 levels was comparable to that observed in cultured calvariae incubated in acid medium. We also found that cortisol inhibits H^+-induced bone resorption through a decrease in osteoblastic PGE_2 production. These results suggest that H^+-induced, cell-mediated Ca efflux from bone is regulated, at least in part, by an increase in endogenous PGE_2 production in the osteoblast leading to an increase in RANKL. Recently it has been shown that PGE_2 mediates induction of RANKL in osteoblasts by periodontal pathogens ultimately leading to increased osteoclastogenesis [70].

Prostaglandin synthesis is regulated by the release of arachidonic acid from membrane phospholipids. *The rate limiting step converting* arachidonic acid to specific prostanoids is catalyzed by prostaglandin G/H synthase, also called cyclooxygenase (COX) [185]. There are two forms of COX: COX1, which is constitutively expressed, and COX2, which is the inducible form of the enzyme. Both forms of COX are expressed in osteoblasts [166]. COX2 expression is regulated by several bone-resorbing factors, including interleukin-1 [114], PTH [114;203], interleukin-6 [196], TGF-α [167], TNF-α [111], and basic fibroblast growth factor [112]. We have found that 1 mM NS-398, a specific COX2 inhibitor [162], significantly inhibits H^+-induced Ca release from calvariae, which supports the hypothesis that this enzyme is stimulated by acidosis. We have tested the effects of COX2 knockout using calvariae from the offspring of matings of COX2 +/- mice and correlating genotype and phenotype. We found that in Ntl, bones from -/- pups (knockouts) released less Ca than did bones from +/+ (wild type) mice. Met stimulated Ca efflux from bones from +/+ and +/- (heterozygotes), but did not stimulate Ca efflux from -/- bones. The extent of Ca release in Met was less from +/- and -/- bones than from +/+ bones and release from -/- bones was less than release from +/- bones. These data indicate that COX2 is necessary for H^+-induced bone Ca efflux and suggest that the gene dosage of COX2 sets the level of both basal and H^+-induced resorption.

Using northern analysis, as well as real-time PCR, initial studies indicate that incubation of primary bone cells in Met causes greater stimulation of COX2 RNA levels than in Ntl, *with no change in COX1.* An initial microarray experiment using RNA from cultured calvariae also found a ~2-fold increase in COX2 mRNA in response to acid compared to control medium. To address a potential acid stimulation of the COX2 promoter, 2T3 osteoblastic cells were transfected with a –371-+70 promoter construct coupled to luciferase. 24h after transfection, the cells were treated with Ntl or Met medium, or with 1mM PMA, or left untreated. After 1h the cells were harvested (3h for PMA) and assayed for luciferase activity, normalized to protein content. In preliminary experiments Met caused an approximately 45% increase in luciferase activity, similar to the increase seen with PMA. A second construct including the sequences from –130-+70 displayed no apparent acid induction of promoter activity.

Although activation of adenylate cyclase has been the best characterized signal transduction pathway activated by PGE_2 in bone [113;174], and we have found partial inhibition of H^+-stimulated Ca release from calvariae in the presence of the PKA inhibitor H89 [69], we have not observed a significant stimulation of cAMP in the calvariae in response to acidosis. Thus we have begun to investigate other signaling pathways. P38, one of the major subfamilies of MAP kinases [68;157;220], may be necessary for osteoblast differentiation [107]; and activation of p38 has been shown to mediate regulation of COX2 and subsequent production of PGE_2 by interleukin-1b in chondrocytes [204] and neuroblastoma cells [83], to regulate stretch activated responses in mouse osteoblasts [155] and mouse podocytes [147] and endothelin-1 stimulation of MC3T3E-1 osteoblastic cells [216]. We tested the effect of 10 mM SB203580, a specific inhibitor of p38 [127], on acidosis-induced bone resorption and found significant inhibition of H^+-mediated Ca efflux as well as a parallel inhibition of PGE_2 synthesis. Preliminary immunoblot experiments in primary calvarial cells indicate a rapid stimulation of p38 phosphoprotein levels in response to Met (A) compared to Ntl (N). Treatment of primary calvarial cells with SB203580 for 6h also inhibited H^+-induced stimulation of COX2 mRNA. These data suggest that activation of p38 mediates the subsequent stimulation of COX2 and prostaglandin synthesis.

To further characterize the mechanism by which PGE_2 mediates acidosis-induced resorption, we found that 1 mM L161,982, a specific inhibitor of the EP4 prostaglandin receptor [145], completely blocked H^+-induced Ca efflux from calvariae at 48h, while an inactive isomer, L161,983, had no effect. As PGE_2 binding to its EP4 receptor may be less potent in stimulating cAMP compared to the EP2 receptor [177], and can activate phosphatidylinositol 3-kinase (PI 3-kinase) in other tissues [94], we tested the effect of 100 nM wortmannin (WTM), a specific PI 3-kinase inhibitor [3;219], on acidosis-induced bone resorption. WTM had no effect on Ntl Ca efflux, but almost completely inhibited Met-induced Ca efflux at 48h. Mechanical stretching of MC3T3-E1 osteoblastic cells has been shown to activate PI 3-kinase by a Ca-dependent process [73] and IGF-1-induced acid efflux from UMR-106 cells was inhibited by WTM [178]. WTM has also been shown to directly inhibit osteoclast activity [154], and PI 3-kinase is suggested to have a direct antiapoptotic effect in osteoclasts [96]. Thus WTM could be inhibitory in either cell type. We do not yet know whether the PI 3-kinase pathway that is activated by acidosis is involved in the signaling events initiated in the osteoblast *before the increase in RANKL or downstream during the* subsequent activation of osteoclasts.

CHRONIC ACIDOSIS – REGULATION OF GENE EXPRESSION

External pH modulates gene expression in several cell types. MA induces rat renal cells to increase ammonia production [109]. As a part of this adaptation, RNA for glutaminase is stabilized by the binding of an AU-rich region in the 3'-untranslated domain to ς-crystallin [180]. Insertion of this motif into a β-globin gene results in its acid-dependent stabilization. A similar ς-crystallin-binding sequence is found in the glutamate dehydrogenase gene. MA also increased RNA expression of the Na/citrate cotransporter NaDC-1 [5] and the Na/H exchangers NHE3 and NHE2 in renal cells [142]. The response of NHE3 to H^+ is dependent on c-src and ERK kinase activities [207]. Transcriptional regulation by external pH of phosphoenolpyruvate carboxykinase (PEPCK) is dependent on the presence of binding sites for hepatic nuclear factor-1 (HNF-1) and accessory factor-1 (AF-1) in the 5' upstream region of the PEPCK gene [64]. Expression of RNA for the gap junction protein connexin 43 is downregulated transcriptionally by lowered pH in osteoblastic MC3T3-E1 cells [218].

Thus, we hypothesized that acidosis would alter specific gene expression in osteoblasts. We examined several immediate early response genes in primary neonatal mouse calvarial cells, including egr-1, junB, c-jun, junD and c-fos. In response to incubation in acidic medium, only the magnitude of egr-1 stimulation was dependent on medium pH [92]. Osteoblasts express type 1 collagen as the major component of the bone extracellular matrix, which subsequently becomes mineralized. Similarly to egr-1, type I collagen RNA synthesis was decreased by acidosis and increased by alkalosis [92].

Primary mouse calvarial cells differentiate in culture to form bone nodules [188]. These osteoblastic cells express a number of bone specific matrix proteins, including bone sialoprotein, osteocalcin, osteonectin (ON), osteopontin (OP), and matrix gla protein (MGP) [188]. Since acidic medium decreases bone nodule number, size and

Ca content [187], we hypothesized that acidosis would alter the pattern of matrix gene expression in these longterm cell cultures. After 3-4 wks in Ntl (N) OP RNA levels increased while Met (A) completely inhibited this increase [89]. The RNA levels of two other proteins, ON and transforming growth factor b_1, as well as the housekeeping gene, GAPDH, did not vary with pH. RNA for MGP was also induced by Ntl differentiation medium while Met almost totally prevented the increase in MGP RNA levels. The inhibition of MGP and OP RNA levels by acidosis was found to be reversible [89].

We hypothesized that the MA-induced bone resorption was a result of alterations in osteoblastic expression of osteoclastogenic factors. Such factors include macrophage colony stimulating factor (M-CSF), a growth factor for osteoclast precursor cells [6;191]; RANKL, the ligand for the osteoclast receptor activator of NFkB (RANK) [6;105;191]; and osteoprotegerin (OPG), a decoy receptor for RANKL that prevents the RANK/RANKL interaction [6;106;191]. Activation of RANK by RANKL initiates a differentiation cascade that culminates in mature, bone-resorbing osteoclasts, as well as stimulation of mature osteoclast activity and inhibition of apoptosis. Analysis of RNA extracted from calvariae incubated for 24 or 48h in Ntl or Met by RT-PCR indicated that expression of RANKL RNA was upregulated by acidosis, while expression of M-CSF, OPG, and b-actin were not altered [91]. Quantitation by northern blotting confirmed that Met induced an increase in RANKL RNA expression. Analysis of culture supernatants by ELISA demonstrated that calvariae in Met produced greater amounts of soluble RANKL protein than calvariae cultured at neutral pH; production of OPG was not affected [93].

To examine the role of PGE_2 synthesis in RANKL expression, calvariae were incubated in the absence or presence of indomethacin (Indo) to inhibit COX activity; Ca flux was determined as well as RANKL RNA content by northern analysis. Indo significantly *inhibited* H^+-induced Ca flux and completely suppressed the induction of RANKL RNA by Met [91]. Thus acidosis-induced synthesis of PGE_2 causes an autocrine or paracrine stimulation of osteoblastic prostaglandin receptors. Activation of these receptors consequently induces an increase in RANKL RNA expression, which in turn increases osteoclastogenesis and activation of mature osteoclasts.

CURRENT MODEL OF THE EFFECTS OF ACID ON BONE

Our studies have shown that MA induces changes in the bone mineral, which are consistent with its purported role as a proton buffer [22;24;27;31;33;34;42;47;48;54; 121;122;135]. The fall in mineral Na, K, carbonate and phosphate will each buffer protons and lead to an increase in systemic pH toward the physiologic normal. These changes in mineral composition come about first through physicochemical mineral dissolution and later through alterations in bone cell function. MA suppresses specific osteoblastic matrix protein synthesis and alkaline phosphatase activity. There is a concomitant acid stimulation of PGE_2 production by the osteoblasts which, acting in a paracrine manner, increases osteoblastic RANKL synthesis. RANKL then stimulates osteoclastic activity and recruitment of new osteoclasts to further promote bone resorption and buffering of the proton load. The apparent protective function of bone to maintain systemic pH, which has a clear survival advantage for mammals, will come, in part, at the expense of its mineral stores.

REFERENCES

1. Adams ND, Gray RW, Lemann J, Jr.: The calciuria of increased fixed acid production in humans: evidence against a role for parathyroid hormone and 1,25(OH)2-vitamin D. Calcif Tissue Int 28:233-238, 1979
2. Adler S, Roy A, Relman AS: Intracellular acid-base regulation. I. The response of muscle cells to changes in CO_2 tension or extra-cellular bicarbonate concentration. J Clin Invest 44:8-20, 1965
3. Arcaro A, Wymann MP: Wortmannin is a potent phosphatidylinositol 3-kinase inhibitor: The role of phosphatidylinositol 3,4,5-triphosphate in neutrophil responses. Biochem J 296:297-301, 1993
4. Arnett TR, Dempster DW: Protons and osteoclasts. J Bone Miner Res 5:1099-1103, 1990
5. Aruga S, Wehrli S, Kaissling B et al.: Chronic metabolic acidosis increases NaDC-1 mRNA and protein abundance in rat kidney. Kid Int 58:206-215, 2000
6. Aubin JE, Bonnelye E: Osteoprotegerin and its ligand: a new paradigm for regulation of osteoclastogenesis and bone resorption. Osteoporos Int 11:905-913, 2000
7. Barzel US: The effect of excessive acid feeding on bone. Calcif Tissue Res 4:94-100, 1969
8. Barzel US: The role of bone in acid base metabolism, in Osteoporosis, edited by Barzel US, New York, Grune and Stratton, 1970, p 199
9. Barzel US: Osteoporosis II: an overview, in Osteoporosis II, edited by Barzel US, New York, Grune and Stratton, 1976, p 1
10. Barzel US: The skeleton as an ion exchange system: Implications for the role of acid-base imbalance in the genesis of osteoporosis. J Bone Min Res 10:1431-1436, 1995
11. Batlle DC: Renal tubular acidosis, in The Regulation of Acid-Base Balance, edited by Seldin DW, Giebisch G, New York, Raven Press, 1989, pp 353-390
12. Bergstrom WH, Ruva FD: Changes in bone sodium during acute acidosis in the rat. Am J Physiol 198:1126-1128, 1960
13. Bettice JA: Skeletal carbon dioxide stores during metabolic acidosis. Am J Physiol (Renal Fluid Electrolyte Physiol 16) 247:F326-F330, 1984
14. Bettice JA, Gamble JL, Jr.: Skeletal buffering of acute metabolic acidosis. Am J Physiol 229:1618-1624, 1975
15. Bhargava U, Bar-Lev M, Bellows CG, Aubin JE: Ultrastructural analysis of bone nodules formed in vitro by isolated fetal rat calvaria cells. Bone 9:155-163, 1988
16. Bishop MC, Ledingham JG: Alkali treatment of renal osteodystrophy. British Medical Journal 4:529, 1972
17. Block GA, Klassen PS, Lazarus JM et al.: Mineral metabolism, mortality, and morbidity in maintenance hemodialysis. J Am Soc Nephrol 15:2208-2218, 2004
18. Boskey AL, Posner AS: Conversion of amorphous calcium phosphate to microcrystalline hydroxyapatite-pH-dependent, solution mediated, solid-solid conversion. J Phys Chem 77:2313-2317, 1973
19. Burnell JM: Changes in bone sodium and carbonate in metabolic acidosis and alkalosis in the dog. J Clin Invest 50:327-331, 1971
20. Bushinsky DA: Effects of parathyroid hormone on net proton flux from neonatal mouse calvariae. Am J Physiol (Renal Fluid Electrolyte Physiol 21) 252:F585-F589, 1987
21. Bushinsky DA: Net proton influx into bone during metabolic, but not respiratory, acidosis. Am J Physiol (Renal Fluid Electrolyte Physiol 23) 254:F306-F310, 1988
22. Bushinsky DA: Internal exchanges of hydrogen ions: Bone, in The Regulation of Acid-Base Balance, edited by Seldin DW, Giebisch G, New York, Raven Press, 1989, pp 69-88
23. Bushinsky DA: Net calcium efflux from live bone during chronic metabolic, but not respiratory, acidosis. Am J Physiol (Renal Fluid Electrolyte Physiol 25) 256:F836-F842, 1989
24. Bushinsky DA: Acidosis and bone. Miner Electrolyte Metab 20:40-52, 1994
25. Bushinsky DA: Metabolic Acidosis, chap. 136, in The Principles and Practice of Nephrology, edited by Jacobson HR, Striker GE, Klahr S, St. Louis, MO, Mosby, 1995, pp 924-932
26. Bushinsky DA: Stimulated osteoclastic and suppressed osteoblastic activity in metabolic but not respiratory acidosis. Am J Physiol (Cell Physiol 37) 268:C80-C88, 1995
27. Bushinsky DA: The contribution of acidosis to renal osteodystrophy. Kidney Int 47:1816-1832, 1995
28. Bushinsky DA: Metabolic alkalosis decreases bone calcium efflux by suppressing osteoclasts and stimulating osteoblasts. Am J Physiol (Renal Fluid Electrolyte Physiol 40) 271:F216-F222, 1996

29. Bushinsky DA: Bone disease in moderate renal failure: cause, nature and prevention. Annual Review of Medicine 48:167-176, 1997
30. Bushinsky DA: Renal Osteodystrophy, chap. 30, in Nephrology, 1 ed., edited by Jamison R, Wilkinson B, London, Chapman and Hall, 1997, pp 369-382
31. Bushinsky DA: Acid-Base Imbalance and the Skeleton, chap. 23, in Nutritional Aspects of Osteoporosis, edited by Burckhardt P, Dawson-Hughes B, Heaney RP, Norwell, Massachusetts, Serono Symposia USA, 1998, pp 208-217
32. Bushinsky DA: High-Turnover Renal Osteodystrophy, chap. 11, in Renal Osteodystrophy, edited by Bushinsky DA, Philadelphia, Lippincott-Raven, 1998, pp 283-303
33. Bushinsky DA: Hydrogen Ions, chap. 5, in Renal Osteodystrophy, edited by Bushinsky DA, Philadelphia, Lippincott-Raven, 1998, pp 103-127
34. Bushinsky DA: Acid-base imbalance and the skeleton. Eur J Nutrition 40:238-244, 2001
35. Bushinsky DA: Acid-Base Balance and Bone Health, chap. 18, in Nutrition and Bone Health, edited by Holick MF, Dawson-Hughes B, Totowa, Humana Press, Inc., 2004, pp 279-304
36. Bushinsky DA: Disorders of calcium and phosphorus homeostasis, chap. 13, in Primer on Kidney Diseases, 4 ed., edited by Greenberg A, San Diego, Academic Press, 2005, pp 120-130
37. Bushinsky DA, Chabala JM, Gavrilov KL, Levi-Setti R: Effects of in vivo metabolic acidosis on midcortical bone ion composition. Am J Physiol (Renal Physiol 46) 277:F813-F819, 1999
38. Bushinsky DA, Chabala JM, Levi-Setti R: Ion microprobe analysis of bone surface elements: effects of $1,25(OH)_2D_3$. Am J Physiol (Endocrinol Met Physiol 20) 257:E815-E822, 1989
39. Bushinsky DA, Chabala JM, Levi-Setti R: Ion microprobe analysis of mouse calvariae in vitro: evidence for a "bone membrane". Am J Physiol (Endocrinol Metab 19) 256:E152-E158, 1989
40. Bushinsky DA, Chabala JM, Levi-Setti R: Comparison of in vitro and in vivo ^{44}Ca labeling of bone by scanning ion microprobe. Am J Physiol (Endocrinol Metab 22) 259:E586-E592, 1990
41. Bushinsky DA, Favus MJ, Schneider AB et al.: Effects of metabolic acidosis on PTH and $1,25(OH)_2D_3$ response to low calcium diet. Am J Physiol (Renal Fluid Electrolyte Physiol 12) 243:F570-F575, 1982
42. Bushinsky DA, Frick KK: The effects of acid on bone. Current Opinion in Nephrology and Hypertension 9:369-379, 2000
43. Bushinsky DA, Gavrilov K, Chabala JM et al.: Effect of metabolic acidosis on the potassium content of bone. J Bone Min Res 12:1664-1671, 1997
44. Bushinsky DA, Gavrilov K, Stathopoulos VM et al.: Effects of osteoclastic resorption on bone surface ion composition. Am J Physiol (Cell Physiol 40) 271:C1025-C1031, 1996
45. Bushinsky DA, Gavrilov KL, Chabala JM, Levi-Setti R: Contribution of organic material to the ion composition of bone. J Bone Min Res 15:2026-2032, 2000
46. Bushinsky DA, Goldring JM, Coe FL: Cellular contribution to pH-mediated calcium flux in neonatal mouse calvariae. Am J Physiol (Renal Fluid Electrolyte Physiol 17) 248:F785-F789, 1985
47. Bushinsky DA, Krieger NS: Role of the Skeleton in Calcium Homeostasis, in The Kidney: Physiology and Pathophysiology, edited by Seldin DW, Giebisch G, New York, Raven Press, 1992, pp 2395-2430
48. Bushinsky DA, Krieger NS: Regulation of Bone Formation and Dissolution, in Kidney Stones: Medical and Surgical Management, edited by Coe F, Favus M, Pak C et al., New York, Raven Press, 1996, pp 239-258
49. Bushinsky DA, Krieger NS, Geisser DI et al.: Effects of pH on bone calcium and proton fluxes in vitro. Am J Physiol (Renal Fluid Electrolyte Physiol 14) 245:F204-F209, 1983
50. Bushinsky DA, Lam BC, Nespeca R et al.: Decreased bone carbonate content in response to metabolic, but not respiratory, acidosis. Am J Physiol (Renal Fluid Electrolyte Physiol 34) 265:F530-F536, 1993
51. Bushinsky DA, Lechleider RJ: Mechanism of proton-induced bone calcium release: calcium carbonate-dissolution. Am J Physiol (Renal Fluid Electrolyte Physiol 22) 253:F998-F1005, 1987
52. Bushinsky DA, Levi-Setti R, Coe FL: Ion microprobe determination of bone surface elements: Effects of reduced medium pH. Am J Physiol (Renal Fluid Electrolyte Physiol 19) 250:F1090-F1097, 1986
53. Bushinsky DA, Nilsson EL: Additive effects of acidosis and parathyroid hormone on mouse osteoblastic and osteoclastic function. Am J Physiol (Cell Physiol 38) 269:C1364-C1370, 1995
54. Bushinsky DA, Ori Y: Effects of metabolic and respiratory acidosis on bone. Current Opinion Nephrol Hyper 2:588-596, 1993
55. Bushinsky DA, Parker WR, Alexander KM, Krieger NS: Metabolic, but not respiratory, acidosis increases bone PGE_2 levels and calcium release. Am J Physiol (Renal Fluid Electrolyte Physiol) 281:F1058-F1066, 2001
56. Bushinsky DA, Riera GS, Favus MJ, Coe FL: Response of serum $1,25(OH)_2D_3$ to variation of ionized calcium during chronic acidosis. Am J Physiol (Renal Fluid Electrolyte Physiol 18) 249:F361-365, 1985
57. Bushinsky DA, Sessler NE: Critical role of bicarbonate in calcium release from bone. Am J Physiol (Renal Fluid Electrolyte Physiol 32) 263:F510-F515, 1992

58. Bushinsky DA, Sessler NE, Glena RE, Featherstone JDB: Proton-induced physicochemical calcium release from ceramic apatite disks. J Bone Miner Res 9:213-220, 1994
59. Bushinsky DA, Sessler NE, Krieger NS: Greater unidirectional calcium efflux from bone during metabolic, compared with respiratory, acidosis. Am J Physiol (Renal Fluid Electrolyte Physiol 31) 262:F425-F431, 1992
60. Bushinsky DA, Smith SB, Gavrilov KL et al.: Chronic acidosis-induced alteration in bone bicarbonate and phosphate. American Journal of Physiology Renal Physiol 285:F532-F539, 2003
61. Bushinsky DA, Smith SB, Gavrilov KL et al.: Acute acidosis-induced alteration in bone bicarbonate and phosphate. Am J Physiol Renal Physiol 283:F1091-F1097, 2002
62. Bushinsky DA, Sprague SM, Hallegot P et al.: Effects of aluminum on bone surface ion composition. J Bone Min Res 10:1988-1997, 1995
63. Bushinsky DA, Wolbach W, Sessler NE et al.: Physicochemical effects of acidosis on bone calcium flux and surface ion composition. J Bone Miner Res 8:93-102, 1993
64. Cassuto H, Olswang Y, Heinemann S et al.: The transcriptional regulation of phosphoenolpyruvate carboxykinase gene in the kidney requires the HNF-1 binding site of the gene. Gene 318:177-184, 2003
65. Centrella M, Casinghino S, McCarthy TL: Differential actions of prostaglandins in separate cell populations from fetal rat bone. Endocrinol 135:1611-1620, 1994
66. Chabala JM, Levi-Setti R, Bushinsky DA: Alteration in surface ion composition of cultured bone during metabolic, but not respiratory, acidosis. Am J Physiol (Renal Fluid Electrolyte Physiol 30) 261:F76-F84, 1991
67. Challa A, Krieg RJJr, Thabet MA et al.: Metabolic acidosis inhibits growth hormone secretion in rats: mechanism of growth retardation. Am J Physiol 265:E547-E553, 1993
68. Chang L, Karin M: Mammalian MAP kinase signalling cascades. Nature 410:37-40, 2001
69. Chijiwa T, Mishima A, Hagiwara M et al.: Inhibition of forskolin-induced neurite outgrowth and protein phosphorylation by a newly synthesized selective inhibitor of cyclic AMP-dependent protein kinase, N-[2-(p-bromocinnamylamino)ethyl]-5-isoquinolinesulfonamide (H-89), of PC12D pheochromocytoma cells. J Biol Chem 265:5267-5272, 1990
70. Choi BK, Moon SY, Cha JH et al.: Prostaglandin E_2 is a main mediator in receptor activator of nuclear factor-kB ligand-dependent osteoclastogenesis induced by Porphyromonas gingivalis, Trepoema denticola and Treponema socranskii. J Periodontology 76:813-820, 2005
71. Cochran M, Wilkinson R: Effect of correction of metabolic acidosis on bone mineralization rates in patients with renal osteomalacia. Nephron 15:98-110, 1975
72. Coe FL, Bushinsky DA: Pathophysiology of hypercalciuria. Am J Physiol (Renal Fluid Electrolyte Physiol) 247:F1-F13, 1984
73. Danciu TE, Adam RM, Naruse K et al.: Calcium regulates the PI3K-Akt pathway in streched osteoblasts. FEBS Letters 536:193-197, 2003
74. Dominguez JH, Raisz LG: Effects of changing hydrogen ion, carbonic acid, and bicarbonate concentrations on bone resorption in vitro. Calcif Tissue Int 29:7-13, 1979
75. Domrongkitchaiporn S, Pongsakul C, Stitchantrakul W et al.: Bone mineral density and histology in distal renal tubular acidosis. Kidney Int 59:1086-1093, 2001
76. Domrongkitchaiporn S, Pongskul C, Sirikulchayanonta V et al.: Bone histology and bone mineral density after correction of acidosis in distal renal tubular acidosis. Kidney Int 62:2160-2166, 2002
77. Ecarot-Charrier B, Glorieux FH, Van Der Rest M, Pereira G: Osteoblasts isolated from mouse calvaria initiate matrix mineralization in culture. J Cell Biol 96:639-643, 1983
78. Ellies LG, Carter JM, Natiella JR et al.: Quantitative analysis of early in vivo tissue response to synthetic apatite implants. J Biomed Mater Res 22:137-148, 1988
79. Ellies LG, Nelson DGA, Featherstone JDB: Crystallographic structure and surface morphology of sintered carbonated apatites. J Biomed Mater Res 22:541-553, 1988
80. Featherstone JDB, Nelson DGA: Recent uses of electron microscopy in the study of physico-chemical processes affecting the reactivity of synthetic and biological apatites. Scanning Microsc 3:815-828, 1989
81. Featherstone JDB, Pearson S, LeGeros RZ: An infrared method for quantification of carbonate in carbonated apatites. Caries Res 18:63-66, 1984
82. Feldman RS, Krieger NS, Tashjian JrAH: Effects of parathyroid hormone and calcitonin on osteoclast formation in vitro. Endocrinology 107:1137-1143, 1980
83. Fiebich GL, Mueksch B, Boehringer M, Hull M: Interleukin-1 beta induces cyclooxygenase-2 and prostaglandin E(2) synthesis in humban neuroblastoma cells: Involvement of p38 mitogen-activated protein kinase and nuclear factor-kappaB. J Neurochem 75:2020-2028, 2000
84. Forrest JNJr, Schneider CJ, Goodman DBP: Role of prostaglandin E_2 in mediating the effects of pH on the hydroosmotic response to vasopressin in the toad urinary bladder. J Clin Invest 69:499-506, 1982
85. Frassetto L, Morris JrRC, Sebastian A: Long-term persistence of the urine calcium-lowering effect of potassium bicarbonate in postmenopausal women. J Clin Endocrinol Metab 90:831-834, 2005

86. Frassetto L, Sebastian A: Age and systemic acid-base equilibrium: analysis of published data. J Gerontol A Biol Sci Med Sci 51:B91-B99, 1996
87. Frassetto LA, Morris RC, Jr., Sebastian A: Effect of age on blood acid-base composition in adult humans: role of age-related renal functional decline. Am J Physiol (Renal Fluid Electrolyte Physiol 40) 271:F1114-F1122, 1996
88. Frazier LW, Yorio T: Prostaglandins as mediators of acidification in the urinary bladder of Bufo marinus. Proc Soc Exp Bio Med 194:10-15, 1990
89. Frick KK, Bushinsky DA: Chronic metabolic acidosis reversibly inhibits extracellular matrix gene expression in mouse osteoblasts. Am J Physiol (Renal Physiol 44) 275:F840-F847, 1998
90. Frick KK, Bushinsky DA: In vitro metabolic and respiratory acidosis selectively inhibit osteoblastic matrix gene expression. Am J Physiol (Renal Physiol 46) 277:F750-F755, 1999
91. Frick KK, Bushinsky DA: Metabolic acidosis stimulates RANK ligand RNA expression in bone through a cyclooxygenase dependent mechanism. J Bone Miner Res 18:1317-1325, 2003
92. Frick KK, Jiang L, Bushinsky DA: Acute metabolic acidosis inhibits the induction of osteoblastic egr-1 and type 1 collagen. Am J Physiol (Cell Physiol 41) 272:C1450-C1456, 1997
93. Frick KK, LaPlante K, Bushinsky DA: RANK Ligand and TNF-a Mediate Acid-Induced Bone Calcium Efflux In Vitro. Am J Physiol Renal Physiol 289:F1005-F1011, 2005
94. Fujino H, Xu W, Regan JW: Prostaglandin E_2 induced functional expression of early growth response factor-1 by EP4, but not EP2, prostanoid receptors via th phosphatidylinositol 3-kinase and extracelular signal-regulated kinases. J Biol Chem 278:12151-12156, 2003
95. Gardner CR, Blanque R, Cottereaux C: Mechanisms involved in prostaglandin-induced increase in bone resorption in neonatal mouse calvaria. Prostaglandins Leukotrienes & Essential Fatty Acids 64:117-125, 2001
96. Gingery A, Bradley E, Shaw A, Oursler MJ: Phosphatidylinositol 3-kinase coordinately activates the MEK/ERK and AKT/NFkappaB pathways to maintain osteoclast survival. J Cell Biochem 89:165-179, 2003
97. Gitterman DP, Wilson J, Randall AD: Functional properties and pharmacological inhibition of ASIC channels in the human SJ-RH30 skeletal muscle cell line. J Physiol (Lond) 562:759-769, 2005
98. Goldhaber P, Rabadjija L: H^+ stimulation of cell-mediated bone resorption in tissue culture. Am J Physiol (Endocrinol Metab 16) 253:E90-E98, 1987
99. Goodman AD, Lemann J, Jr., Lennon EJ, Relman AS: Production, excretion, and net balance of fixed acid in patients with renal acidosis. J Clin Invest 44:495-506, 1965
100. Goodman WG, Coburn JW, Slatopolsky E, Salusky IB: Renal osteodystrophy in adults and children, chap. 69, in Primer on the Metabolic Bone Diseases and Disorders of Mineral Metabolism, 4 ed., edited by Favus MJ, Philadelphia, Lippincott-Raven, 1999, pp 347-363
101. Green J, Kleeman CR: Role of bone in regulation of systemic acid-base balance. Kidney Int 39:9-26, 1991
102. Grynpas MD, Bonar LC, Glimcher MJ: Failure to detect an amorphous calcium-phosphate solid phase in bone mineral. A radial distribution function study. Calcif Tissue Int 36:291-301, 1984
103. Hallegot P, Girod C, Levi-Setti R: Scanning ion microprobe assessment of biological sample preparation techniques. Scanning Microsc 4:605-612, 1990
104. Ho ML, Chang JK, Chuang LY et al.: Effects of nonsteroidal anti-inflammatory drugs and prostaglandins on osteoblastic functions. Biochem Pharm 58:983-990, 1999
105. Hofbauer LC, Heufelder AE: Role of receptor activator of nuclear factor-Kappa B ligand and osteoprotegerin in bone cell biology. J Mol Med 79:243-253, 2001
106. Horowitz MC, Xi Y, Wilson K, Kacena MA: Control of osteoclastogenesis and bone resorption by members of the TNF family of receptors and ligands. Cytokine Growth Factor Reviews 12:9-18, 2001
107. Hu Y, Chan E, Wang SX, Li B: Activation of p38 Mitogen-activated protein kinase is required for osteoblast differentiation. Endocrinol 144:2068-2074, 2003
108. Ishii S, Kihara Y, Shimizu T: Identification of T cell death-associated gene 8 (TDAG8) as a novel acid sensing G-Protein-copled receptor. J Biol Chem 280:9083-9087, 2005
109. Jones ER, Beck TR, Kapoor S et al.: Prostaglandins inhibit renal ammoniagenesis in the rat. J Clin Invest 74:992-1002, 1984
110. Kaneki H, Takasugi I, Fujieda M et al.: Prostaglandin E_2 stimulates the formation of mineralized bone nodules by a cAMP-independent mechanism in the culture of adult rat calvarial osteoblasts. J Cell Biochem 73:36-48, 1999
111. Kawaguchi H, Nemoto K, Raisz LG et al.: Interleukin-4 inhibits prostaglandin G/H synthase-2 and cytosolic phospholipase A_2 induction in neonatal mouse parietal bone cultures. J Bone Miner Res 11:358-366, 1996
112. Kawaguchi H, Pilbeam CC, Gronowicz G et al.: Transcriptional induction of prostaglandin G/H synthase-2 by basic fibroblast growth factor. J Clin Invest 96:923-930, 1995
113. Kawaguchi H, Pilbeam CC, Harrison JR, Raisz LG: The role of prostaglandins in the regulation of bone metabolism. Clin Orth Rel Res 313:36-46, 1995

114. Kawaguchi H, Raisz LG, Voznesensky OS et al.: Regulation of the two prostaglandin G/H synthases by parathyroid hormone, interleukin-1, cortisol and prostaglandin E_2 in cultured neonatal mouse calvariae. Endocrinol 135:1157-1164, 1994

115. Kaye M, Frueth AJ, Silverman M: A study of vertebral bone powder from patients with chronic renal failure. J Clin Invest 49:442-453, 1970

116. Kerstetter JE, O'Brian KO, Insogna KL: Dietary protein, calcium metabolism, and skeletal homeostasis revisited. American Journal of Clinical Nutrition 78:584S-592S, 2003

117. Kerstetter JE, O'Brian KO, Insogna KL: Dietary protein affects intestinal calcium absorption. American Journal of Clinical Nutrition 68:859-865, 2004

118. Klein DC, Raisz LG: Prostaglandins: stimulation of bone resorption in tissue culture. Endocrinol 86:1436-1440, 1970

119. Komarova SV, Pereverzev A, Shum JW et al.: Convergent signaling by acidosis and receptor activator of NF-{kappa}B ligand (RANKL) on the calcium/calcineurin/NFAT pathway in osteoclasts. PNAS 102:2643-2648, 2005

120. Kraut JA, Mishler DR, Kurokawa K: Effect of colchicine and calcitonin on calcemic response to metabolic acidosis. Kidney Int 25:608-612, 1984

121. Krieger NS, Bushinsky DA, Frick KK: Cellular mechanisms of bone resorption induced by metabolic acidosis. Semin Dial 16:463-466, 2003

122. Krieger NS, Frick KK, Bushinsky DA: Mechanism of acid-induced bone resorption. Current Opin in Nephrol Hypertens 13:423-436, 2004

123. Krieger NS, Hefley TJ: Differential effects of parathyroid hormone on protein phosphorylation in two osteoblast-like cell populations isolated from neonatal mouse calvaria. Calc Tiss Int 44:192-199, 1989

124. Krieger NS, Parker WR, Alexander KM, Bushinsky DA: Prostaglandins regulate acid-induced cell-mediated bone resorption. Am J Physiol Renal Physiol 279:F1077-F1082, 2000

125. Krieger NS, Sessler NE, Bushinsky DA: Acidosis inhibits osteoblastic and stimulates osteoclastic activity in vitro. Am J Physiol (Renal Fluid Electrolyte Physiol 31) 262:F442-F448, 1992

126. Kurtz I, Maher T, Hulter HN et al.: Effect of diet on plasma acid-base composition in normal humans. Kidney Intl 24:670-680, 1983

127. Lee JC, Kassis S, Kumar S et al.: p38 mitogen-activated protein kinase inhibitors - mechanisms and therapeutic potentials. Pharmacol Ther 82:389-397, 1999

128. Lefebvre A, de Vernejoul MC, Gueris J et al.: Optimal correction of acidosis changes progression of dialysis osteodystrophy. Kidney Int 36:1112-1118, 1989

129. Lemann J, Jr.: The urinary excretion of calcium, magnesium and phosphorus, in Primer on the Metabolic Bone Diseases and Disorders of Mineral Metabolism, edited by Favus MJ, Kelseyville, California, American Society for Bone and Mineral Research, 1990, pp 36-39

130. Lemann J, Jr., Adams ND, Gray RW: Urinary calcium excretion in human beings. N Engl J Med 301:535-541, 1979

131. Lemann J, Jr., Gray RW, Pleuss JA: Potassium bicarbonate, but not sodium bicarbonate, reduces urinary calcium excretion and improves calcium balance in healthy men. Kidney Intl 35:688-695, 1989

132. Lemann J, Jr., Litzow JR, Lennon EJ: The effects of chronic acid loads in normal man: Further evidence for the participation of bone mineral in the defense against chronic metabolic acidosis. J Clin Invest 45:1608-1614, 1966

133. Lemann J, Jr., Litzow JR, Lennon EJ: Studies of the mechanism by which chronic metabolic acidosis augments urinary calcium excretion in man. J Clin Invest 46:1318-1328, 1967

134. Lemann JJr, Adams ND, Wilz DR, Brenes LG: Acid and mineral balances and bone in familial proximal renal tubular acidosis. Kidney Int 58:1267-1277, 2000

135. Lemann JJr, Bushinsky DA, Hamm LL: Bone buffering of acid and base in humans. Am J Physiol Renal Physiol 285:F811-F832, 2003

136. Lennon EJ, Lemann J, Jr., Litzow JR: The effects of diet and stool composition on the net external acid balance of normal subjects. J Clin Invest 45:1601-1607, 1966

137. Levi-Setti R, Chabala JM, Smolik S: Nucleotide and protein distribution in BrdU-labelled polytene chromosomes revealed by ion probe mass spectrometry. Journal of Microscopy 175:44-53, 1994

138. Levitt MF, Turner LB, Sweet AY, Pandiri D: The response of bone, connective tissue, and muscle to acute acidosis. J Clin Invest 35:98-105, 1956

139. Lin W, Burks CA, Hansen DR et al.: Taste Receptor Cells Express pH-Sensitive Leak K+ Channels. J Neurophysiol 92:2909-2919, 2004

140. Litzow JR, Lemann J, Jr., Lennon EJ: The effect of treatment of acidosis on calcium balance in patients with chronic azotemic renal disease. J Clin Invest 46:280-286, 1967

141. Liu XH, Kirschenbaum A, Yao S, Levine AC: Cross-talk between the iInterleukin-6 and prostaglandin E_2 signaling systems results in enhancement of osteoclastogenesis through effects on the osteoprotegerin/receptor activator of nuclear factor-{kappa}B (RANK) ligand/RANK system. Endocrinology 146:1991-1998, 2005
142. Lucioni A, Womack C, Musch MW et al.: Metabolic acidosis in rats increases intestinal NHE2 and NHE3 expression and function. Am J Physiol Gastrointest Liver Physiol 283:G51-G56, 2002
143. Ludwig MG, Vanek M, Gueirine D et al.: Proton-sensing G-protein-coupled receptors. Nature 425:93-98, 2003
144. Lundgren T, Engstrom EU, Levi-Setti R et al.: The use of the stable isotope 44Ca in studies of calcium incorporation into dentin. Journal of Microscopy 173:149-154, 1994
145. Machwate M, Harada S, Leu CT et al.: Prostaglandin receptor EP_4 mediates the bone anabolic effects of PGE2. Mol Pharm 60:36-41, 2001
146. Madias NE, Kraut JA: Uremic acidosis, in The Regulation of Acid-Base Balance, edited by Seldin DW, Giebisch G, New York, Raven Press, 1989, pp 285-317
147. Martineau LC, McVeigh LI, Jasmin BJ, Kennedy CRJ: MAP kinase mediates mechanically induced COX-2 and PG EP_4 receptor expression in podocytes: implications for the actin cytoskeleton. Am J Physiol 286:F693-F701, 2004
148. McSherry E: Acidosis and growth in nonuremic renal disease. Kidney Int 14:349-354, 1978
149. McSherry E, Morris RC: Attainment and maintenance of normal stature with alkali therapy in infants and children with classic renal tubular acidosis. J Clin Invest 61:509-527, 1978
150. Meghji S, Morrison MS, Henderson B, Arnett TR: pH dependence of bone resorption: mouse calvarial osteoclasts are activated by acidosis. Am J Physiol Endocrinol Metab 280:E112-E119, 2001
151. Mogi C, Tomura H, Tobo M et al.: Sphingosylphosphorylcholine antagonized proton-sensing ovarian cancer G-protein coupled receptor 1 (OGR1)-mediated inositol phosphate production and cAMP accumulation. J Pharmacol Sci 99:160-167, 2005
152. Mora Palma FJ, Ellis HA, Cook DB et al.: Osteomalacia in patients with chronic renal failure before dialysis or transplantation. Q J Med 52:332-348, 1983
153. Murakami N, Yokomizo T, Okuno T, Shimizu T: G2A is a proton-sensing G-protein-coupled receptor antagonized by lysophosphatidylcholine. J Biol Chem 279:42484-42491, 2004
154. Nakamura I, Takahashi N, Sasaki T et al.: Wortmannin, a specific inhibitor of phosphatidylinositol-3 kinase, blocks osteoclastic bone resorption. FEBS Letters 361:79-84, 1995
155. Naruse K, Miyauchi A, Itoman M, Mikuni-Takagaki Y: Distinct anabolic response of osteoblast to low-intensity pulsed ultrasound. J Bone Min Res 18:360-369, 2003
156. National Kidney Foundation: K/DOQI clinical practice guidelines for bone metabolism and disease in chronic kidney disease. Am J Kidney Dis 42:S1-S201, 2003
157. Nebreda A, Porras A: p38 MAP kinases: beyond the stress response. TIBS 25:257-260, 2000
158. Nelson DGA, Barry JC, Shields CP et al.: Crystal morphology, composition, and dissolution behavior of carbonated apatites prepared at controlled pH and temperature. J Colloid Interface Sci 130:467-479, 1989
159. Nelson DGA, Featherstone JDB: Preparation, analysis and characterization of carbonated apatites. Calcif Tiss Intl 34:S69-S81, 1982
160. Nelson DGA, Featherstone JDB, Duncan JF, Cutress TW: Effect of carbonate and fluoride on the dissolution behavior of synthetic apatites. Caries Res 17:200-211, 1983
161. Neuman WF, Neuman MW: The Chemical Dynamics of Bone Mineral. Chicago, University Chicago Press, 1958
162. O'Neill GP, Kennedy BP, Mancini JA et al.: Selective inhibitors of COX-2. Agents Actions Suppl 46:159-168, 1995
163. Pasquale SM, Messier AA, Shea ML, Schaefer KE: Bone CO_2-titration curves in acute hypercapnia obtained with a modified titration technique. J Appl Physiol 48:197-201, 1980
164. Pellegrino ED, Blitz RM: The composition of human bone in uremia. Medicine 44:397-418, 1965
165. Pellegrino ED, Blitz RM, Letteri JM: Inter-relationships of carbonate, phosphate, monohydrogen phosphate, calcium, magnesium, and sodium in uraemic bone: Comparison of dialyzed and non-dialyzed patients. Clin Sci Mol Med 53:307-316, 1977
166. Pilbeam CC, Kawaguchi H, Hakeda Y et al.: Differential regulation of the inducible and constitutive prostaglandin endoperoxide synthase in osteoblastic MC3T3-E1 cells. J Biol Chem 268:25643-25649, 1993
167. Pilbeam CC, Kawaguchi H, Voznesensky O et al.: Regulation of inducible prostaglandin G/H synthase by interleukin-1, transforming growth factors-a and -b, and prostaglandins in bone cells. Adv Exp Med Biol 400B:617-623, 1997
168. Poole-Wilson PA, Cameron IR: Intracellular pH and K^+ of cardiac and skeletal muscle in acidosis and alkalosis. Am J Physiol 229:1305-1310, 1975

169. Qin L, Raggatt J, Partridge NC: Parathyroid hormone: a double-edged sword for bone metabolism. Trends in Endocrinology and Metabolism 15:60-65, 2004
170. Radu CG, Nijagal A, McLaughlin J et al.: Differential proton sensitivity of related G protein-coupled receptors T cell death-associated gene 8 and G2A expressed in immune cells. Proc Natl Acad Sci USA 102:1632-1637, 2005
171. Raisz LG: Physiologic and pathologic roles of prostaglandins and other eicosanoids in bone metabolism. J Nutr 125:2024S-2027S, 1995
172. Raisz LG: Prostaglandins and bone: physiology and pathophysiology. Osteoarthritis Cartilage 7:419-421, 1999
173. Raisz LG, Fall PM, Petersen DN et al.: Prostaglandin E_2 inhibits alpha 1(1) procollagen gene transcription and promoter activity in the immortalized rat osteoblastic clonal cell line Py1a . Mol Endocrin 7:17-22, 1993
174. Raisz LG, Martin TJ: Prostaglandins in bone and mineral metabolism, in Bone and Mineral Research Annual 2, edited by Peck WA, Amsterdam, Elsevier Science Publishers, 1984, pp 286-310
175. Rizzoli R, Bonjour JP: Dietary Protein and Bone Health. Journal of Bone & Mineral Research 19:527-531, 2004
176. Sakhaee K, Nicar M, Hill K, Pak CY: Contrasting effects of potassium citrate and sodium citrate therapies on urinary chemistries and crystallization of stone-forming salts. Kidney Intl 24:348-352, 1983
177. Sakuma Y, Li Z, Pilbeam CC et al.: Stimulation of cAMP production and cyclooxygenase-2 by prostaglandin E_2 and selective prostaglandin rceptor agonists in murine osteoblastic cells. Bone 34:827-834, 2004
178. Santhanagopal A, Dixon SJ: Insulin-like growth factor I rapidly enhances acid efflux from osteoblastic cells. Am J Physiol 277:E423-E432, 1999
179. Schelling SH, Wolfe HJ, Tashjian JrAH: Role of the osteoclast in prostaglandin E_2-stimulated bone resorption. A correlative morphometric and biochemical analysis. Lab Invest 42:290-295, 1980
180. Schroeder JM, Liu W, Curthoys NP: pH-responsive stabilization of glutamate dehydrogenase mRNA in LLX-PK1-F+ cells. Am J Physiol Renal Plysiol 285:F258-F265, 2003
181. Schwartz WB, Hall PW, III, Hays RM, Relman AS: On the mechanism of acidosis in chronic renal disease. J Clin Invest 38:39-52, 1959
182. Schwartz WB, Relman AS: Acidosis in renal disease. N Eng J Med 256:1184-1186, 1957
183. Sebastian A, Harris ST, Ottaway JH et al.: Improved mineral balance and skeletal metabolism in postmenopausal women treated with potassium bicarbonate. N Engl J Med 330:1776-1781, 1994
184. Slatopolsky E, Delmez J: Bone Disease in Chronic Renal Failure and After Renal Transplantation, chap. 39, in Disorders of Bone and Mineral Metabolism, edited by Coe F, Favus M, New York, NY, Raven Press, 1992, pp 905-934
185. Smith WL: Prostanoid biosynthesis and mechanisms of action. Am J Physiol 263:F181-F191, 1992
186. Sprague SM, Krieger NS, Bushinsky DA: Aluminum inhibits bone nodule formation and calcification in vitro. Am J Physiol (Renal Fluid Electrolyte Physiol 33) 264:F882-F890, 1993
187. Sprague SM, Krieger NS, Bushinsky DA: Greater inhibition of in vitro bone mineralization with metabolic than respiratory acidosis. Kidney Int 46:1199-1206, 1994
188. Stein GS, Lian JB, Stein JL et al.: Transcriptional control of osteoblast growth and differentiation. (Review). Physiol Rev 76:593-629, 1996
189. Stern PH, Krieger NS, Nissenson RA et al.: Human transforming growth factor-alpha stimulates bone resorption in vitro. J Clin Invest 76:2016-2019, 1985
190. Stern PH, Raisz LG: Organ culture of bone, in Skeletal Research, edited by Simmons DJ, Kunin AS, New York, Academic Press, 1979, pp 21-59
191. Suda T, Takahashi N, Udagawa N et al.: Modulation of osteoclast differentiation and function by the new members of the tumor necrosis factor receptor and ligand families. Endo Rev 20:345-357, 1999
192. Sudo H, Kodama HA, Amagai Y et al.: In vitro differentiation and calcification in a new clonal osteogenic cell line derived from newborn mouse calvaria. J Cell Biol 96:191-198, 1983
193. Sutton RAL, Wong NLM, Dirks JH: Effects of metabolic acidosis and alkalosis on sodium and calcium transport in the dog kidney. Kidney Int 15:520-533, 1979
194. Swan RC, Pitts RF: Neutralization of infused acid by nephrectomized dogs. J Clin Invest 34:205-212, 1955
195. Swarthout JT, D'Alonzo RC, Selvamurugan N, Partridge NC: Parathyroid hormone-dependent signaling pathways regulating genes in bone cells. Gene 282:1-17, 2002
196. Tai H, Miyaura C, Pilbeam CC et al.: Transcriptional induction of cyclooxygenase-2 in osteoblasts is involved in interleukin-6-induced osteoclast formation. Endocrinol 138:2372-2379, 1997
197. Tang LY, Kimmel DB, Jee WSS, Yee JA: Functional characterization of prostaglandin E_2 inducible osteogenic colony forming units in cultures of cells isolated from the neonatal rat calvarium. J Cell Physiol 166:76-83, 1996

198. Tashjian JAH, Hohmann EL, Antoniades HN, Levine L: Platelet-derived growth factor stimulates bone resorption via a prostaglandin-mediated mechanism. Endocrinol 111:118-124, 1982
199. Tashjian JrAH, Levine L: Epidermal growth factor stimulates prostaglandin production and bone resorption in cultured mouse calvaria. Bioch Biophys Res Commun 85:966-975, 1978
200. Tashjian JrAH, Voelkel EF, Lazzaro M et al.: Tumor necrosis factor-a (cachectin) stimulates bone resorption in mouse calvaria via a prostaglandin-mediated mechanism. Endocrinol 120:2029-2036, 1987
201. Tashjian JrAH, Voelkel EF, Lazzaro M et al.: Alpha and beta human transforming growth factors stimulated prostaglandin production and bone resorption in cultured mouse calvaria. Proc Nat Acad Sci 82:4535-4538, 1985
202. Tashjian JrAH, Voelkel EF, Levine L, Goldhaber P: Evidence that the bone resorption-stimulating factor produced by mouse fibrosarcoma cells is prostaglandin E2. J Exp Med 136:1329-1343, 1972
203. Tetradis S, Pilbeam CC, Liu Y, Kream BE: Parathyroid hormone induces prostaglandin G/H synthase-2 expression by a cyclic adenosine 3',5'-monophosphate-mediated pathway in the murine osteoblastic cell line MC3T3-E1. Endocrinol 137:5435-5440, 1996
204. Thomas B, Thirion S, Humbert L et al.: Differentiation regulates interleukin-1B-induced cyclo-oxgenase-2 in human articular chondrocytes: role of p38 mitogen-activated protein kinase. Biochem J 362:367-373, 2002
205. Tomura H, Mogi C, Sato K, Okajima F: Proton-sensing and lysolipid-sensitive G-protein-coupled receptors: A novel type of multi-functional receptors. Cellular Signalling 17:1466-1476, 2005
206. Tomura H, Wang JQ, Komachi M et al.: Prostaglandin I2 Production and cAMP Accumulation in Response to Acidic Extracellular pH through OGR1 in Human Aortic Smooth Muscle Cells. Journal of Biological Chemistry 280:34458-34464, 2005
207. Tsuganezawa H, Sato S, Yamaji Y et al.: Role of c-SRC and ERK in acid-induced activation of NHE3. Kidney Int 62:41-50, 2002
208. Ugawa S: Identification of sour-taste receptor genes. Anat Sci Int 78:205-210, 2003
209. Ugawa S, Ueda T, Ishida Y et al.: Amiloride-blockable acid-sensing ion channels are leading acid sensors expressed in human nociceptors. J Clin Invest 110:1185-1190, 2002
210. Voelkel EF, Tashjian JrAH, Levine L: Cyclooxygenase products of arachidonic acid metabolism by mouse bone in organ culture. Biochim Biophys Acta 620:418-428, 1980
211. Vrotsos Y, Miller SC, Marks SC, Jr.: Prostaglandin E - A powerful anabolic agent for generalized or site-specific bone formation. Critical Reviews in Eurkaryotic Gene Expression 13:255-263, 2003
212. Wang JQ, Kon J, Mogi C et al.: TDAG8 is a proton-sensing and psychosine-sensitive G-protein-coupled receptor. J Biol Chem 279:45626-45633, 2004
213. Weber HP, Gray RW, Dominguez JH, Lemann J, Jr.: The lack of effect of chronic metabolic acidosis on 25-OH vitamin D metabolism and serum parathyroid hormone in humans. J Clin Endocrinol Metab 43:1047-1055, 1976
214. Widdowson EM, Dickerson JWT: Chemical composition of the body, in Mineral Metabolism, edited by Comar CL, Bronner F, New York, Academic Press, Inc., 1964, pp 1-247
215. Widdowson EM, McCance RA, Spray CM: The chemical composition of the human body. Clin Sci 10:113-125, 1951
216. Windischhofer W, Zach D, Fauler GRG et al.: Involvement of rho and p38 MAPK in endothelin-1-induced expression of PGHS-2 mRNA in ostoblast-like cells. J Bone Min Res 17:1774-1784, 2002
217. Woodiel FN, Fall PM, Raisz LG: Anabolic effects of prostaglandins in cultured fetal rat calvariae: structure-activity relations and signal transduction pathway. J Bone Miner Res 11:1249-1255, 1996
218. Yamaguchi DT, Ma D: Mechanism of pH regulation of connexin 43 expression in MC3T3-E1 cells. Bioch Biophys Res Commun 304:736-739, 2003
219. Yano H, Nakanishi S, Kimura K et al.: Inhibition of histamine secretion by wortmannin through the blockade of phosphatidylinositol 3-kinase in RBL-2H3 cells. J Biol Chem 268:25846-25856, 1993
220. Zarubin T: Activation and signaling of the p38 MAP kinase pathway. Cell Research 15:11-18, 2005

Pyrophosphate Transport and Stones

John A. Sayer,[a,b] Georgina Carr,[b] Shabbir H. Moochhala[b] and Nicholas L. Simmons[b]

[a]*Institute of Human Genetics, International Centre for Life, Newcastle University, NE1 3BZ, United Kingdom.*
[b]*Epithelial Research Group, Institute for Cell and Molecular Bioscience, Medical School, Newcastle University, NE2 4HH, United Kingdom.*

Abstract. Since the 1960's, inorganic pyrophosphate (PPi) has been known to inhibit apatite precipitation. Recent findings suggest that PPi plays a central role in the control of normal bone mineralization. Knockout mice have established the functional importance of PPi trans-membrane transport, via the pyrophosphate transporter ANKH. The molecular nature and transport function of ANKH are reviewed. PPi is present in urine and ANKH is expressed in the cortical collecting duct where PPi transport to both the tubular lumen and renal interstitium may occur. Arginine vasopressin stimulation of cortical collecting duct cells grown on semi-permeable supports appears to upregulate apical ANKH expression, which we postulate may be a mechanism of stone inhibition during urinary concentration and supersaturation of calcium salts. Hypopyrophosphaturia may be a forgotten metabolic risk factor for stone formation and polymorphisms of the ANKH gene may underlie this defect. The physiological importance and clinical significance of PPi generation and transport in preventing idiopathic renal stone disease and nephrocalcinosis now needs to be established.

Keywords: pyrophosphate; mineralization; apatite; cortical collecting duct; aquaporins; vasopressin
PACS: 87.15.nt

PYROPHOSPHATE: THE FIRST STONE INHIBITOR

Since the seminal work of Fleisch and Bisaz in 1962, inorganic pyrophosphate (PPi) has been recognized as a potent inhibitor of crystallization [1,2]. Indeed they noted at that time that industry utilized polyphosphates to prevent boilers from limescale deposits. The modern day use of pyrophosphates is as an additive to tartar control toothpaste. Serum and plasma PPi levels were estimated to be in the micromolar range, with a greater concentration in the urine than plasma [2]. Fleisch *et al.* postulated that delivery of urinary pyrophosphate was achieved via glomerular filtration. PPi inhibits crystallization by binding to the surface of basic calcium phosphate (this includes hydroxyapatite) crystals and blocking further crystal growth [3]. The chemical structure of pyrophosphates is two phosphates bound together via an ester bond. Pyrophosphate has chemical analogues in the form of bisphosphonates, where a carbon atom replaces the oxygen (Figure 1).

PPi is involved in many aspects of cellular physiology, with roles in intracellular calcium traffic and modification of enzyme function, as well as being a metabolic by-

CP1049, *Renal Stone Disease 2, 2nd International Urolithiasis Research Symposium,*
edited by A. P. Evan, J. E. Lingeman, J. A. McAteer, and J. C. Williams, Jr.

product, for example in the hydrolysis of adenosine triphosphate by adenylate cyclase [4]. *In vivo* pyrophosphate turnover studies suggest that most pyrophosphate metabolism is intracellular [5]; however recent work emphasizes its extracellular role in inhibition of bone mineralization [6]. In fact, the ratio of extracellular matrix phosphate to PPi determines whether mineralization via hydroxyapatite crystal formation is promoted or inhibited.

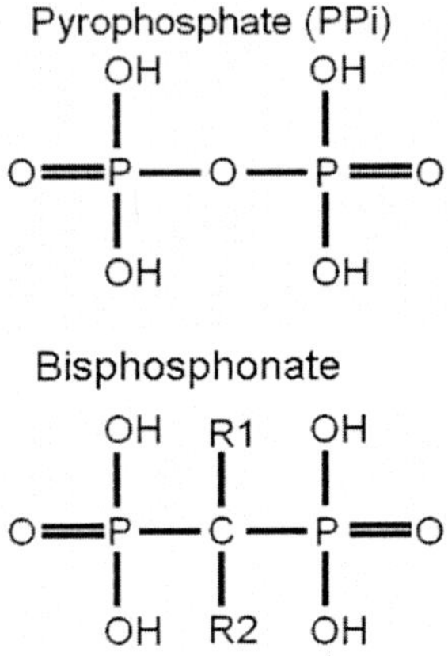

FIGURE 1: Chemical structure of pyrophosphate and generic bisphosphonate.

URINARY PYROPHOSPHATE

Pyrophosphate in urine was first measured using anion separation followed by acid hydrolysis and the measurement of Pi by colorimetric formation of a molybdate complex. Using this assay urinary PPi was estimated to be 10 μM [2]. Subsequently a variety of PPi dependent enzyme reactions (e.g., PPi-dependent conversion by fructose-6-phosphate kinase of fructose-6-phosphate to fructose-1-6-diphosphate coupled to disappearance of NADH [7] or glucose-1-phosphate formation from UDPP-glucose catalyzed by UDPG-pyrophosphorylase and ultimately to reduction of NADP [8]) have been developed with increasing sensitivity achieved by a radiometric separation of UDP-glucose from 6-phosphogluconate [9]. Where urine PPi has been measured, estimates fall within the range described by Fleisch (i.e., 8-16 μM [10]).

In order to make consistent and repeatable measurements of urinary pyrophosphate, it is necessary to know its stability. March *et al.* concluded that PPi was relatively stable in urine with complete recovery of added PPi from urine samples. The mean output rate of PPi in normal males was 45 μmol/24 hours. In addition, 24 h urinary PPi are positively correlated with urine volumes [7], but PPi is elevated in most concentrated (low volume) urines. Pyrophosphate is also subject to rapid hydrolysis by alkaline phosphatases (see Figure 4). Given that the proximal tubule has strong expression of alkaline phosphatase, intratubular hydrolysis is likely to eliminate PPi arising from glomerular filtration and by inference suggest that PPi arises from and has its main action in distal segments. Increased levels of urinary enzymes, as is found in renal tubular injury may confound measurements of urinary PPi levels, especially in established stone disease.

Given the hypothesis that pyrophosphate is a urinary inhibitor of calcification, we must consider whether hypopyrophosphaturia is a metabolic risk factor for stone formation. Some clinical studies have shown that hypopyrophosphaturia may be present in idiopathic stone formers [7,11,12]. For example, in a group of 107 patients with recurrent calcium stones, 48% had reduced urinary pyrophosphate:creatinine ratios compared with control subjects [13]. Other studies, however, are also small and are inconclusive.

MOLECULAR GENETICS OF PYROPHOSPHATE TRANSPORT

The interest in pyrophosphate as a modifier of mineralization has suddenly increased since a molecular candidate for pyrophosphate transport was identified in 2000. Ho *et al.* studied a mouse model of arthritis known as *progressive ankylosis* or *ank* [14]. They were able to define the genetic lesion in this long-studied mouse model as a premature stop codon at position 440 in a gene they named *ank*. Using fibroblasts cultured from *ank* mice they showed an increase in intracellular PPi levels, together with a decrease in extracellular PPi levels. Transfection of wild type ANKH protein rescued the defect, consistent with ANKH-mediated PPi transport from cell to medium [14]. The postulated pathophysiology was that decreased extracellular pyrophosphate led to extra-articular crystal deposition leading to inflammation and ultimately arthrosis. Interestingly, the authors comment *"we have observed increased calcification in kidneys of adults"* which leads to our speculation that this was due to urinary/interstitial PPi deficiency, promoting nephrocalcinosis.

The *ank* gene is highly conserved in vertebrates, with the human homologue known as *ANKH* being virtually identical to the mouse (98%). This conservation exists in other vertebrates, with the *Danio rerio* showing 82% amino acid identity with the human ANKH [15]. In humans *ANKH* is on the short arm of Chromosome 5, and encodes a 492 amino acid protein. Human ANKH protein domain analysis depicts the whole amino acid sequence as an "ANKH" domain which is unique to the human genome (SMART sequence analysis: http://smart.embl-heidelberg.de/). Depending on criteria used for hydropathy plots, ANKH may have between 8 and 12 transmembrane spanning domains [16], which may form a pore like structure [15].

More recently, further definitive evidence that ANKH acts as a pyrophosphate transporter has been obtained. Expression of ANKH in *Xenopus* oocytes has confirmed the transport of ^{32}PPi; interestingly ^{32}PPi influx into the oocytes was enhanced by ANKH suggesting that bi-directional transport of PPi is possible [17]. ^{32}PPi influx showed saturation with an apparent K_m of 1.3μM, suggesting that ANKH is not simply an anion channel but functions as a facilitated transporter, symporter or antiporter. It is possible that ANKH may transport other anions (suggested in [18]) such as phosphate or even ATP.

ANKH AND HUMAN DISEASE

Mutations in *ANKH* have been described in two separate human disorders of calcification, craniometaphyseal dysplasia (OMIM 123000) and a subtype of familial calcium pyrophosphate dihydrate deposition disease (CCAL2; OMIM 118600) [14,15,19]. Craniometaphyseal dysplasia (CMD) is an autosomal dominant disorder which causes a generalized increase in bone density, leading to disability such as facial palsy and deafness due to nerve compression when this occurs in the bones of the skull. There is abnormal modeling of long bone metaphyses but there are no major effects on joints. Reichenberger [20] demonstrated loss of function mutations (two in-frame single amino acid deletions (F376del, S375del) and one insertion (A380ins) caused by a splicing defect) in *ANKH* leading to CMD. Nurnberg *et al.* described additional human *ANKH* mutations (W292R, C331R, F377del, P380insA, G389R) [15]. Mostly, these mutations cluster in a small region of the protein on a cytoplasmic domain.

In contrast, autosomal dominant calcium pyrophosphate dihydrate deposition (CPPD) disease is caused by "activating" mutations of *ANKH*. Four mutations mostly clustered at the N-terminal (P5T, M48T, E490del and -11CT) of *ANKH* cause the familial CCAL2 form of CPPD [21]. The -11CT mutation results in an alternative ATG initiation codon that adds four amino acids to the highly conserved N-terminus of the ANKH protein. It is thought that CCAL2 mutations result in gain of function and increased PPi export and ultimately pyrophosphate precipitation. Pendleton reconstructed these mutations in an expression construct followed by transfection into COS-7 cells [21]. One mutation, -11CT, caused a reduction in intracellular PPi suggesting a gain of function. However, the M48T mutation caused no significant change in intracellular PPi and direct measurement of ^{32}PPi influx in control and coding mutants P5T and M48T expressed in *Xenopus* oocytes showed no elevation above control levels [17].

Polymorphisms in the 5' non-coding region and the promoter region of the *ANKH* gene have been associated with ankylosing spondylitis (AS) [22]. These alleles were significantly associated with disease in affected family members with AS, compared to unaffected family members. These results are in contrast to findings by Timms *et al.* where they found no association with disease in 233 AS patients following genotyping of 5 SNPs (including three known promoter variants) [23]. Subsequently, SNP variants in the *TNAP* gene have been associated with AS [24].

Given a possible universal role in calcification, *ANKH* is a candidate gene for osteoporosis. Using this approach, Kiel *et al.* found that two intronic SNPs within the *ANKH* gene (rs2454873 and rs379016) were associated with femoral neck section modulus. This candidate approach however may be biased, as *ANKH* was not identified to be associated with loss of bone mineral density on a genome wide screen using 100K SNP GeneChip markers [25].

ANKH EXPRESSION IN RENAL CELLS AND TISSUES

Work we have performed in our laboratory has confirmed expression of ANKH in murine and human kidney cell lines and tissues. Using RT-PCR we have confirmed expression in mIMCD-3 cells, a renal inner medullary collecting duct cell line (Figure 2).

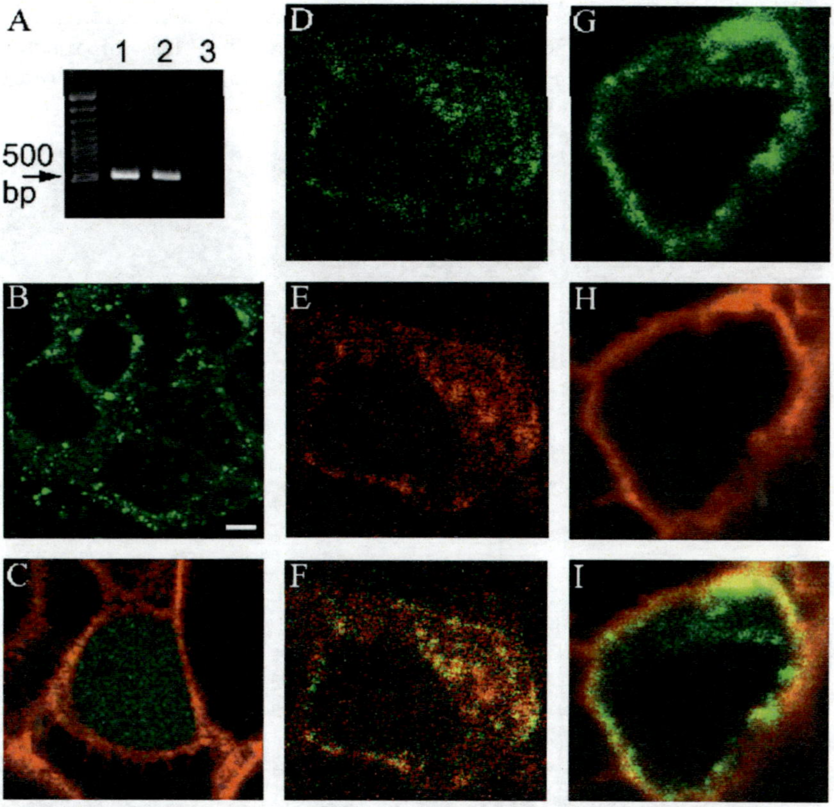

FIGURE 2. (A) RT-PCR of an internal (490bp) *Ankh* product. PCR products are seen in the mouse terminal collecting duct epithelial cell line (mIMCD-3, lane 1) as well as whole murine kidney (lane 2); lane 3 water control. PCR products were confirmed as *Ankh* by direct sequencing. (B) Cellular localisation of ANKH in mIMCD-3cells; *x-y* mid-cell confocal section showing ANKH staining using the primary antibody Ab3 and AF 488 goat anti-rabbit Ig. (C) *x-y* mid-cell confocal section showing GFP transfected cell, counterstained with TRITC-WGA lectin. (D) *x-y* mid-cell confocal section of ANK-NT-GFP transfected cell, (E) same cell counterstained with primary antibody Ab3/ and secondary AF 568. (F) Overlay of D+E. (G) *x-y* mid-cell confocal section of ANK-NT-GFP transfected cell, (H) same cell counterstained with TRITC-WGA lectin. (I) Overlay of G+H showing co-localisation at the plasma membrane. Scale bars=5μm. (Reprinted from figure 1 of ref [26], used with permission).

Using these cells we have been able to demonstrate plasma membrane localization for wild-type ANKH using both antibodies and transfection with N-terminal GFP tagged ANKH constructs (Figure 2). Using site directed mutagenesis, we have mimicked an "activating" mutation of ANKH (M48T) which gives rise to chondrocalcinosis. Similarly, we have mimicked the *ank* mouse mutation (*progressive ankylosis*) by introducing a premature stop codon in ANKH at position 440X. These constructs, with an N-terminal tag were transfected into mIMCD-3 cells (Figure 3). Expression of M48T-ANKH mimics wild type, with plasma membrane expression, consistent with the phenotype of a postulated upregulation of PPi export form the cell. In contrast ANK-R440X fails to traffic to the plasma membrane and remains trapped intracellularly (Figure 3) [26]. This is consistent with a loss of function and intracellular accumulation of PPi [14], and the fact that this mutation fails to reach the plasma membrane in *Xenopus* oocytes [17].

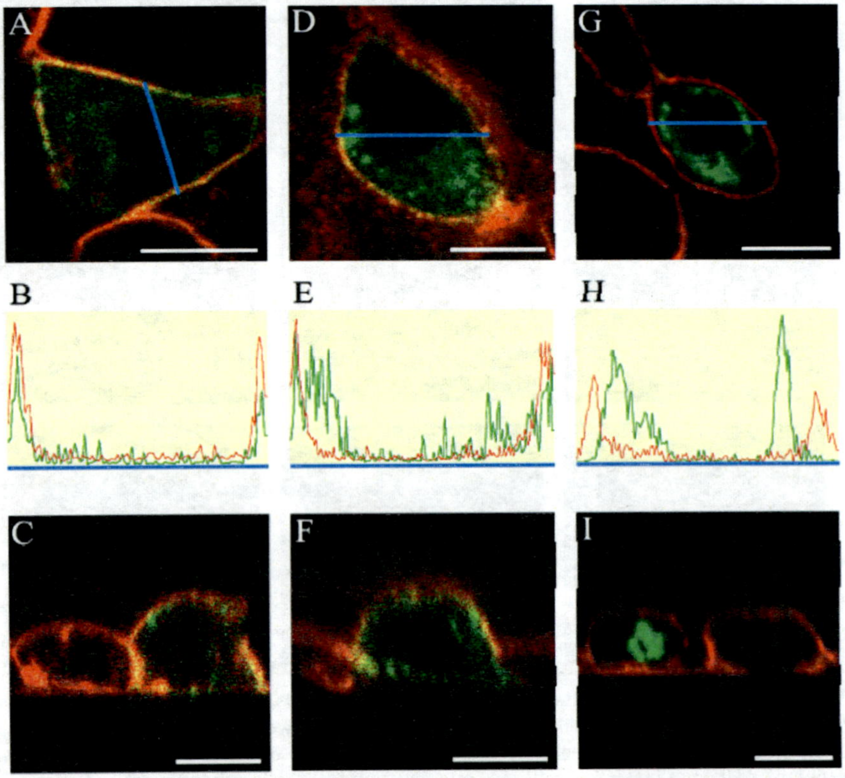

FIGURE 3. Effect of the Met48Thr and Glu440X mutations on the membrane localization of ANK. Mid-cell x-y confocal sections of ANK-NT-GFP (A), Met48Thr ANK-NT-GFP (D) and Glu440X ANK-NT-GFP (G) showing the comparison between wild type and mutant cells stained with the plasma membrane marker TRITC-WGA lectin after 2 min incubation. Blue bars indicate mid-cell transect used to compare the pixel intensity of GFP fluorescence intensity with that of TRITC-WGA lectin (A, D, G for B, E, H respectively). Note the co-incidence of peak fluorescence for GFP and TRITC-WGA for wild type ANK-NT-GFP and Met48Thr ANK-NT-GFP, but not for Glu440X ANK-NT-GFP. x-z section showing prominent lateral localisation of ANK-NT-GFP (C) and Met48Thr ANK-NT-GFP (F) but note absence of membrane staining for Glu440X ANK-NT-GFP I). Scale bars = 10μm. (Reprinted from figure 2 of ref [26], used with permission).

Since we have shown endogenous expression of ANKH in mIMCD-3 cells and that we have demonstrated plasma membrane expression of ANKH, we wished to ascertain whether PPi was exported from confluent monolayers of mIMCD-3 cells, cultured in serum free conditions in the absence of phenol red. Using an enzymatic assay, PPi was quantified using PPi-dependent fructose-6-phosphate kinase activity coupled to the disappearance of NADH [26]. After 24 h the apical concentration of PPi attained ~12 μM and the basolateral concentration ~4 μM. This correlates well with known urine concentration of PPi and is consistent with ANKH functioning as a PPi transporter at both apical and basolateral membranes. The half life of PPi is limited at cell surfaces by actions of alkaline phosphatase and ectonucleotide pyrophosphatases, and thus quantification of PPi in cell culture systems (and indeed patients' urine) is hampered.

Using the anti-ANKH antibody (ab3) gifted from the Kingsley laboratory, we have assessed the distribution of ANKH in murine and human kidney sections. Immunofluorescent staining showed clearly that ANKH expression was limited to a subset of distal tubules. There was co-staining of ANKH-positive tubules with aquaporin-2 antibodies, correlating with a collecting duct expression pattern. In these cortical collecting duct (CCD) segments, both the majority cell population (aquaporin-2 positive, principal cells) and the minority aquaporin-2 negative cells (intercalated cells) stained positively with ANKH antibodies [26]. ANKH staining was present at both apical and basolateral plasma membranes, suggesting a role in PPi delivery to both the lumen and the interstitium, respectively. We have recently confirmed similar findings in human kidney sections, where ANKH shows a similar distribution in collecting duct segments expressing aquaporin-2 [27].

Given that we have shown expression at collecting duct sites, and that PPi is in greater quantities in the urine than the plasma, we should consider the delivery rates and destruction rates of PPi in the kidney. We postulate a model of delivery of PPi to the final urine (Figure 4). Here glomerular filtrate delivers PPi to the proximal tubule.

Within the proximal tubule, there is additional PPi production from ATP via local enzymes such as nucleotide pyrophosphatase phosphodiesterase-3 (NPP3). Proximal tubule brush borders are however rich in alkaline phosphatases (TNAP) and hydrolyze PPi to phosphate. In the collecting duct there is further PPi production from apically located enzymes which include nucleoside triphosphate diphosphohydrolases. At this location, we suggest that PPi delivery to the lumen and interstitium is facilitated by ANKH. This nephron segment is the point of maximal urinary concentration, where crystaluria develops and the delivery of stone inhibitors may play an important physiological role [28]. Interstitial delivery of PPi at this location may also prevent the development of Randall's plaques and nephrocalcinosis. Given this hypothesis, is there evidence for regulation of ANKH in this nephron segment?

In accordance with the nephron localization of ANKH, we have chosen to study an immortalized cell-line derived from mouse cortical collecting tubule (mpkCCDcl4) (kindly provided by A. Vandewalle [29]). mpkCCDcl4 cells show aquaporin-2 protein expression regulated in the long term by both vasopressin (via V2 receptor stimulation) and by raised extracellular tonicity [30,31]. We have confirmed ANKH expression in mpkCCDcl4 cells. Immunofluorescence using ab3 shows both intracellular and limited plasma membrane expression at apical and basal membranes. Incubation of cells for 24 h in either arginine vasopressin (AVP, 10^{-8}M) or forskolin (10^{-5}M) results in marked expression of aquaporin-2 at the apical membrane in a subset of cells, as previously shown [30]. ANKH expression shows a similar increase in apically expressing cells, but the population is distinct from that showing raised aquaporin-2 expression. These data suggest that ANKH may be subject to physiologically relevant regulation by AVP and requires investigation within the renal tubule *in vivo*.

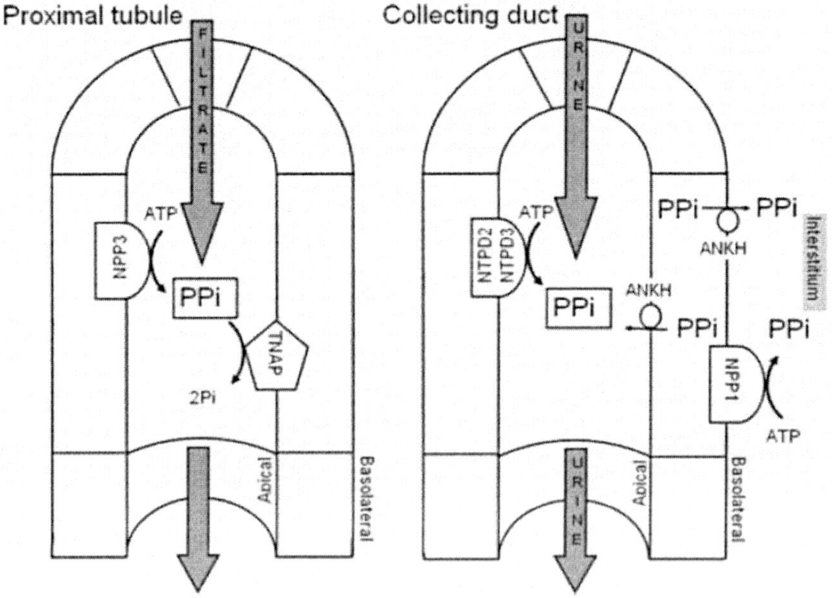

FIGURE 4. Pyrophosphate production in the proximal and distal nephron (collecting duct). In the proximal nephron, PPi, arising both from glomerular filtration and from ATP via nucleotide pyrophosphatase phosphodiesterase-3 (NPP3) action, is degraded by alkaline phosphatase (TNAP). In the distal nephron, tubular secretion of ATP contributes to the extracellular pool of PPi by the action of NPP1 at the basolateral membrane and by nucleoside triphosphate diphosphohydrolases (NTPD) 2 and 3 at the apical membrane. The protein ANKH is expressed in aquaporin-2-positive cortical collecting ducts at both apical and basolateral cell membranes to transport PPi from cytoplasm to both tubular lumen and interstitium. Extracellular PPi, together with protein crystal inhibitors such as osteopontin, limits intraluminal and interstitial stone formation. (Reprinted from figure 2 of ref [16], used with permission).

CONCLUSIONS

The perhaps forgotten inhibitor of renal stone formation, pyrophosphate, has been brought into the molecular age. It is now clear that there is a dynamic relationship between ANKH, TNAP and NPP1 in regulating calcification. This has been investigated most vigorously in bone, but we suggest that similar mechanisms may be present in the kidney to limit both luminal and interstitial calcification. It now remains to be seen whether polymorphisms in ANKH or dysregulation of ANKH traffic and activity may contribute to hypopyrophosphaturia and stone formation. More robust methods of measuring urinary pyrophosphate need to be developed, so that clinicians may identify hypopyrophosphaturia as an underlying metabolic risk factor in stone formation.

ACKNOWLEDGMENTS

JAS is a Clinician Scientist funded by GlaxoSmithKline. GC is a Fellow funded by Kidney Research UK. SM is a Research Training Fellow funded by the Wellcome Trust.

REFERENCES

1. Fleisch, H., S. Bisaz, Mechanism of calcification: inhibitory role of pyrophosphate. Nature. 195, 911 (1962).
2. Fleisch, H., S. Bisaz, Isolation from urine of pyrophosphate, a calcification inhibitor. Am J Physiol. 203, 671-5 (1962).
3. Jung, A., S. Bisaz, P. Bartholdi, H. Fleisch, Influence of pyrophosphate on the exchange of calcium and phosphate ions on hydroxyapatite. Calcif Tissue Res. 13, 27-40 (1973).
4. Rachow, J.W., L.M. Ryan, Inorganic pyrophosphate metabolism in arthritis. Rheum Dis Clin North Am. 14, 289-302 (1988).
5. Jung, A., R.G. Russel, S. Bisaz, D.B. Morgan, H. Fleisch, Fate of intravenously injected pyrophosphate-32P in dogs. Am J Physiol. 218, 1757-64 (1970).
6. Harmey, D., L. Hessle, S. Narisawa, K.A. Johnson, R. Terkeltaub, J.L. Millan, Concerted regulation of inorganic pyrophosphate and osteopontin by akp2, enpp1, and ank: an integrated model of the pathogenesis of mineralization disorders. Am J Pathol. 164, 1199-209 (2004).
7. Roberts, N.B., J. Dutton, T. Helliwell, P.J. Rothwell, J.P. Kavanagh, Pyrophosphate in synovial fluid and urine and its relationship to urinary risk factors for stone disease. Ann Clin Biochem. 29 (Pt 5), 529-34 (1992).
8. Lust, G., J.E. Seegmiller, A rapid, enzymatic assay for measurement of inorganic pyrophosphate in biological samples. Clin Chim Acta. 66, 241-9 (1976).
9. McGuire, M.B., C.H. Colman, N. Baghat, R.G. Russell, Radiometric measurement of pyrophosphate in cell cultures. Biochem Soc Trans. 8, 529-30 (1980).
10. March, J.G., B.M. Simonet, F. Grases, Determination of pyrophosphate in renal calculi and urine by means of an enzymatic method. Clin Chim Acta. 314, 187-94 (2001).
11. Baumann, J.M., S. Bisaz, R. Felix, H. Fleisch, U. Ganz, R.G. Russell, The role of inhibitors and other factors in the pathogenesis of recurrent calcium-containing renal stones. Clin Sci Mol Med. 53, 141-8 (1977).
12. Wikstrom, B., U. Backman, B.G. Danielson, B. Fellstrom, G. Johansson, S. Ljunghall, Ambulatory diagnostic evaluation of 389 recurrent renal stone formers. A proposal for clinical classification and investigation. Klin Wochenschr. 61, 85-90 (1983).
13. Laminski, N.A., A.M. Meyers, M.I. Sonnekus, A.E. Smyth, Prevalence of hypocitraturia and hypopyrophosphaturia in recurrent calcium stone formers: as isolated defects or associated with other metabolic abnormalities. Nephron. 56, 379-86 (1990).
14. Ho, A.M., M.D. Johnson, D.M. Kingsley, Role of the mouse ank gene in control of tissue calcification and arthritis. Science. 289, 265-70 (2000).
15. Nurnberg, P., H. Thiele, D. Chandler, W. Hohne, M.L. Cunningham, H. Ritter, G. Leschik, K. Uhlmann, C. Mischung, K. Harrop, J. Goldblatt, Z.U. Borochowitz, D. Kotzot, F. Westermann, S. Mundlos, H.S. Braun, N. Laing, S. Tinschert, Heterozygous mutations in ANKH, the human ortholog of the mouse progressive ankylosis gene, result in craniometaphyseal dysplasia. Nat Genet. 28, 37-41 (2001).
16. Moochhala, S.H., J.A. Sayer, G. Carr, N.L. Simmons, Renal calcium stones: Insights from the control of bone mineralisation. Exp Physiol. 93, 43-9 (2008).

17. Gurley, K.A., R.J. Reimer, D.M. Kingsley, Biochemical and genetic analysis of ANK in arthritis and bone disease. Am J Hum Genet. 79, 1017-29 (2006).
18. Ryan, L.M., The ank gene story. Arthritis Res. 3, 77-9 (2001).
19. Andrew, L.J., V. Brancolini, L.S. de la Pena, M. Devoto, F. Caeiro, R. Marchegiani, A. Reginato, A. Gaucher, P. Netter, P. Gillet, D. Loeuille, D.J. Prockop, A. Carr, B.F. Wordsworth, M. Lathrop, S. Butcher, E. Considine, K. Everts, A. Nicod, S. Walsh, C.J. Williams, Refinement of the chromosome 5p locus for familial calcium pyrophosphate dihydrate deposition disease. Am J Hum Genet. 64, 136-45 (1999).
20. Reichenberger, E., V. Tiziani, S. Watanabe, L. Park, Y. Ueki, C. Santanna, S.T. Baur, R. Shiang, D.K. Grange, P. Beighton, J. Gardner, H. Hamersma, S. Sellars, R. Ramesar, A.C. Lidral, A. Sommer, C.M. Raposo do Amaral, R.J. Gorlin, J.B. Mulliken, B.R. Olsen, Autosomal dominant craniometaphyseal dysplasia is caused by mutations in the transmembrane protein ANK. Am J Hum Genet. 68, 1321-6 (2001).
21. Pendleton, A., M.D. Johnson, A. Hughes, K.A. Gurley, A.M. Ho, M. Doherty, J. Dixey, P. Gillet, D. Loeuille, R. McGrath, A. Reginato, R. Shiang, G. Wright, P. Netter, C. Williams, D.M. Kingsley, Mutations in ANKH cause chondrocalcinosis. Am J Hum Genet. 71, 933-40 (2002).
22. Tsui, F.W., H.W. Tsui, E.Y. Cheng, M. Stone, U. Payne, J.D. Reveille, M.J. Shulman, A.D. Paterson, R.D. Inman, Novel genetic markers in the 5'-flanking region of ANKH are associated with ankylosing spondylitis. Arthritis Rheum. 48, 791-7 (2003).
23. Timms, A.E., Y. Zhang, L. Bradbury, B.P. Wordsworth, M.A. Brown, Investigation of the role of ANKH in ankylosing spondylitis. Arthritis Rheum. 48, 2898-902 (2003).
24. Tsui, H.W., R.D. Inman, J.D. Reveille, F.W. Tsui, Association of a TNAP haplotype with ankylosing spondylitis. Arthritis Rheum. 56, 234-43 (2007).
25. Kiel, D.P., S. Demissie, J. Dupuis, K.L. Lunetta, J.M. Murabito, D. Karasik, Genome-wide association with bone mass and geometry in the Framingham Heart Study. BMC Med Genet. 8 Suppl 1, S14 (2007).
26. Carr, G., J.A. Sayer, N.L. Simmons, Expression and localisation of the pyrophosphate transporter, ANK, in murine kidney cells. Cell Physiol Biochem. 20, 507-16 (2007).
27. Moochhala, S.H., G. Carr, J.A. Sayer, N.L. Simmons, The Pyrophosphate Transporter, ANK, Is Expressed in Mouse and Human Kidney and Co-Localises with Aquaporin-2 in Renal Collecting Ducts. J Am Soc Nephrol. 18, 595A (2007).
28. Sayer, J.A., G. Carr, N.L. Simmons, Nephrocalcinosis: molecular insights into calcium precipitation within the kidney. Clin Sci (Lond). 106, 549-61 (2004).
29. Bens, M., V. Vallet, F. Cluzeaud, L. Pascual-Letallec, A. Kahn, M.E. Rafestin-Oblin, B.C. Rossier, A. Vandewalle, Corticosteroid-dependent sodium transport in a novel immortalized mouse collecting duct principal cell line. J Am Soc Nephrol. 10, 923-34 (1999).
30. Hasler, U., D. Mordasini, M. Bens, M. Bianchi, F. Cluzeaud, M. Rousselot, A. Vandewalle, E. Feraille, P.Y. Martin, Long term regulation of aquaporin-2 expression in vasopressin-responsive renal collecting duct principal cells. J Biol Chem. 277, 10379-86 (2002).
31. Hasler, U., M. Vinciguerra, A. Vandewalle, P.Y. Martin, E. Feraille, Dual effects of hypertonicity on aquaporin-2 expression in cultured renal collecting duct principal cells. J Am Soc Nephrol. 16, 1571-82 (2005).

Distal Renal Tubular Acidosis and Calcium Nephrolithiasis

Orson W. Moe,[a,b,c] Daniel G. Fuster[a,b] and Xiao-Song Xie[d]

University of Texas Southwestern Medical Center, [a]Department of Internal Medicine, Division of Nephrology, [b]Department of Physiology, [c]Charles and Jane Pak Center of Mineral Metabolism and Clinical Research, [d]McDermot Center for Human Growth and Development, Dallas, TX, 75380, USA

Abstract. Calcium stones are commonly encountered in patients with congenital distal renal tubular acidosis, a disease of renal acidification caused by mutations in either the vacuolar H^+-ATPase (B1 or a4 subunit), anion exchanger-1, or carbonic anhydrase II. Based on the existing database, we present two hypotheses. First, heterozygotes with mutations in B1 subunit of H^+-ATPase are not normal but may harbor biochemical abnormalities such as renal acidification defects, hypercalciuria, and hypocitraturia which can predispose them to kidney stone formation. Second, we propose at least two mechanisms by which mutant B1 subunit can impair H^+-ATPase: defective pump assembly and defective pump activity.

Keywords: membrane transport; proton ATPase; anion exchanger; carbonic anhydrase
PACS: 87.14.ep; 87.19.xk

INTRODUCTION

It is well recognized and accepted that there is a hereditary component of nephrolithiasis and it is in the form of a complex polygenic trait [1,2]. While an *en face* tackle of this problem constitutes a formidable challenge, the study of monogenic causes of nephrolithiasis has been most informative in unraveling its genetic components [2-4]. Calcium stones are commonly encountered in patients with congenital distal renal tubular acidosis (dRTA) but dRTA is considered a rare cause of calcium stones due to the low prevalence of the disease [5-7]. Congenital dRTA is a disease of renal acidification caused by mutations in either the vacuolar (V) H^+-ATPase (B1 or a4 subunit), anion exchanger-1 (AE1), or carbonic anhydrase II (CAII) [5-7]. With the exception of a form of AE1 mutation associated with spherocytosis, all congenital dRTAs are generally believed to be autosomal recessive. Based on the existing database, we present two hypotheses. First, heterozygotes with mutations in B1 subunit of H^+-ATPase are not normal but may harbor biochemical abnormalities such as renal acidification defects, hypercalciuria, and hypocitraturia which can predispose them to kidney stone formation. Second, we propose at least two mechanisms by which mutant B1 subunit can impair H^+-ATPase: defective pump assembly and defective pump activity.

CP1049, *Renal Stone Disease 2, 2nd International Urolithiasis Research Symposium,*
edited by A. P. Evan, J. E. Lingeman, J. A. McAteer, and J. C. Williams, Jr.

KIDNEY STONES AND dRTA

The literature in kidney stones and dRTA can be approximately partitioned into camps. On one end, decades of well-designed and executed population and metabolic studies have attempted to define the frequency of dRTA in stone formers using subnormal urinary acidification as the criteria for RTA without genetic information. On the other end, elegant human genetic studies of kindreds with Mendelian dRTA have identified candidate genes that cause dRTA. Unfortunately, there is a paucity of cross fertilization between these two disciplines.

Wrong *et al.* first recognized that defective distal renal acidification can be associated with a normal plasma [HCO_3^-] [8] and set the precedent for using the acute acid loading test to uncover limited ability to lower their urinary pH (UpH)—a condition deemed to be a *forme fruste* of the RTA, termed incomplete dRTA. While most patients with calcium oxalate stones can maximally acidify their urine, 20-30% of patients with calcium phosphate stones have restricted ability to lower their UpH [9-12]. This is not limited to calcium phosphate stone formers. Impaired maximal acidification is also more common in recurrent stone formers and those with bilateral disease [12-20]. Decades of patient data have suggested that there is evidence for impaired renal acidification in the general stone-forming population without frank dRTA or obvious Mendelian inheritance. No genotypic data were presented in these studies so the genetic basis for these cases remains elusive.

Human genetic studies in well defined kindreds have led to the identification of several candidate genes for dRTA [5]. This will be presented below. Targeted gene deletion experiments in animals have revealed other candidates but no human equivalent disease states have yet been identified to date. What is somewhat surprising is that the two lines of investigation—metabolic studies and human genetics—never really synergize each other in a bidirectional fashion. In addition to metabolic studies and human genetics, there are sophisticated biochemical and cell biology studies of the V-ATPase using purified proteins and heterologous systems that have advanced the understanding of the structure and function of this protein further than many other ion transporters [21-24]. On the disappointing side is that one has not witnessed a lot of assimilation of this highly sophisticated discipline to human diseases of acidification.

Nephrocalcinosis and nephrolithiasis are common in dRTA [25,26]. The pathophysiology of calcium stone formation in dRTA is multifactorial. The major abnormalities are high UpH, hypocitraturia, and hypercalciuria stemming from the low plasma pH and [HCO_3^-] (Figure 1) [8, 27-32]. In the incomplete form where plasma [HCO_3^-] is normal, urinary abnormalities can still be present [33]. Low plasma pH and [HCO_3^-] alter the balance of bone formation and resorption resulting in increased mineral mobilization [34,35]. There is some evidence for increased intestinal Ca^{2+} absorption in dRTA with alkali therapy but the mechanism is unknown [36]. In addition to increased Ca^{2+} released from bone, acidosis directly inhibits renal Ca^{2+} reabsorption leading to hypercalciuria [37,38]. Defective urinary acidification elevates UpH and escalates the risk for Ca^{2+} phosphate precipitation. The marked hypocitraturia from the systemic acidosis further aggravates precipitation of all Ca^{2+} salts (both phosphate and calcium oxalate) [39,40]. Some degree of hyperphosphaturia occurs due to increased bone release or from the acidosis *per se* [34].

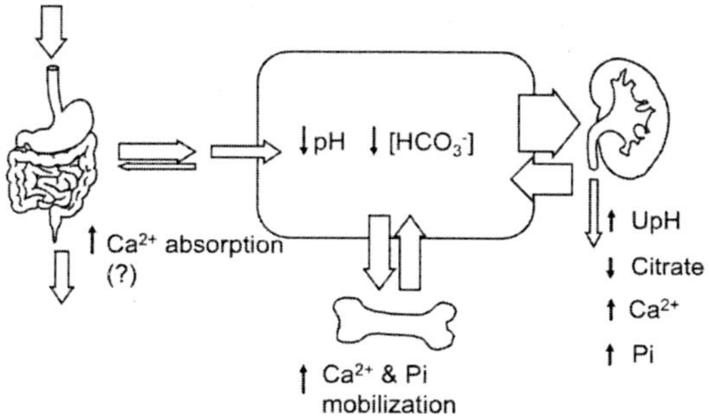

FIGURE 1. Pathophysiology of calcium stone predisposition in distal renal tubular acidosis. The primary abnormalities are believed to be low extracellular pH and bicarbonate concentration leading to a series of secondary effects on bone, kidney and possibly gut. The final urinary chemical abnormalities are hypocitraturia, alkaline urine, and hypercalciuria. Hyperphosphaturia may occur to some extent.

GENETICS AND MOLECULAR PHYSIOLOGY OF CONGENITAL dRTA

Congenital dRTA in humans can result from inactivating mutations of one of three genes which encode the three critical proteins for H+ extrusion into the urinary lumen in the distal nephron (Figure 2): the apical membrane V-ATPase, the basolateral anion exchanger-1, and carbonic anhydrase II, which catalyzes the segregation of intracellular H+ from HCO_3^- to furnish substrate for the two transporters [41,42]. Mutations of all three of these proteins have been associated with dRTA [5]. Table 1 summarizes the current known genetic mutations associated with congenital dRTA in humans. These candidate loci were identified in a series of seminal papers by applying classical human genetic techniques on kindreds derived from probands identified by clinicians. Phenotypic definition of these subjects is limited to clinical data and the biochemical diagnosis of RTA is based on non-anion gap hypobicarbonatemia and unduly alkaline urine pH. More detailed characterization of stone risk and analysis of the phenotype of heterozygotes are generally not available.

Table 2 lists the known mutations of ATP6V1B1 associated with congenital dRTA [43-48] which encompasses missense, nonsense, frameshift, and splice site mutations. We discovered a novel frame-shift mutation in our functional analysis of the B1 subunit (F468fsX487), and found a previously described polymorphic allele (E161K) to be actually an inactivating mutation [46].

The mechanisms by which mutant V-ATPase, AE1 or CAII cause dRTA is not entirely clear. Some progress has been made for each of these three proteins. A brief summary is presented.

Anion Exchanger 1. This anion exchanger is critical for basolateral base exit from the α-intercalated cell and its dysfunction will clearly disrupt distal acidification. AE1 is also known as Band 3 in the erythrocyte membrane, where in addition to its Cl^- /HCO_3^- exchange function also provides a membrane anchor for the cytoskeleton. Mutations of AE1 cause dRTA as well as a variety of erythrocyte disorders [49-55]. Impaired trafficking to the cell membrane is a well-documented mechanism of impaired distal acidification and the genetically dominant effect has been explained by mutant protein undergoing apical membrane mistargeting or non-polarized targeting to both membranes, in essence creating a cell that secretes base to the lumen [45, 56-60]. The limited renal involvement with red cell sparing in some forms of dRTA (mutant G701D AE1) is explained by rescue of the targeting defect by the chaperone protein glycophorin A in erythrocytes but no such rescue is possible in renal epithelia, which do not express glycophorin A [61, 62].

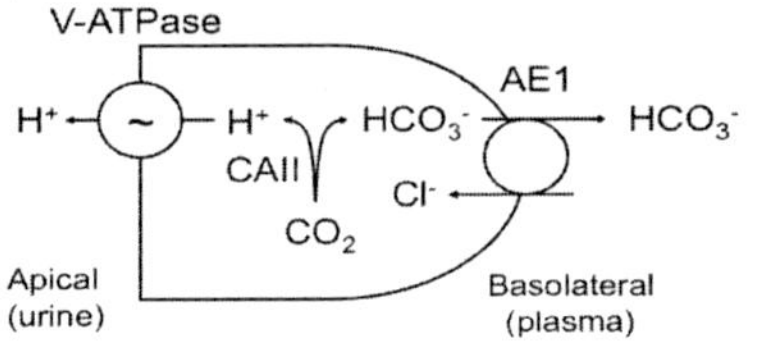

FIGURE 2. Acid-secreting intercalated cell in the distal nephron. V-ATPase: Vacuolar H^+-ATPase; AE1: Anion exchanger-1; CAII: Carbonic anhydrase II.

TABLE 1. Congenital forms of distal renal tubular acidosis

Protein	Gene	OMIM	Inheritance	Additional Features
Humans				
AE1 (Anion exchanger 1)	*SLC4A1*	602722	Recessive	Hemolytic anemia, SE Asians
AE1 (Anion exchanger 1)	*SLC4A1*	179800	Dominant	Erythrocytosis; older age presentation
B1 (Subunit of V-ATPase)	*ATP6V1B1*	267300	Recessive	Hearing loss
a4 (Subunit of V-ATPase)	*ATP6V0A4*	602722	Recessive	Later onset milder hearing loss
CAII (carbonic anhydrase)	*CA2*	259730	Recessive	Osteopetrosis; CNS disease; Proximal RTA

Protein	Finding	Possible explanation
Animals		
B1 deletion	Normal baseline plasma values but inability to maximally acidifiy urine	Possible redundancy from other acidification mechanisms
*ClC-5 channel	proximal tubule V-ATPase mistargeting	Possible targeting defect in proximal tubule
*KCl cotransporter	dRTA	Possible impaired basolateral Cl^- recycling

*In some animal models of targeted gene deletion, unexpected findings emerged There is no evidence to date to suggest equivalent human mutations exist in these loci that are associated with dRTA.

Carbonic Anhydrase II. Inactivating mutations of CAII will place H^+-secreting cells at a kinetic disadvantage by reducing available H^+ substrate from CO_2 and is expected to cause dRTA. In addition, CAII function is also vital in the proximal tubule, in osteoclasts and in the brain. Hence the phenotype of this disorder includes proximal RTA, osteopetrosis, conductive deafness, and cerebral calcification [63-65].

V-ATPase. Inactivating mutations of two subunits B1 and a4 have been associated with congenital autosomal recessive dRTA with sensorineural hearing loss [44,45,47, 66,67]. The mechanism of dysregulated acidification was unclear until a recent important paper from the Schwartz lab [68]. Yang and coworkers first demonstrated disrupted V-ATPase assembly as the mechanism for seven known ATP6V1B1 missense mutations using mammalian cells [68]. Based on the fact that overexpressed mutant B1 subunits can lower Na^+-independent cell pH recovery after acid load in a rat IMCD cell line, these investigators proposed a dominant-negative mechanism of the transfected mutant B1 subunits over the native wild-type B1 subunit. In contrast, we have not been able to show dominant negative effect of several mutant B1 subunits over wild type (see below). A handful of recessive families with dRTA do not link to either ATP6V1B1 or ATP6V0A4 [66] suggesting potential additional loci and mechanisms for congenital dRTA.

TABLE 2. Human mutations of *ATP6V1B1*

Mutation type	Nucleotide Change	Amino Acid Change
	c.232G>A	G78R
	c.242T>C	L81P
	c.368G>T	G123V
	c.370C>T	R124W
	c.469C>T	R157C
	c.481G>A	E161K
Missense	c.521T>G	M174R
	c.823A>C	T275P
	c.947G>A	G316E
	c.988G>A	E330K
	c.1037C>G	P346R
	c.1090G>A	G364S
	c.1181G>A	R394Q
	c.1449G>A	R465H
Nonsense	c.91C>T	R31X
	c.497delC	T166fsX174
Frameshift	c.1155-1156delC	I386fsX395
	c.1155-1156insC	I386fsX441
	c.1401-1402dupGT	F468fsX487
	Intron 2: gt>ct	*splicing defect*
	Intron 6: gt>at	*splicing defect*
Splice-site	Intron 7: gt>tt	*splicing defect*
	Intron 8: gt>at	*splicing defect*
	Intron 9: ag>tg	*splicing defect*

V-ATPASE BIOLOGY

V-ATPases belong to a family of ATP-driven H^+-translocating ion pumps. The ubiquitous function of V-pumps within cells is to acidify intracellular organelles, which is essential for receptor-mediated endocytosis, lysosomal hydrolase activities, intracellular protein targeting, processing of hormones, and uptake and storage of neurotransmitters [69-75]. In cells with certain specialized functions, V-pumps are localized in the plasma membrane and are instrumental in the regulation of intracellular pH, acid secretion, bone resorption, synaptic transmission, endolymph pH regulation of the inner ear, and whole organism acid-base homeostasis by participating in renal acid excretion [44,76].

V-ATPases are complex proteins containing at least 13 different subunits and are organized into two distinct functional domains—a peripheral catalytic sector 560 kDa V_1 $(A_3B_3C_1D_1E_1F_1G_2H_1)$ and a membranous 260 kDa proteolipid V_0 $(a_1d_1c''_1[c',c]_6)$ —similar to the F_1F_0 complex of bacterial and mitochondrial ATP synthases. The left panel of Figure 3 is a cartoon of this enzyme. The right panel shows a recent 3-D reconstruction of the V-ATPase using cryo-electron microscopy and single particle analysis [77]. In mammals, there are two different B subunits in the V_1 domain, of which the B2 subunit is ubiquitous whereas the B1 subunit is restricted to epithelia of the inner ear, epididymis and the distal renal tubule [78-81]. As discussed above, mutations in the B1 subunit gene *ATP6V1B1* are responsible for autosomal-recessive dRTA with deafness [44,45]. The molecular mechanisms by which some B1 subunit mutations lead to V-ATPase dysfunction were unknown until recently [46,68].

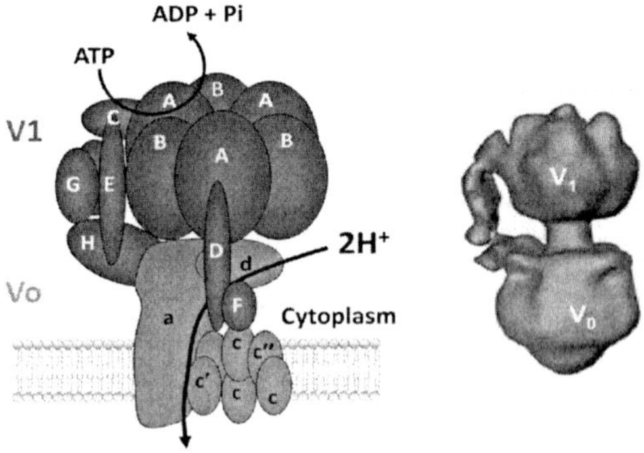

FIGURE 3. Structural model of the V-ATPase. The left panel shows the V_1 domain in red and V_0 domain in green. Individual subunits are indicated by their letters. The right panel shows a three dimensional reconstruction of the holoenzyme based on cryo-electron microscopy.

In the kidney, in addition to intracellular vesicular acidification, V-ATPase is responsible for luminal acidification and HCO_3^- absorption [6,24,82]. It is expressed in the proximal tubule at the base of the microvilli on the apical membrane; in the collecting duct, it is on the apical membrane of the α-intercalated acid-secreting cells and on the basolateral membrane of the β-intercalated base-secreting cells [83]. Some subunits have restricted tissue distribution: B1 (kidney, eye, inner ear), a4 (kidney), C2 (kidney, lung, placenta), G3 (kidney), d2 (kidney, osteoclasts, dendritic cells). Renal V-ATPase is regulated by a variety of physiologic stimuli including acid-base status and the renin-angiotensin system [6,24,82].

V-ATPases are regulated at various levels including transcription, translation, direct modulation of enzymatic activity by activators, and by a reversible sulfhydryl-disulfide bond inter-conversion [84]. Pump activity is also indirectly controlled through the activity of a parallel chloride channel [85,86]. But a regulatory mechanism that is unique to V-ATPases is the reversible dissociation and association of V_1 and V_0 in response to energy demand; this mechanism has been well studied in yeast and in tobacco hornworm. In yeast, a heterotrimeric complex called RAVE (**R**egulator of the **A**TPase of **V**acuolar and **E**ndosomal membranes) has been shown to associate with the V_1 domain and to promote glucose-triggered assembly of V-ATPase [87]. In mammals, interaction between V-ATPase and the glycolytic enzyme aldolase has been observed in osteoclasts and kidney cells, implying coupling between glucose metabolism and pump activity similar to that described in yeast [88].

Recently, there is evidence that direct physical interactions between aldolase and the B, H and a subunits of V-ATPase are essential for the assembly and activity of the pump [89]. Therefore in addition to the notion that the V-ATPase may "serve glycolysis" by pumping out the generated H^+, this raises the converse notion that glycolytic enzymes such as aldolase may "serve the pump" by facilitating its assembly. The synergistic role of aldolase and V-ATPase, however, is blurred by the observation that the enzymatic activity of aldolase is not essential for the activation of V-ATPase but the ability of aldolase to bind to B subunit is (Xie, personal communication). The current model is thus incomplete.

Mere physical association between V_1 and V_0 is not sufficient for function of V-pumps, which in addition has an unequivocal requirement for subunit H. Subunit H is a key regulatory element of V-ATPase that is not required for the assembly of V_1V_0 but is absolutely essential for the function of V-type H^+ pumps as shown both *in vivo* and *in vitro* [86,90]. It remains to be determined how subunit H regulates the functional coupling of V-ATPases, and it is equally unclear what role other subunits, subunit B1 or its disease-causing mutants for example, may play in this process.

MECHANISM OF V-ATPASE DYSFUNCTION ASSOCIATED WITH B1 MUTATIONS IN AUTOSOMAL-RECESSIVE dRTA

We studied a novel frameshift mutation in *ATP6V1B1* (exon 14 GT insertion at nt. 1402) in a Mexican kindred [91]. In contrast to all the reported *ATP6V1B1* mutations, this novel mutation results in insertion of 19 amino acids near the C-terminus of B1 followed by a stop codon (F468fsX487). Figure 4 compares this mutant (M), wild type B1, B2, and the yeast ortholog Vma2p.

We examined V_1 domain assembly as a potential basis of pump dysfunction. We expressed epitope-tagged human wild-type and disease-associated F468fsX487 (mutant) B1 subunits in distal tubule-derived MDCK cells. Wild-type, but not mutant (M) B1 subunits, co-immunoprecipitated with the endogenous V_1 domain E subunit in MDCK cells, demonstrating assembly of the wild-type but not the mutant B1 subunit into the V_1 domain (Figure 4). Identical results were obtained when the constructs

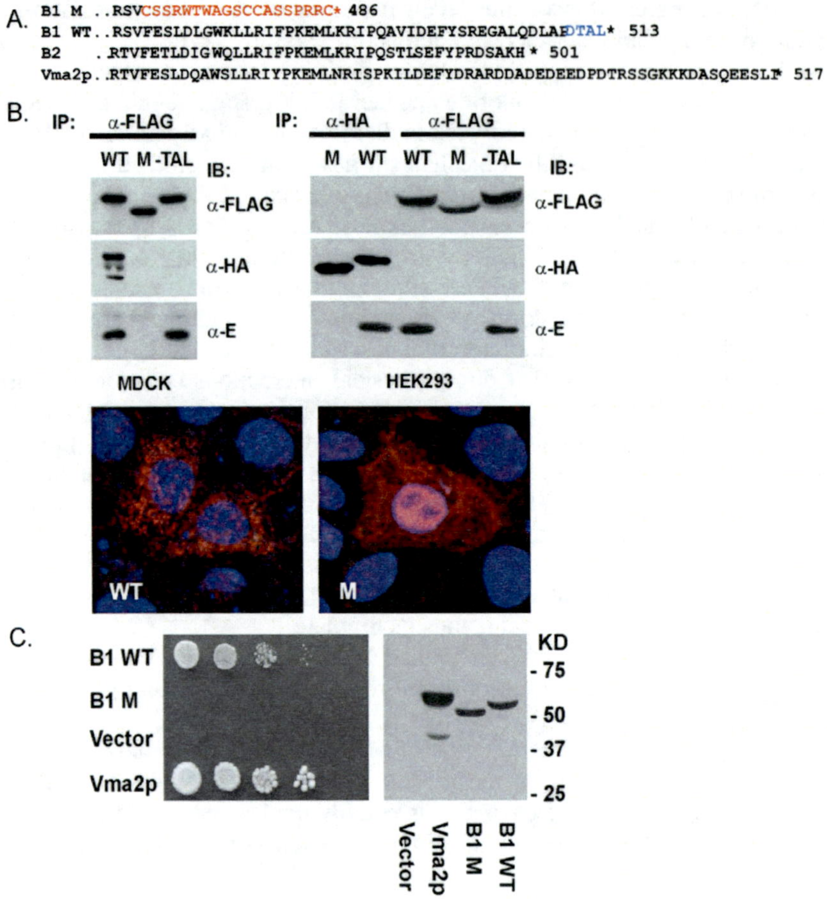

FIGURE 4. Characterization of mutant B1 subunit. **(A)** Frameshift-truncation mutation in ATP6V1B1 (exon 14 GT insertion at nt. 1402) of B1 subunit. M= mutant. For comparison: Human wild type B1 (WT), human wild type B2 (B2), yeast ortholog (Vma2p). **(B)** Epitope-tagged human wild-type and disease-associated F468fsX487 (mutant) B1 subunits were expressed in MDCK or HEK293 cells. Wild-type, but not mutant (M) B1 subunits, co-immunoprecipitated with the endogenous V_1 domain E subunit in MDCK cells, demonstrating assembly of the wild-type but not the mutant B1 subunit into the V_1 domain. Identical results were obtained in HEK293 or when the tag was relocated (N-terminal FLAG vs. C-terminal HA). A PDZ-binding motif at the C-terminus of the B1 subunit binds to NHERF-1. Truncation of the PDZ-binding motif (-TAL) abolished interaction with NHERF-1 but integration into V1 remains intact. We next analyzed the intracellular localization of wild-type or mutant B1 subunits by immunocytochemistry in MDCK cells overexpressing wild-type or mutant B1 subunits with laser confocal microscopy. WT B1 subunit had a characteristic intracellular vesicular pattern, suggesting incorporation into the V-ATPase. In contrast, the mutant B1 subunit (M) had a diffuse cytoplasmic and nuclear staining. **(C)** Yeast complementation assay. HA-tagged human B1 wild type (WT), F468fsX487 (M),Yeast B1 ortholog Vma2p were transformed in to Vma2p null strain. Presence of yeast colonies indicates intact pump function. Left panel shows dilution series of growth at non-permissive pH 7.5. Right panel is immunoblot of yeast lysate with anti-HA showing equivalent expression of recombinant proteins. Figure reproduced by permission from *Kidney International*, ref 46.

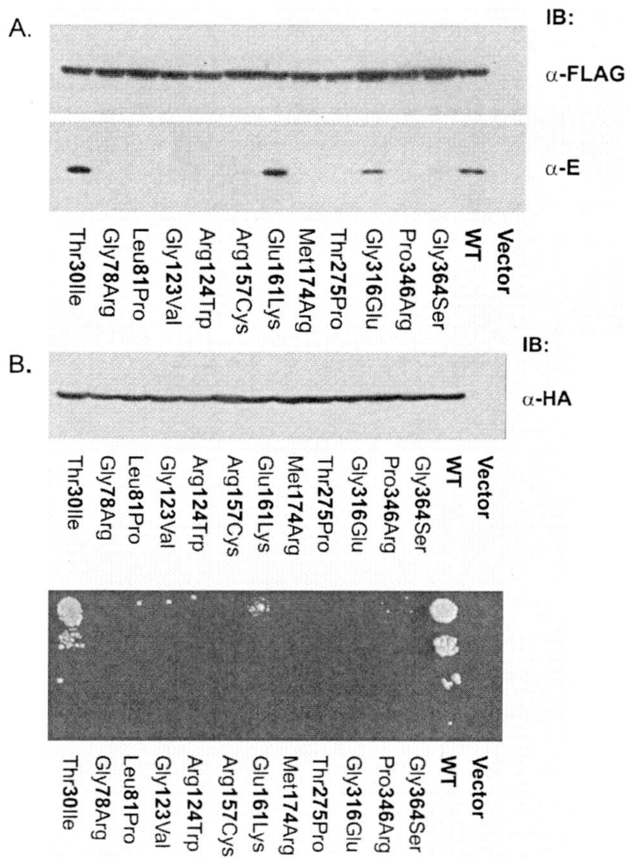

FIGURE 5. WT and point B1 mutants transfected into MDCK cells (A; FLAG-B1; top panel) and Vma2p null yeast (B; HA-B1; bottom 2 panels). **(A)** Assembly assay by co-immuniprecipitation. Human wild type and different mutant B1 subunits were FLAG-tagged and co-expressed and intact assembly is indicated by the ability to co-precipitate native E subunit. **(B)** Top panel shows equivalence of expression. Bottom panel shows H^+-pump function which manifests as complementation of null yeast resulting in colony growth. Figure reproduced by permission from *Kidney International*, ref 46.

were expressed in a different host (HEK293) or when the tag was relocated (N-terminal FLAG vs. C-terminal HA) (Figure 4). With the exception of a PDZ-binding motif at the C-terminus of the B1 subunit which binds to the adaptor protein NHERF-1, little is known about the function of the last ~30 amino acids of B subunits [92,93]. Since the mutation abolishes the PDZ-binding motif in B1, we tested if deletion of this domain accounts for defective assembly possibly via disruption of PDZ interaction. Truncation of the PDZ-binding motif (-TAL) abolished interaction with NHERF-1 but integration into V_1 remains intact (Figure 4). Truncation of the PDZ domain is insufficient to disrupt V_1 assembly. Under laser confocal microscopy, the WT B1 subunit had a characteristic intracellular vesicular pattern, suggesting incorporation into the V-ATPase; compatible with our biochemical findings. In contrast, the mutant B1 subunit (M) had a diffuse cytoplasmic and nuclear staining.

Because of the universal presence of V-ATPase B subunits in mammalian cells, we employed a Saccharomyces cerevisiae strain devoid of the endogenous yeast B subunit (Vma2p) for functional assessment of wild-type and mutant human B1 subunits. The Vma2p null strain is able to grow at acidic pH (5.5) but fails to grow at neutral or alkaline pH. Growth at 7.5 can be rescued by expression of Vma2p [92-94]. Figure 4 shows transformed yeast (dilution series pH 7.5 YEPD) [95]. Expression of constructs was driven by the high-copy p426TEF vector [96]. Complementation of the deleted endogenous yeast Vma2p subunit (growth at pH 7.5) was observed in yeast expressing WT-B1 or Vma2p but not in mutant human B1 subunits expressed at the same level. No dominant-negative effect was observed when wild-type and mutant B1 subunits were co-expressed (data not shown).

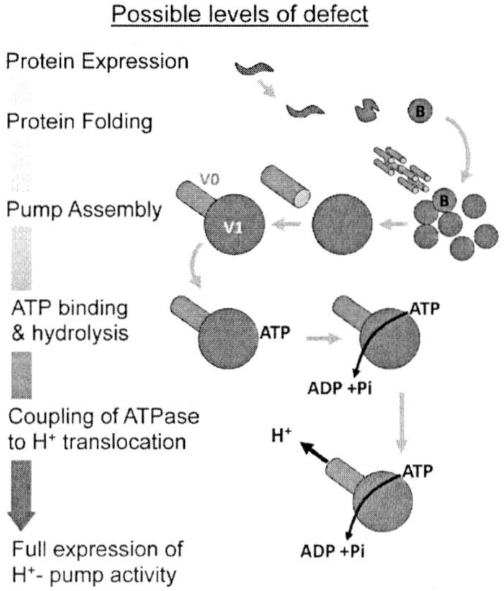

FIGURE 6. Theoretical consideration of the possible mechanisms of disrupting H^+-pumping in the V-ATPase. The final common pathway is defective H^+ pumping although the primary defect can occur at highly varied levels

We next screened 12 naturally occurring point B1 mutants using the mammalian cell assay of V_1 assembly by co-immunoprecipitation and the yeast assay of functional H^+ pumping (bottom two panels Figure 5). Expression in yeast was confirmed by immunoblot of yeast lysate (Figure 5). Three distinct patterns emerged from this screen: **1**. Intact assembly and intact H^+ pump. Therefore T30I is a true polymorphism. **2**. Intact assembly but defective H^+ pumping. These will be E161K and G316E. **3**. Defective pump assembly and defective H^+ pump which represents the rest of the point mutants screened. We found lack of V_1 assembly of F468fsX487 B1 subunit mutation as the molecular mechanism of V-ATPase dysfunction. Furthermore, we demonstrate the importance of the B1 subunit C-terminus in V-ATPase assembly. V-ATPase is a complex multisubunit protein and hence the possible means of disrupting its function will be protean. Figure 6 summarizes the possible lesions one can place on this hierarchy that can all potentially converge onto the final outcome of impaired H^+ pumping.

A HYPOTHESIS: B1 DYSFUNCTION IN THE GENERAL CALCIUM STONE FORMING POPULATION

One of premises on which we based our conjecture is that the E161K allele is rather common in the general population. The lack of overt clinical dRTA misled previous investigators into believing that EK heterozygotes are normal individuals. We have shown in the yeast complementation assay that this particular amino acid substitution, although not disruptive to V-ATPase assembly, clearly impaired pump function. There are a number remaining questions. Do these individuals have a sub-clinical predisposition to forming stones and if they do, what percentage of them actually have kidney stones? Finally, can B1 subunit alleles be one of the many genes whose polymorphism contributes to the complex polygenic trait of calcium nephrolithiasis?

It is an enigma why the high prevalence of calcium phosphate stones described in patients with classical dRTA [10] was not seen with high frequency in the B1 heterozygous mutants studied to date. Based on the preliminary data, disturbances in urinary chemistry is highly variable from one heterozygous individual to another. Figure 7 is a theoretical consideration and a proposed explanation. Three main pathophysiologic factors are expressed heterogeneously in different patients. If the defect involves primarily high UpH (which is frequently the case with complete dRTA), the stones will be mostly calcium phosphate. If the defect is mostly hypercalciuria or hypocitraturia, calcium oxalate stones may be encountered more frequently.

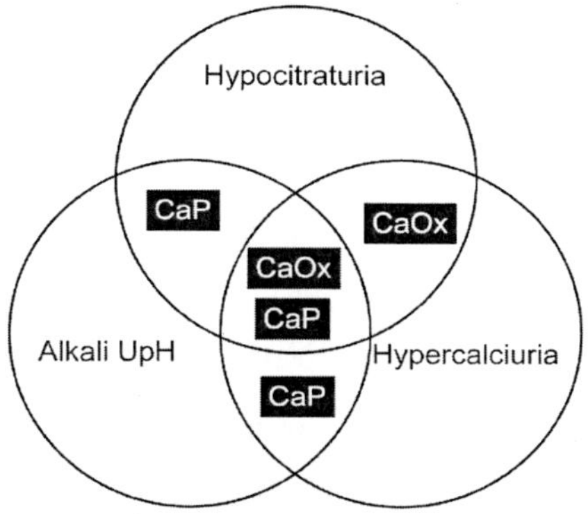

FIGURE 7. Theoretical spectrum of pathophysiologic abnormalities in heterozygous inactivating mutations of B1.

Patients with heterozygous mutations of V-ATPase subunits are clearly very unlikely to present themselves in a doctor's office with complaints. If they gather attention, they may present themselves as a garden variety calcium stone former which will not alert the practitioner to pursue genetic causes. What then should be our tools to probe? To fully understand how abnormalities in urine chemistry increase kidney stone risk, we have to expand beyond the usual computer-based programs such as EQUIL2 and undertake physicochemical exploration. High UpH and hypocitraturia, commonly encountered in dRTA, are believed to be important in calcium phosphate stone formation. High urinary pH may increase the propensity for calcium phosphate crystallization by enhancing phosphate dissociation and saturation of brushite. Hypocitraturia further exaggerates the crystallization, since citrate is believed to be an inhibitor of calcium phosphate crystal growth [39].

We conducted preliminary studies where crystal growth (CG) of brushite was measured *in vitro*, with or without added citrate at various pH's [97]. In a fresh whole urine sample from normal subjects, urinary pH was adjusted to 5.65, 6.0, 6.35, and 6.7. In an alternate set of urine samples at the same pH's, 2.8 mEq $citrate^{3-}$ (citric acid) was added per L of urine which corresponded to the expected increase in urinary citrate during potassium citrate therapy (60 mEq/day) assuming urine volume of 1.5 L/day [98].

Urinary saturation of brushite was obtained by a semi-empirical method (CPR; concentration product ratio), by calculating dissolution or growth of excess solid phase added to urine [99]. CPR increased progressively as the pH rose. At corresponding pH's, CPR was lower when citrate was added. Crystal growth (CG) of brushite was determined after seeding of urine with 0.25 mg brushite per ml. Without added citrate, CG of brushite increased curvi-linearly as the pH rose. When citrate was added, the relationship was still curvi-linear but shifted lower at higher pH's. This study shows that high UpH increases both urinary saturation and crystal growth of brushite. Added citrate attenuates these effects. Thus, hypocitraturia is expected to exaggerate the propensity for calcium phosphate crystallization at high pH. Citrate's attenuation of pH-dependent increase in saturation and crystal growth of brushite is probably due to ion pair formation.

Table 3. Physicochemical properties of brushite in dilute fasting urine samples (0.25 mg seed per ml) in four non-stone-formers with two different genotypes at aa161.

EE Wild type EK heterozygote	pH	[Ca] mg/L	Concentration Product Ratio	Crystal Growth or Dissolution mg Ca + P
Heterozygote #1	6.86	45	0.43	-6
Heterozygote #2	6.63	47	0.86	+5
Wild type #1	6.79	16	0.03	-62
Wild type #2	5.96	26	0.13	-43

In another study, we examined 2-h fasting urine from two heterozygous (E161K) non-stone formers and two non-stone formers with wild type B1 after generous hydration (Table 3). We determined CPR (saturation) and CG or crystal dissolution (CD) of brushite. Heterozygotes had higher fasting urinary calcium and tendency toward higher pH (Table 3). All 4 samples were under-saturated with respect to brushite (CPR<1); but much more so in the wild type. One heterozygote showed slight brushite crystal dissolution (CD; negative value) while the other displayed a slight growth (CG; positive value). In contrast, wild type subjects showed substantial CD. This preliminary study shows that in subjects with liberal water consumption, fasting urine samples may normally be undersaturated with brushite, and incapable of supporting crystal growth. However, in heterozygotes, fasting urines are only marginally undersaturated and are more susceptible to crystal growth. These differences are expected to be exaggerated without high fluid intake.

SUMMARY OF POTENTIAL IMPACT ON THE FIELDS OF NEPHROLITHIASIS AND V-ATPASE BIOLOGY

It is quite conceivable that we can use the B1 subunit as a portal of entry to examine how allelic variants in individual genes, even in its heterozygous state can confer risk in calcium stones. Although the hereditary basis of nephrolithiasis is complex polygenic, the inheritance of a given candidate gene is still Mendelian. These studies provide the foundation for us to test the hypothesis that monogenic predisposition of nephrolithiasis is actually not rare in the general stone-forming population. Stone formers may harbor mutations in B1 that predispose them to kidney stones. Since the allelic variants confer predisposition rather than disease, there may not be easily recognizable Mendelian inheritance patterns and the pathophysiology may not be uniform as in dRTA. This is especially true if the genetic variants of B1 cause only mild V-ATPase dysfunction due to partial protein malfunction, partial haploinsufficiency, or both. If we set this precedence, other monogenic predisposition may begin to emerge. From the cell biology and biochemistry point of view, these studies will significantly advance the understanding of V-ATPase function by defining the mechanisms of V-ATPase dysfunction due to specific mutations of B1. These data will provide valuable structure-function information on the biology of V-ATPase.

ACKNOWLEDGEMENTS

The authors were supported by National Institutes of Health Grants DK-48482 and DK-20543, a stipend from the Swiss National Science Foundation, and a Fellowship from the Charles and Jane Pak Center of Mineral Metabolism and Clinical Research. The authors are grateful to the assistance of Ms Vicki Perkins in the preparation of the manuscript.

REFERENCES

1. Coe FL, Evan A, Worcester E. Kidney stone disease. J Clin Invest 2005;115(10):2598-608.
2. Moe OW, Bonny O. Genetic hypercalciuria. J Am Soc Nephrol 2005;16(3):729-45.
3. Gambaro G, Vezzoli G, Casari G, Rampoldi L, D'Angelo A, Borghi L. Genetics of hypercalciuria and calcium nephrolithiasis: from the rare monogenic to the common polygenic forms. Am J Kidney Dis 2004;44(6):963-86.
4. Langman CB. The molecular basis of kidney stones. Curr Opin Pediatr 2004;16(2):188-93.
5. Fry AC, Karet FE. Inherited renal acidoses. Physiology (Bethesda) 2007;22:202-11.
6. Karet FE. Physiological and metabolic implications of V-ATPase isoforms in the kidney. J Bioenerg Biomembr 2005;37(6):425-9.
7. Laing CM, Unwin RJ. Renal tubular acidosis. J Nephrol 2006;19 Suppl 9:S46-52.
8. Dedmon RE, Wrong O. The excretion of organic anion in renal tubular acidosis with particular reference to citrate. Clin Sci 1962;22:19-32.

9. Gault MH, Chafe LL, Morgan JM, et al. Comparison of patients with idiopathic calcium phosphate and calcium oxalate stones. Medicine (Baltimore) 1991;70(6):345-59.
10. Pak CY, Poindexter JR, Adams-Huet B, Pearle MS. Predictive value of kidney stone composition in the detection of metabolic abnormalities. Am J Med 2003;115(1):26-32.
11. Pak CY, Poindexter JR, Peterson RD, Heller HJ. Biochemical and physicochemical presentations of patients with brushite stones. J Urol 2004;171(3):1046-9.
12. Backman U, Danielson BG, Johansson G, Ljunghall S, Wikstrom B. Incidence and clinical importance of renal tubular defects in recurrent renal stone formers. Nephron 1980;25(2):96-101.
13. Cintron-Nadal E, Lespier LE, Roman-Miranda A, Martinez-Maldonado M. Renal acidifying ability in subjects with recurrent stone formation. J Urol 1977;118(5):704-6.
14. D'Angelo A, Pagano F, Ossi E, et al. Renal tubular defects in recurring bilateral nephrolithiasis. Clin Nephrol 1976;6(2):352-60.
15. Konnak JW, Kogan BA, Lau K. Renal calculi associated with incomplete distal renal tubular acidosis. J Urol 1982;128(5):900-2.
16. Osther PJ, Hansen AB, Rohl HF. Renal acidification defects in patients with their first renal stone episode. Scand J Urol Nephrol Suppl 1988;110:275-8.
17. Osther PJ, Hansen AB, Rohl HF. Screening renal stone formers for distal renal tubular acidosis. Br J Urol 1989;63(6):581-3.
18. Singh PP, Pendse AK, Ahmed A, Ramavataram DV, Rajpurohit SK. A study of recurrent stone formers with special reference to renal tubular acidosis. Urol Res 1995;23(3):201-3.
19. Szendröi Z, Simon K, Kiss L. Renal tubular acidosis: its types and role in renal calculosis. Int Urol Nephrol 1982;14(3):247-57.
20. Tessitore N, Ortalda V, Fabris A, et al. Renal acidification defects in patients with recurrent calcium nephrolithiasis. Nephron 1985;41(4):325-32.
21. Drory O, Nelson N. The emerging structure of vacuolar ATPases. Physiology 2006;21:317-25.
22. Inoue T, Wang Y, Jefferies K, Qi J, Hinton A, Forgac M. Structure and regulation of the V-ATPases. J Bioenerg Biomembr 2005;37(6):393-8.
23. Kane PM. Close-up and genomic views of the yeast vacuolar H+-ATPase. J Bioenerg Biomembr 2005;37(6):399-403.
24. Breton S, Brown D. New insights into the regulation of V-ATPase-dependent proton secretion. Am J Physiol Renal Physiol 2007;292(1):F1-10.
25. Courey WR, Pfister RC. The radiographic findings in renal tubular acidosis: analysis of 21 cases. Radiology 1972;105(3):497-503.
26. Van den Berg CJ, Harrington TM, Bunch TW, Pierides AM. Treatment of renal lithiasis associated with renal tubular acidosis. Proc Eur Dial Transplant Assoc 1983;20:473-6.
27. Batlle DC, Sehy JT, Roseman MK, Arruda JA, Kurtzman NA. Clinical and pathophysiologic spectrum of acquired distal renal tubular acidosis. Kidney Int 1981;20(3):389-96.
28. Brenner RJ, Spring DB, Sebastian A, et al. Incidence of radiographically evident bone disease, nephrocalcinosis, and nephrolithiasis in various types of renal tubular acidosis. N Engl J Med 1982;307(4):217-21.
29. Buckalew VM, Jr., Purvis ML, Shulman MG, Herndon CN, Rudman D. Hereditary renal tubular acidosis. Report of a 64 member kindred with variable clinical expression including idiopathic hypercalciuria. Medicine (Baltimore) 1974;53(4):229-54.
30. Caruana RJ, Buckalew VM, Jr. The syndrome of distal (type 1) renal tubular acidosis. Clinical and laboratory findings in 58 cases. Medicine 1988;67(2):84-99.
31. Coe FL, Parks JH. Stone disease in hereditary distal renal tubular acidosis. Ann Intern Med 1980;93(1):60-1.
32. Lee DB, Drinkard JP, Gonick HC, Coulson WF, Cracchiolo A. Pathogenesis of renal calculi in distal renal tubular acidosis. Possible role of parathyroid hormone. Clin Orthop Relat Res 1976;121:234-42.
33. Osther PJ, Bollerslev J, Hansen AB, Engel K, Kildeberg P. Pathophysiology of incomplete renal tubular acidosis in recurrent renal stone formers: evidence of disturbed calcium, bone and citrate metabolism. Urol Res 1993;21(3):169-73.
34. Krieger NS, Frick KK, Bushinsky DA. Mechanism of acid-induced bone resorption. Curr Opin Nephrol Hypertens 2004;13(4):423-36.
35. Lemann J, Jr., Bushinsky DA, Hamm LL. Bone buffering of acid and base in humans. Am J Physiol Renal Physiol 2003;285(5):F811-32.
36. Preminger GM, Sakhaee K, Pak CY. Hypercalciuria and altered intestinal calcium absorption occurring independently of vitamin D in incomplete distal renal tubular acidosis. Metabolism 1987;36(2):176-9.
37. Moe OW, Huang CL. Hypercalciuria from acid load: renal mechanisms. J Nephrol 2006;19(9):S53-61.

38. Sutton RA, Wong NL, Dirks JH. Effects of metabolic acidosis and alkalosis on sodium and calcium transport in the dog kidney. Kidney Int 1979;15(5):520-33.
39. Moe SM, O'Neill KD, Fineberg N, et al. Assessment of vascular calcification in ESRD patients using spiral CT. Nephrol Dial Transplant 2003;18(6):1152-8.
40. Moe OW, Preisig PA. Dual role of citrate in mammalian urine. Curr Opin Nephrol Hypertens 2006;15(4):419-24.
41. Geibel JP. Distal tubule acidification. J Nephrol 2006;19(9):S18-26.
42. Schwartz GJ. Physiology and molecular biology of renal carbonic anhydrase. J Nephrol 2002;15(5):S61-74.
43. Borthwick KJ, Kandemir N, Topaloglu R, et al. A phenocopy of CAII deficiency: a novel genetic explanation for inherited infantile osteopetrosis with distal renal tubular acidosis. J Med Genet 2003;40(2):115-21.
44. Karet FE, Finberg KE, Nelson RD, et al. Mutations in the gene encoding B1 subunit of H+-ATPase cause renal tubular acidosis with sensorineural deafness. Nat Genet 1999;21(1):84-90.
45. Stover EH, Borthwick KJ, Bavalia C, et al. Novel ATP6V1B1 and ATP6V0A4 mutations in autosomal recessive distal renal tubular acidosis with new evidence for hearing loss. J Med Genet 2002;39(11):796-803.
46. Fuster DG, Zhang J, Xie XS, Moe OW. The vacuolar-ATPase B1 subunit in distal tubular acidosis: novel mutations and mechanisms for dysfunction. Kidney Int 2008;73(10):1151-1158.
47. Vargas-Poussou R, Houillier P, Le Pottier N, et al. Genetic investigation of autosomal recessive distal renal tubular acidosis: evidence for early sensorineural hearing loss associated with mutations in the ATP6V0A4 gene. J Am Soc Nephrol 2006;17(5):1437-43.
48. Ruf R, Rensing C, Topaloglu R, et al. Confirmation of the ATP6B1 gene as responsible for distal renal tubular acidosis. Pediatr Nephrol 2003;18(2):105-9.
49. Bruce LJ, Cope DL, Jones GK, et al. Familial distal renal tubular acidosis is associated with mutations in the red cell anion exchanger (Band 3, AE1) gene. J Clin Invest 1997;100(7):1693-707.
50. Bruce LJ, Wrong O, Toye AM, et al. Band 3 mutations, renal tubular acidosis and South-East Asian ovalocytosis in Malaysia and Papua New Guinea: loss of up to 95% band 3 transport in red cells. Biochem J 2000;1:41-51.
51. Cheidde L, Vieira TC, Lima PR, Saad ST, Heilberg IP. A novel mutation in the anion exchanger 1 gene is associated with familial distal renal tubular acidosis and nephrocalcinosis. Pediatrics 2003;112(6 Pt 1):1361-7.
52. Jarolim P, Shayakul C, Prabakaran D, et al. Autosomal dominant distal renal tubular acidosis is associated in three families with heterozygosity for the R589H mutation in the AE1 (band 3) Cl^- /HCO_3^- exchanger. J Biol Chem 1998;273(11):6380-8.
53. Karet FE, Gainza FJ, Gyory AZ, et al. Mutations in the chloride-bicarbonate exchanger gene AE1 cause autosomal dominant but not autosomal recessive distal renal tubular acidosis. Proc Natl Acad Sci U S A 1998;95(11):6337-42.
54. Sritippayawan S, Sumboonnanonda A, Vasuvattakul S, et al. Novel compound heterozygous SLC4A1 mutations in Thai patients with autosomal recessive distal renal tubular acidosis. Am J Kidney Dis 2004;44(1):64-70.
55. Yenchitsomanus PT, Vasuvattakul S, Kirdpon S, et al. Autosomal recessive distal renal tubular acidosis caused by G701D mutation of anion exchanger 1 gene. Am J Kidney Dis 2002;40(1):21-9.
56. Cordat E, Kittanakom S, Yenchitsomanus PT, et al. Dominant and recessive distal renal tubular acidosis mutations of kidney anion exchanger 1 induce distinct trafficking defects in MDCK cells. Traffic 2006;7(2):117-28.
57. Devonald MA, Smith AN, Poon JP, Ihrke G, Karet FE. Non-polarized targeting of AE1 causes autosomal dominant distal renal tubular acidosis. Nat Genet 2003;33(2):125-7.
58. Quilty JA, Cordat E, Reithmeier RA. Impaired trafficking of human kidney anion exchanger (kAE1) caused by hetero-oligomer formation with a truncated mutant associated with distal renal tubular acidosis. Biochem J 2002;368(Pt 3):895-903.
59. Sawasdee N, Udomchaiprasertkul W, Noisakran S, Rungroj N, Akkarapatumwong V, Yenchitsomanus PT. Trafficking defect of mutant kidney anion exchanger 1 (kAE1) proteins associated with distal renal tubular acidosis and Southeast Asian ovalocytosis. Biochem Biophys Res Commun 2006;350(3):723-30.
60. Toye AM, Banting G, Tanner MJ. Regions of human kidney anion exchanger 1 (kAE1) required for basolateral targeting of kAE1 in polarised kidney cells: mis-targeting explains dominant renal tubular acidosis (dRTA). J Cell Sci 2004;117(Pt 8):1399-410.
61. Tanphaichitr VS, Sumboonnanonda A, Ideguchi H, et al. Novel AE1 mutations in recessive distal renal tubular acidosis. Loss-of-function is rescued by glycophorin A. J Clin Invest 1998;102(12):2173-9.
62. Toye AM, Bruce LJ, Unwin RJ, Wrong O, Tanner MJ. Band 3 Walton, a C-terminal deletion associated with distal renal tubular acidosis, is expressed in the red cell membrane but retained internally in kidney cells. Blood 2002;99(1):342-7.

63. Hu PY, Roth DE, Skaggs LA, et al. A splice junction mutation in intron 2 of the carbonic anhydrase II gene of osteopetrosis patients from Arabic countries. Hum Mutat 1992;1(4):288-92.
64. Shah GN, Bonapace G, Hu PY, Strisciuglio P, Sly WS. Carbonic anhydrase II deficiency syndrome (osteopetrosis with renal tubular acidosis and brain calcification): novel mutations in CA2 identified by direct sequencing expand the opportunity for genotype-phenotype correlation. Hum Mutat 2004;24(3):272.
65. Sly WS, Hewett-Emmett D, Whyte MP, Yu YS, Tashian RE. Carbonic anhydrase II deficiency identified as the primary defect in the autosomal recessive syndrome of osteopetrosis with renal tubular acidosis and cerebral calcification. Proc Natl Acad Sci U S A 1983;80(9):2752-6.
66. Smith AN, Skaug J, Choate KA, et al. Mutations in ATP6N1B, encoding a new kidney vacuolar proton pump 116-kD subunit, cause recessive distal renal tubular acidosis with preserved hearing. Nat Genet 2000;26(1):71-5.
67. Stehberger PA, Schulz N, Finberg KE, et al. Localization and regulation of the ATP6V0A4 (a4) vacuolar H+-ATPase subunit defective in an inherited form of distal renal tubular acidosis. J Am Soc Nephrol 2003;14(12):3027-38.
68. Yang T. Regulation of cyclooxygenase-2 in renal medulla. Acta Physiol Scand 2003;177(4):417-21.
69. Al-Awqati Q. Proton-translocating ATPases. Annu Rev Cell Biol 1986;2:179-99.
70. Gluck S. V-ATPases of the plasma membrane. J Exp Biol 1992;172:29-37.
71. Harvey WR, Wieczorek H. Animal plasma membrane energization by chemiosmotic H+ V-ATPases. J Exp Biol 1997;200(Pt 2):203-16.
72. Nelson N, Klionsky DJ. Vacuolar H(+)-ATPase: from mammals to yeast and back. Experientia 1996;52(12):1101-10.
73. Nishi T, Forgac M. The vacuolar (H+)-ATPases--nature's most versatile proton pumps. Nat Rev Mol Cell Biol 2002;3(2):94-103.
74. Stevens TH, Forgac M. Structure, function and regulation of the vacuolar (H+)-ATPase. Annu Rev Cell Dev Biol 1997;13:779-808.
75. Stone DK, Xie XS. Proton translocating ATPases: issues in structure and function. Kidney Int 1988;33(4):767-74.
76. Bacic D, Capuano P, Baum M, et al. Activation of dopamine D1-like receptors induces acute internalization of the renal Na+/phosphate cotransporter NaPi-IIa in mouse kidney and OK cells. Am J Physiol Renal Physiol 2005;288(4):F740-7.
77. Gregorini M, Wang J, Xie XS, Milligan RA, Engel A. Three-dimensional reconstruction of bovine brain V-ATPase by cryo-electron microscopy and single particle analysis. J Struct Biol 2007;158(3):445-54.
78. Gluck S, Al-Awqati Q. An electrogenic proton-translocating adenosine triphosphatase from bovine kidney medulla. J Clin Invest 1984;73(6):1704-10.
79. Gluck S, Kelly S, Al-Awqati Q. The proton translocating ATPase responsible for urinary acidification. J Biol Chem 1982;257(16):9230-3.
80. Miller RL, Zhang P, Smith M, et al. V-ATPase B1-subunit promoter drives expression of EGFP in intercalated cells of kidney, clear cells of epididymis and airway cells of lung in transgenic mice. Am J Physiol Cell Physiol 2005;288(5):C1134-44.
81. Smith AN, Lovering RC, Futai M, Takeda J, Brown D, Karet FE. Revised nomenclature for mammalian vacuolar-type H+ -ATPase subunit genes. Mol Cell 2003;12(4):801-3.
82. Valles P, Lapointe MS, Wysocki J, Batlle D. Kidney vacuolar H+ -ATPase: physiology and regulation. Semin Nephrol 2006;26(5):361-74.
83. Brown D, Hirsch S, Gluck S. Localization of a proton-pumping ATPase in rat kidney. J Clin Invest 1988;82(6):2114-26.
84. Feng Y, Forgac M. A novel mechanism for regulation of vacuolar acidification. J Biol Chem 1992;267(28):19769-72.
85. Mulberg AE, Tulk BM, Forgac M. Modulation of coated vesicle chloride channel activity and acidification by reversible protein kinase A-dependent phosphorylation. J Biol Chem 1991;266(31):20590-3.
86. Fuster DG, Zhang J, Xie X-S, Moe OW. The vacuolar-ATPase B1 subunit in distal tubular acidosis: novel mutations and mechanisms for dysfunction. Kidney Int 2008;73(10):1151-1158.
87. Seol JH, Shevchenko A, Shevchenko A, Deshaies RJ. Skp1 forms multiple protein complexes, including RAVE, a regulator of V-ATPase assembly. Nat Cell Biol 2001;3(4):384-91.
88. Lu M, Holliday LS, Zhang L, Dunn WA, Jr., Gluck SL. Interaction between aldolase and vacuolar H+-ATPase: evidence for direct coupling of glycolysis to the ATP-hydrolyzing proton pump. J Biol Chem 2001;276(32):30407-13.
89. Hruska KA, Saab G, Mathew S, Lund R. Renal osteodystrophy, phosphate homeostasis, and vascular calcification. Semin Dial 2007;20(4):309-15.

90. Ho MN, Hirata R, Umemoto N, et al. VMA13 encodes a 54-kDa vacuolar H(+)-ATPase subunit required for activity but not assembly of the enzyme complex in Saccharomyces cerevisiae. J Biol Chem 1993;268(24):18286-92.
91. Bajaj G, Quan A. Renal tubular acidosis and deafness: report of a large family. Am J Kidney Dis 1996;27(6):880-2.
92. Liu W, Morimoto T, Kondo Y, et al. Analysis of NaCl transport in thin ascending limb of Henle's loop in CLC-K1 null mice. Am J Physiol Renal Physiol 2002;282(3):F451-7.
93. Vasilyeva E, Liu Q, MacLeod KJ, Baleja JD, Forgac M. Cysteine scanning mutagenesis of the noncatalytic nucleotide binding site of the yeast V-ATPase. J Biol Chem 2000;275(1):255-60.
94. Yamashiro CT, Kane PM, Wolczyk DF, Preston RA, Stevens TH. Role of vacuolar acidification in protein sorting and zymogen activation: a genetic analysis of the yeast vacuolar proton-translocating ATPase. Mol Cell Biol 1990;10(7):3737-49.
95. Schiestl RH, Gietz RD. High efficiency transformation of intact yeast cells using single stranded nucleic acids as a carrier. Curr Genet 1989;16(5-6):339-46.
96. Mumberg D, Muller R, Funk M. Yeast vectors for the controlled expression of heterologous proteins in different genetic backgrounds. Gene 1995;156(1):119-22.
97. Pak CYC. New methods for assessing crystal growth and saturation of brushite in whole urine: effect of pH, calcium and citrate. J Urol 2008(In Press).
98. Wabner CL, Pak CY. Effect of orange juice consumption on urinary stone risk factors. J Urol 1993;149(6):1405-8.
99. Pak CY, Holt K. Nucleation and growth of brushite and calcium oxalate in urine of stone-formers. Metabolism 1976;25(6):665-73.

II. MEDULLARY AND PAPILLARY CELL BIOLOGY

H^+, Water and Urea Transport in the Inner Medullary Collecting Duct and Their Role in the Prevention and Pathogenesis of Renal Stone Disease

Susan M. Wall[a,b] and Janet D. Klein[a]

Departments of [a]Medicine and [b]Physiology, Emory University School of Medicine, Atlanta, GA 30322

Abstract. The inner medullary collecting duct (IMCD) is the final site within the kidney for the reabsorption of urea, water and electrolytes and for the secretion of H^+ before the luminal fluid becomes the final urine. Transporters expressed in the IMCD contribute to the generation of the large ion gradients that exist between the interstitium and the collecting duct lumen. Thus, the luminal fluid within the human IMCD can reach an osmolality of 1200 mOsm/kg H_2O and a pH of 4. This ability of the human nephron to concentrate and acidify the urine might predispose to stone formation. However, under treatment conditions that predispose to stone formation, such as during hypercalciuria, the kidney mitigates stone formation by reducing solute concentration by reducing H_2O reabsorption. Moreover, the kidney attenuates stone formation by tightly controlling acid-base balance, which prevents the bone loss, hypocitraturia and hypercalciuria observed during metabolic acidosis by augmenting net H^+ excretion by tightly regulating H^+ transporter function and through luminal buffering, particularly with NH_3. This article will review the ion transporters present in the mammalian IMCD and their role in the prevention and in the pathogenesis of renal stone formation.

Keywords: inner medullary collecting duct, intercalated cell, net acid excretion, urea, aquaporins, H^+-ATPase, AE1, Na,K-ATPase, H,K-ATPase
PACS: 87.18.–h

SUBSEGMENTS OF THE INNER MEDULLARY COLLECTING DUCT

The inner medullary collecting duct (IMCD) is the terminal portion of the collecting duct, and represents the most distal portion of the nephron. It is divided into 2 subsegments, the initial IMCD or the most proximal 20% of the IMCD and the terminal IMCD, or the last 80% of this segment [1,2]. These 2 subsegments have distinct cell types with distinct ultrastructure and distinct transporter expression and function. The initial IMCD (Figure 1) resembles the OMCD in that it consists of type A intercalated cells that mediate net H^+ secretion [1,2] and principal cells, which absorb Na^+ and H_2O through the epithelial Na^+ channel, ENaC, and through water channels, such as aquaporins (AQP) 2, 3 and 4 [2,3]. In contrast, the terminal IMCD

CP1049, *Renal Stone Disease 2, 2nd International Urolithiasis Research Symposium,*
edited by A. P. Evan, J. E. Lingeman, J. A. McAteer, and J. C. Williams, Jr.

(Figure 2) consists of a unique cell type, called the "IMCD" cell [2], which secretes H^+ equivalents and absorbs Na^+, Cl^-, water and urea.

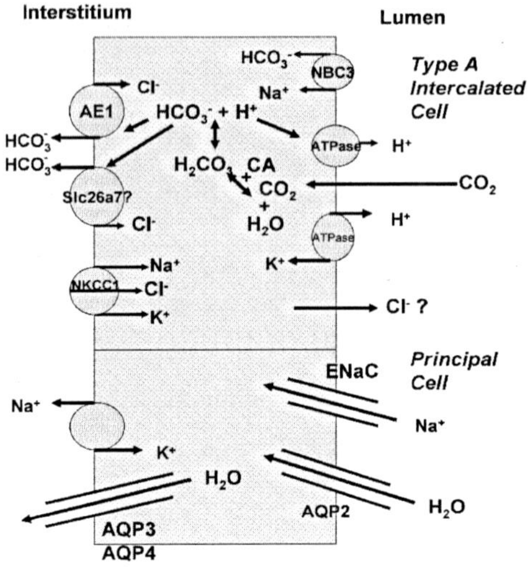

Initial IMCD

Figure 1. *Transporter expression in the rat initial IMCD*. The initial 20% of the IMCD is composed of 2 cell types, principal cells and type A intercalated cells. Secretion of H^+ and Cl^- occur across A cells through AE1 and NKCC1 which localize to the basolateral membrane, which act in series with the H^+-ATPase and possibly NBC3 [97] that localize to the apical plasma membrane. Carbonic anhydrase II (CA) catalyzes the production of H_2CO_3 from CO_2 and H_2O. In turn, H_2CO_3 forms H^+ and HCO_3^-, thus enabling CO_2 to serve as a source of H^+. The mechanism of apical Cl^- secretion and the physiological function of Slc26a7 is unknown. Principal cells mediate net reabsorption of Na^+ through the ENaC on the apical plasma membrane acting in tandem with the Na,K-ATPase in the basolateral plasma membrane. Water is absorbed through AQP2 in the apical membrane and then exits the cell through AQP 3 and 4 (see text).

FUNCTION OF TYPE A INTERCALATED CELLS WITHIN THE INITIAL IMCD

Net H^+ secretion into the luminal fluid of the initial IMCD is thought to occur through the action of Type A intercalated cells. Type A cells are expressed not only within the initial IMCD, but also in the distal convoluted tubule (DCT), the connecting tubule (CNT), the cortical collecting duct (CCD), and the OMCD [4-6], whereas the other intercalated cell subtypes (type B and non-A, non-B intercalated cells) are found only in the CCD, CNT and DCT [5,6]. Transporters expressed in type A intercalated cells of the rat OMCD and initial IMCD are shown in Figure 1. Across the apical plasma membrane, type A intercalated cells secrete Cl^- through a poorly understood mechanism and secrete H^+ equivalents through the vacuolar H^+-ATPase (V-ATPase, H^+-ATPase). In A cells, secretion of H^+ and Cl^- into the luminal fluid acts in series with Cl^- uptake and HCO_3^- efflux across the basolateral membrane. Basolateral Cl^- uptake in A cells occurs through a truncated splice variant of the red cell Cl^-/HCO_3^- exchanger, AE1 (kAE1) [7-12], and also through the Na^+-K^+-$2Cl^-$ exchanger, NKCC1 [10] and the Cl^-/HCO_3^- exchanger *Slc26a7* [13,14].

The apical H^+-ATPase is a multi-subunit enzyme that mediates active H^+ secretion through energy derived from the hydrolysis of ATP [15]. Many of the V-ATPase subunits are encoded by separate genes [15], which can have tissue-specific distribution [15]. Of the subunits that make up the various H^+-ATPase isoforms, the $\alpha4$ and B1 subunits have a kidney-specific distribution, whereas the $\alpha1$ subunit is ubiquitous [15]. Other mechanisms of apical H^+ secretion in addition to the V-ATPases have been described in A cells such as the H,K$\alpha1$ and H,K$\alpha2$ isoforms of the H,K-ATPase [16,17]. However, the functional significance of these transporters is not appreciated fully (vide infra).

The source of H^+ for luminal acidification in A cells is CO_2 [10, 18]. Intracellular CO_2 combines with H_2O to produce H_2CO_3, a reaction catalyzed by carbonic anhydrase type II. H_2CO_3 dissociates to H^+ and HCO_3^-. HCO_3^- exits the cell across the basolateral plasma membrane, whereas H^+ generated in this reaction is secreted into the luminal fluid. In the absence of carbonic anhydrase, luminal acidification is markedly attenuated [10,18], presumably because CO_2 cannot serve as a source of H^+.

The importance of these A cell transporters has been demonstrated in transport and balance studies. With pharmacological inhibition or with genetic disruption of the apical H^+-ATPase or basolateral kAE1-mediated Cl^-/HCO_3^- exchange, net H^+ secretion along the medullary collecting duct is markedly reduced [19, 20], which results in metabolic acidosis [7, 21].

ROLE OF TYPE A INTERCALATED CELLS IN THE PROCESS OF NEPHROLITHIASIS

An inability to fully acidify the urine or a "distal renal tubular acidosis" (type 1 RTA) is not uncommon in persons with nephrolithiasis. In fact, distal RTA is observed in 22% of all persons that suffer from recurrent stone formation [22]. These distal RTAs result from a reduced ability to secrete H^+ equivalents and can be acquired or inherited as inactivation mutations in transporters that participate in H^+ secretion. Inactivation mutations in A cell transporters, such as the H^+-ATPase, AE1 and carbonic anhydrase type II produce acidification defects either through autosomal recessive or autosomal dominant inheritance, although disease is generally milder in autosomal dominant forms [23]. Autosomal recessive distal RTA is seen with inactivation mutations in either the B1 or the $\alpha4$ subunits of the H^+-ATPase [24-27], whereas mutations in the transmembrane domain of the kidney-specific splice variant of AE1 (kAE1, *SLC4A1*) present as either autosomal recessive or dominant disease [23,24,28]. Inactivation mutations in carbonic anhydrase type II generate a mixed proximal and distal (type 3) renal tubular acidosis in addition to osteopetrosis and mental retardation [23, 24]. These A cell transporter mutations are all associated with metabolic acidosis in addition to rickets, failure to thrive, nephrolithiasis and hypokalemia.

Metabolic acidosis of any etiology causes calcium phosphate and calcium oxalate stone formation [29] by increasing urinary calcium excretion through enhanced bone resorption [24]. In addition, metabolic acidosis increases mitochondrial citrate consumption [30], which increases the propensity for calcium oxalate stones by reducing urinary citrate excretion [29].

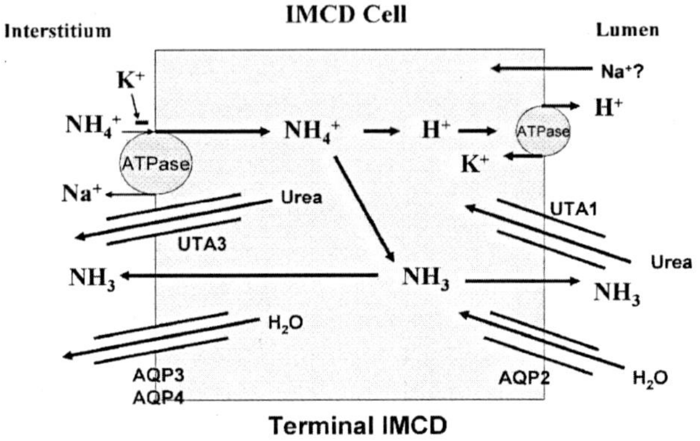

Figure 2: Transporter function in rat terminal IMCD. The terminal 80% of the IMCD is composed of "IMCD" cells, which are distinct morphologically and functionally from other cells along the nephron. ENaC and H^+-ATPase abundance in this cell type is extremely low [98,99]. Instead, Na^+ reabsorption and H^+ secretion occur through mechanisms not fully understood, although H^+ secretion occurs, at least in part, through isoforms of the H,K-ATPase. This cell type absorbs urea and water through highly vasopressin-sensitive mechanisms. Net urea and water reabsorption occur across the apical plasma membrane through UTA-1 and AQP2, respectively, both of which are highly regulated by vasopressin. Urea and water exit across the basolateral membrane through AQP 3 and 4 and UTA-3. Of these UTA-1, UTA-3, and AQP2, but not AQP3 and 4, are vasopressin-sensitive (see text).

FUNCTION OF THE TERMINAL IMCD IN H^+ SECRETION

Robust rates of net H^+ secretion are observed along the terminal IMCD in vivo [31], such that the H^+ concentration in the lumen of the collecting duct can exceed that in the interstitium by more than 1000-fold [32]. However, the mechanism of H^+ secretion in the terminal IMCD is less well understood than in more proximal portions of the collecting duct. Unlike the initial IMCD, the H^+-ATPase is not thought to participate in H^+ secretion in the terminal IMCD since H^+-ATPase immunoreactivity is not observed in this subsegment and since H^+ secretion is not reduced with H^+-ATPase inhibitors [2,33,34]. Nevertheless, in vivo and in vitro studies support the conclusion that H^+ secretion within the terminal IMCD occurs through an active transport mechanism [1,2], such as through isoforms of the H,K-ATPase.

H,K-ATPase expression and function have been detected in the IMCD. H,K-α1 and both splice variants of H,K-α2 (H,K-α2a and H,K-α2b) [35] have been detected at the mRNA and protein levels in the terminal IMCD and within intercalated cells of the initial IMCD [16,17,36-38]. In terminal IMCD tubules perfused in vitro, H^+ secretion is reduced with removal of K^+ from the luminal fluid [33] and with inhibitors of both the colonic H,K-ATPase (H,Kα2) and gastric H,K-ATPase (H,Kα1) [33,39]. Moreover, H^+ secretion is increased in tubules perfused in vitro from K^+-restricted rats [39], a treatment condition that upregulates H,K-α2 -mediated expression and transport [35]. Thus, in rat terminal IMCD, H^+ secretion and K^+ reabsorption are mediated, at least in part, by the colonic (H,K α2) and the gastric (H,Kα1) isoforms of the H,K-ATPase. However, the physiological role of the H,K-ATPase in acid-base balance is controversial since abnormalities in acid-base balance are not observed in mice with genetic disruption of either H,K-α1 or H,K-α2 [40,41].

NH_4^+ SECRETION BY THE TERMINAL IMCD

Acid is excreted by the kidney as NH_4^+ and titratable acid, which is mainly PO_4. However, NH_4^+ is the major regulatable component of net acid excretion [42, 43]. Ammonia (NH_3) is a weak base with a pK of 9.03. Thus at a pH 7.4, 99% of total ammonia (NH_3 + NH_4^+) is NH_4^+. Excretion of acid as NH_4^+ greatly enhances the capacity of the kidney to excrete net H^+ equivalents.

Ammonium (NH_4^+) is synthesized in the proximal tubule through a highly regulated process, and then preferentially secreted in to the luminal fluid [44]. NH_4^+ is absorbed downstream by the thick ascending limb Na-K-2Cl cotransporter, NKCC2 [45-47]. NKCC2 acts in series with the Na^+,K^+-ATPase to generate the "single effect" of countercurrent multiplication. Through countercurrent multiplication, NH_4^+ is concentrated within the interstitium forming an axial gradient from the superficial cortex to the papillary tip [48]. Thus, while interstitial total ammonia concentration is ~0.1 mM in the superficial cortex [49], it reaches nearly 10 mM in the interstitium at the papillary tip [50]. IMCD cells are therefore in a unique environment in that they are exposed to the highest NH_4^+ concentration of any cell in the body.

Of the total ammonia excreted in the urine, only ~20% is present in the luminal fluid of the superficial distal tubule [51]. The remaining 80% of total ammonia present in the final urine is secreted along the length of the collecting duct into the luminal fluid through transepithelial transport [51]. For the past 50 years total ammonia secretion along the collecting duct lumen was thought to occur through the non-ionic diffusion of NH_3. This model predicts that increasing the NH_3 gradient from the interstitium to the collecting duct lumen will increase total ammonia secretion into the luminal fluid of the collecting duct. However, rates of total ammonia secretion in vivo do not always correlate with the NH_3 gradient measured directly in micropuncture studies. For example, total ammonia secretion is not observed at the papillary tip during hyperkalemia, despite a substantial NH_3 gradient between the interstitium and the collecting duct lumen at that level [50]. Thus hyperkalemia reduces NH_3 transfer from the interstitium to the collecting duct lumen [50].

This observation raised the possibility that the increase in interstitial K^+ observed during hyperkalemia inhibits NH_4^+ uptake in IMCD cells. In 1960 Jens Skou observed in crab neuron that NH_4^+ and K^+ compete for binding and thus for transport on the Na,K-ATPase [52]. Over the subsequent 50 years, K^+ and NH_4^+ have been observed to compete for binding on a number of transporters. Since the major pathway for K^+ uptake in the terminal IMCD is through the Na,K-ATPase [53], our laboratory explored the interaction of NH_4^+ and K^+ on the Na,K-ATPase and observed that NH_4^+ and K^+ are competitive inhibitors for the extracellular binding site [53]. We then explored the role of NH_4^+ transport by the Na,K-ATPase in net acid secretion in terminal IMCD tubules perfused in vitro and observed that net acid secretion is higher in tubules perfused in the presence than in the absence of NH_4^+. Moreover, the Na,K-ATPase inhibitor, ouabain, reduced net acid secretion and increased intracellular pH (pH_i) only when NH_4^+ was present in the perfusate and bath [54]. In the absence of NH_4^+, ouabain had no effect on pH_i or net acid secretion [54]. Thus, NH_4^+ enters the cell across the basolateral membrane through the Na,K-ATPase where it provides a source of H^+ for luminal secretion [54, 55] (Figure 2). NH_3 exits the cell through both the apical and basolateral plasma membranes. NH_3/NH_4^+ recycling across the basolateral membrane thus generates a H^+ source for luminal acidification (Figure 2).

However, these experiments were performed with an extracellular K^+ concentration of 3-5 mM [54,55], which is much lower than concentrations observed in the inner medullary interstitium in vivo under basal conditions [56]. Following normal dietary K^+ intake, interstitial K^+ concentration in the rat inner medulla is ~36 mM [56]. However, with 3 days of dietary K^+ restriction, interstitial K^+ concentration at the papillary tip falls to 8 mM [56]. Because K^+ and NH_4^+ are competitive inhibitors for extracellular binding to the Na^+ pump, we hypothesized that NH_4^+ uptake is much greater during K^+ restriction because interstitial K^+ concentration is reduced. Thus, net acid secretion was measured in terminal IMCDs perfused in vitro from K^+-replete and K^+-depleted rats [48, 57]. In these experiments NH_4^+ concentration in the perfusate and bath was 6 mM, while K^+ concentration was 10 or 30 mM, the interstitial K^+ concentrations expected following a K^+-restricted or a K^+-replete diet, respectively. In terminal IMCDs from K^+-restricted rats perfused in vitro in the presence of 10 mM K^+, both the total and the ouabain-sensitive component of net H^+ secretion were at least 2-fold higher than in tubules from K^+-replete rats perfused in the presence of 30 mM K^+. Thus, NH_4^+ uptake by the Na,K-ATPase is physiologically significant in the process of net acid secretion at K^+ and NH_4^+ concentrations expected in the inner medulla in vivo during hypokalemia.

These data suggest that the NH_4^+ transfer defect observed during hyperkalemia occurs from reduced uptake of NH_4^+ by the Na,K-ATPase. During hyperkalemia, interstitial K^+ rises, whereas interstitial NH_4^+ stays the same or falls. This increased interstitial K^+ concentration reduces the ability of NH_4^+ to compete with K^+ for uptake by the Na^+ pump thereby reducing the proton source for luminal acidification.

More recently, other NH_4^+ transporters, such as RhBG and RhCG have been described within the IMCD [58]. However, the contribution of these transporters to net acid secretion in the native IMCD remains to be determined.

RELEVANCE OF THESE TERMINAL IMCD H^+ AND NH_4^+ TRANSPORT PATHWAYS TO THE PATHOGENESIS OF NEPHROLITHIASIS

In persons with uric acid nephrolithiasis urinary pH is reduced, which lowers uric acid solubility [59]. The lower urinary pH observed in uric acid stone formers occurs from reduced urinary total ammonia (NH_4^++NH_3) excretion [59], which limits urinary buffering. As described elsewhere in this symposium, the reduced NH_4^+ excretion observed in uric acid stone formers has been attributed to reduced NH_4^+ synthesis in the proximal tubule. However, these persons frequently have a higher serum K^+ than non-stone formers [59], which may contribute to their inappropriately low urinary NH_4^+ excretion, since hyperkalemia suppresses not only the synthesis of NH_4^+ in the proximal tubule [60,61], but also reduces the transfer of NH_4^+ from the interstitium to the collecting duct lumen [48,50,53,57].

Whereas hyperkalemia might predispose to stone formation, hypokalemia should reduce uric acid stone formation through several mechanisms. Hypokalemia increases NH_4^+ synthesis in the proximal tubule [60,62] and increases NH_4^+ transfer from the interstitium to the collecting duct lumen [50]. Thus, urinary NH_3 concentration increases during hypokalemia, which increases uric acid solubility by raising luminal pH [48]. Second, severe hypokalemia induces nephrogenic diabetes insipidus, which increases urinary flow [63], thus attenuating stone formation.

UREA MOVEMENT IN THE INNER MEDULLA

While urea was initially considered to be freely membrane permeable, urea transport in native IMCD cells is slower than one would expect for a freely permeable solute [64,65]. Urea is a polar molecule that requires a facilitated transporter for rapid movement across lipid bilayers [65]. In the IMCD, urea permeability increases markedly following the application of vasopressin, which results in rapid urea reabsorption and accumulation within the medullary interstitium [64]. In this way, urea reabsorption in the IMCD contributes to the generation of a hyperosmotic medullary interstitium within the renal inner medulla. Moreover, reabsorption of urea within the IMCD prevents the accumulation of urea within the tubular lumen, which would attenuate ongoing water reabsorption [66]. Urea reabsorption in the terminal IMCD, thus allows continued water reabsorption driven by the solute gradient between the interstitium and the collecting duct lumen [66].

These data raised the possibility that a facilitated urea transporter is expressed in native IMCD cells. Facilitated urea transporters and the genes encoding these transporters have since been cloned and characterized. The facilitated urea transporters are gene products of *Slc14a2* and its splice variants (UT-A1 to UT-A6) [67-71]. Of these, only UT-A1 and UT-A3 are present in the IMCD [72]. UT-A2, expressed in the thin descending limb of the loop of Henle and UT-B, expressed in the vasa recta, participate in urea recycling, which is critical to the maintenance of the high osmolality observed at the tip of the renal inner medulla [73].

The largest urea transporter is UT-A1, which is a glycoprotein that is activated by phosphorylation of serine residues [74,75] and by its regulated trafficking between the subapical regions and the apical plasma membrane [76]. UT-A3, a truncated splice variant of UT-A1, is also a glycoprotein and a phosphoprotein [77]. In contrast to UT-A1, UT-A3 localizes to either the basolateral or the apical surface of the IMCD in response to vasopressin [77,78].

ROLE OF UREA TRANSPORTERS IN RENAL STONE DISEASE

Urea transporters are critical in urinary concentration. However, changes in urea transporter abundance or function do not appear to modulate the risk of stone formation [79,80].

THE ROLE OF WATER CHANNELS IN URINARY CONCENTRATION

In the inner medulla, water flow occurs down its concentration gradient from the collecting duct lumen into the hypertonic medullary interstitium. The hypertonic interstitium observed within the inner medulla is generated by the thick ascending limb Na-K-2Cl cotransporter (NKCC2) in the outer medulla, which absorbs NaCl and NH_4^+, and through the urea transporters (discussed above) and the countercurrent arrangement of the vasa recta and loops of Henle [81]. Through the action of these transporters Na^+, Cl^- , NH_4^+ and urea are concentrated in the medullary interstitium, creating an axial gradient for these solutes from the outer medulla to the papillary tip [73,81,82]. Vasopressin increases water permeability along the entire collecting duct, which allows transepithelial reabsorption of water down its concentration gradient from the collecting duct lumen into the hypertonic inner medullary interstitium.

In most epithelia, including kidney, transport of water across the plasma membrane occurs through water channels. The first cloned water channel was aquaporin 1 (AQP1), which localizes to the renal proximal tubule and red cells [83]. To date, 13 water channels have been cloned [84-88]. In the collecting duct, including the terminal IMCD, water is absorbed through the vasopressin-sensitive water channel, aquaporin 2 (AQP2), which localizes to the apical plasma membrane, and then exits the cell across the basolateral membrane through aquaporins 3 and 4 (AQP3, AQP4) [3]. However, the rate-limiting step in vasopressin-stimulated water absorption occurs through the regulation of AQP2 [3, 89]. AQP2 is regulated through both changes in the subcellular distribution of the protein and through changes in total protein abundance [3]. Apical plasma membrane AQP2 expression increases following water restriction, through the action of vasopressin. The importance of AQP2 to urinary concentrating ability is underscored by the observation that both people [90, 91] and mice [90, 92] with genetic disruption of the gene encoding AQP2 have severe polyuria, polydipsia and hypernatremia.

THE ROLE OF WATER TRANSPORT IN THE PATHOGENESIS OF NEPHROLITHIASIS

Increased urinary flow generally inhibits stone formation by reducing the concentration of urinary solutes. Thus, polyuria can be an appropriate renal response to limit stone formation. Increased urine flow can occur from reduced release of vasopressin, from a reduced renal response to vasopressin, from reduced medullary urea recycling or from an inability of the kidney to generate a hypertonic medullary interstitium [93]. In rodent models of hypercalciuria, mild to severe polyuria is observed [93]. This polyuria is caused from decreased AQP2 protein abundance and by the blunted targeting of AQP2 into the apical plasma membrane, mediated by the calcium sensing receptor in the IMCD apical membrane [94]. The mechanism by which hypercalcemia reduces water reabsorption is unclear but may be cAMP-dependent since inhibition of phosphodiesterases IV and III corrected the polyuria and restored apical plasma membrane AQP2 targeting. [95]. However, hypercalcemia may also increase AQP2 degradation [96]. Although the cause of the impaired apical plasma membrane AQP2 targeting and reduced protein abundance observed during hypercalcemia is not explained fully, it is clear that this response is appropriate in that it should be at least partially protective against nephrolithiasis.

CONCLUSIONS

The IMCD is subdivided into the initial 20% and the terminal 80%. The cell types within each of these subsegments have distinct morphology, function and transporter expression. The IMCD functions, in part, to absorb NaCl, water and urea and to secrete H^+ equivalents. However, urinary concentration and a reduced ability to excrete H^+ equivalents can predispose to stone formation. Under treatment conditions that predispose to nephrolithiasis, such as during hypercalciuria, the kidney mitigates stone formation by increasing urinary flow, which reduces urinary concentration, and by maintaining acid-base balance through its robust ability to regulate the excretion of NH_4^+.

ACKNOWLEDGEMENTS

This work was supported by Projects 2 (to S.M. Wall) and 4 (to J.M. Sands) of P01 061521. We thank V. Pech and J.M. Sands for their helpful comments.

REFERENCES

1. Wall, S. M., Sands, J. M., Flessner, M. F., Nonoguchi, H., Spring, K. R. & Knepper, M. A. (1990) *Am. J. Physiol.* **258**, F75-F84.
2. Wall, S. M. & Knepper, M. A. (1990) *Seminars in Nephrology* **10**, 148-158.
3. Nielsen, S., Frokiaer, J., Marples, D., Kwon, T.-H., Agre, P. & Knepper, M. A. (2002) *Physiol. Rev.* **82**, 205-244.
4. Kim, J., Kim, Y.-H., Cha, J.-H., Tisher, C. C. & Madsen, K. M. (1999) *J. Am. Soc. Nephrol.* **10**, 1-12.

5. Teng-ummnuay, P., Verlander, J. W., Yuan, W., Tisher, C. C. & Madsen, K. M. (1996) *J. Am. Soc. Nephrol.* **7**, 260-274.
6. Madsen, K. M. & Tisher, C. C. (1986) *Am. J. Physiol.* **250**, F1-F15.
7. Stone, D. K., Seldin, D. W., Kokko, J. P. & Jacobson, H. R. (1983) *J. Clin. Invest.* **71**, 1505-1508.
8. Alper, S. L., Natale, J., Gluck, S., Lodish, H. F. & Brown, D. (1989) *Proc. Natl. Acad. Sci. USA* **86**, 5429-5433.
9. Hays, S. R. & Alpern, R. J. (1990) *J. Gen. Physiol.* **95**, 347-367.
10. Wall, S. M., Fischer, M. P., Mehta, P., Hassell, K. A. & Park, S. J. (2001) *Am. J. Physiol.* **280**, F913-F921.
11. Kudrycki, K. E. & Shull, G. E. (1989) *J. Biol. Chem.* **264**, 8185-8192.
12. Kudrycki, K. E. & Shull, G. E. (1993) *Am. J. Physiol.* **264**, F540-F547.
13. Barone, S., Amlal, H., Xu, J., Kujala, M., Kere, J., Petrovic, S. & Soleimani, M. (2004) *J. Am. Soc. Nephrol.* **15**, 2002-2011.
14. Xu, J., Nakamura, S., Wang, Z., Barone, S. & Soleimani, M. (2006) *J. Am. Soc. Nephrol.* **17**, 578A. (Abstract)
15. Breton, S. & Brown, D. (2007) *Am. J. Physiol.* **292**, F1-F10.
16. Ahn, K. Y. & Kone, B. C. (1995) *Am. J. Physiol.* **268**, F99-F109.
17. Ahn, K. Y., Park, K. Y., Kim, K. K. & Kone, B. C. (1996) *Am. J. Physiol.* **271**, F314-F321.
18. Wall, S. M. & Fischer, M. P. (2002) *J. Am. Soc. Nephrol.* **13**, 827-835.
19. Tsuruoka, S. & Schwartz, G. J. (1997) *J. Clin. Invest.* **99**, 1420-1431.
20. Weiner, I. D., Frank, A. E. & Wingo, C. S. (1999) *Am. J. Physiol.* **276**, F606-F613.
21. Stehberger, P. A., Shmukler, B. E., Stuart-Tilley, A. K., Peters, L. L., Alper, S. L. & Wagner, C. A. (2007) *J. Am. Soc. Nephrol.* **18**, 1408-1418.
22. Singh, P. P., Pendse, A. K., Ahmed, A., Ramavataram, D. V. & Rajpurohit, S. K. (1995) *Urol. Res.* **23**, 201-203.
23. Alper, S. L. (2002) *Annu. Rev. Physiol.* **64**, 899-923.
24. Feldman, M., Prikis, M., Athanasiou, Y., Elia, A., Pierides, A. & Deltas, C. C. (2006) *Clin. Genet.* **69**, 135-144.
25. Karet, F. E., Finberg, K. E., Nelson, R. D., Nayir, A., Mocan, H., Sanjad, S. A., Rodriguez-Soriano, J., Santos, F., Cremers, C. W. R. J., Di Pietro, A. *et al.* (1999) *Nature Genetics* **21**, 84-90.
26. Karet, F. E., Finberg, K. E., Nayir, A., Bakkaloglu, A., Ozen, S., Hulton, S. A., Sanjad, S. A., Al-Sabban, E. A., Medina, J. F. & Lifton, R. P. (1999) *Am. J. Hum. Genet.* **65**, 1656-1665.
27. Smith, A. N., Skaug, J., Choate, K. A., Nayir, A., Bakkaloglu, A., Ozen, S., Hulton, S. A., Sanjad, S. A., Al-Sabban, E. A., Lifton, R. P. *et al.* (2000) *Nature Genetics* **26**, 71-75.
28. Devonald, M. A. J., Smith, A. N., Poon, J. P., Ihrke, G. & Karet, F. E. (2003) *Nature Genetics* **33**, 125-127.
29. Domrongkitchaiporn, S., Khositseth, S., Stitchantrakul, W., Tapaneya-olarn, W. & Radinahamed, P. (2002) *Am. J. KidneyDis.* **39**, 383-391.
30. Asplin, J. R., Favus, M. J. & Coe, F. L. (2000) in *The Kidney*, ed. Brenner, B. M. (W.B. Saunders Co., Philadelphia), pp. 1774-1819.
31. Graber, M. L., Bengele, H. H., Schwartz, J. H. & Alexander, E. A. (1981) *Am. J. Physiol.* **241**, F659-F668.
32. Graber, M. L., Bengele, H. H., Mroz, E., Lechene, C. & Alexander, E. A. (1981) *Am. J. Physiol.* **241**, F669-F676.
33. Wall, S. M., Truong, A. V. & DuBose, T. D., Jr. (1996) *Am. J. Physiol.* **271**, F1037-F1044.
34. Bastani, B. & Haragsim, L. (1996) *Miner. Electrolyte Metab.* **22**, 382-395.
35. Kone, B. C. & Higham, S. C. (1998) *J. Biol. Chem.* **273**, 2543-2552.
36. Wingo, C. S., Madsen, K. M., Smolka, A. & Tisher, C. C. (1990) *Kidney Int.* **38**, 985-990.
37. Bastani, B. (1995) *J. Am. Soc. Nephrol.* **5**, 1476-1482.
38. Verlander, J. W., Moudy, R. M., Campbell, W. G., Cain, B. D. & Wingo, C. S. (2001) *Am. J. Physiol.* **281**, F357-F365.
39. Wall, S. M., Mehta, P. & DuBose, T. D., Jr. (1998) *Am. J. Physiol.* **275**, F543-F549.
40. Spicer, Z., Miller, M. L., Andringa, A., Riddle, T. M., Duffy, J. J., Doetschman, T. & Shull, G. E. (2000) *J. Biol. Chem.* **275**, 21555-21565.
41. Meneton, P., Schultheis, P. J., Greeb, J., Nieman, M. L., Liu, L. H., Clarke, L. L., Duffy, J. J. & Doetschman, T. (1998) *J. Clin. Invest.* **101**, 536-542.
42. Relman, A. S., Lennon, E. J. & Lemann, J. Jr. (1961) *J. Clin. Invest.* **40**, 1621-1630.
43. Lemann, J., Jr., Lennon, E. J., Goodman, A. D., Litzow, J. R. & Relman, A. S. (1965) *J. Clin. Invest.* **44**, 507-517.
44. DuBose, T. D., Jr., Good, D. W., Hamm, L. L. & Wall, S. M. (1991) *J. Am. Soc. Nephrol.* **1**, 1193-1203.
45. Garvin, J. L., Burg, M. B. & Knepper, M. A. (1988) *Am. J. Physiol.* **255**, F57-F65.
46. Good, D. W., Knepper, M. A. & Burg, M. B. (1984) *Am. J. Physiol.* **247**, F35-F44.
47. Good, D. W. (1988) *Am. J. Physiol.* **255**, F78-F87.
48. Wall, S. M., Davis, B. S., Hassell, K. A., Mehta, P. & Park, S. J. (1999) *Am. J. Physiol.* **277**, F866-F874.
49. Kurtz, I. & Balaban, R. S. (1986) *Am. J. Physiol.* **250**, F497-F502.

50. DuBose, T. D., Jr. & Good, D. W. (1992) *J. Clin. Invest.* **90**, 1443-1449.
51. Sajo, I. M., Goldstein, M. B., Sonnenberg, H., Stinebaugh, B. J., Wilson, D. R. & Halperin, M. L. (1981) *Kidney Int.* **20**, 353-358.
52. Skou, J. C. (1960) *Biochim. Biophys. Acta* **42**, 6-23.
53. Wall, S. M. & Koger, L. M. (1994) *Am. J. Physiol.* **267**, F660-F670.
54. Wall, S. M. (1996) *Am. J. Physiol.* **270**, F432-F439.
55. Wall, S. M. (1997) *Am. J. Physiol.* **273**, F857-F868.
56. Dobyan, D. C., Lacy, F. B. & Jamison, R. L. (1979) *Kidney Int.* **16**, 704-709.
57. Wall, S. M., Fischer, M. P., Kim, G.-H., Nguyen, B.-M. & Hassell, K. A. (2002) *Am. J. Physiol.* **282**, F91-F102.
58. Verlander, J. W., Miller, R. T., Frank, A. E., Royaux, I. E., Kim, Y.-H. & Weiner, I. D. (2003) *Am. J. Physiol.* **284**, F323-F337.
59. Cameron, M. A., Maalouf, N. M., Adams-Huet, B., Moe, O. W. & Sakhaee, K. (2006) *J. Am. Soc. Nephrol.* **17**, 1422-1428.
60. Tannen, R. L. (1977) *Kidney Int.* **11**, 453-465.
61. Sleeper, R. S., Balanger, P., Lemieux, G. & Preuss, H. G. (1982) *Kidney Int.* **21**, 345-353.
62. Nonoguchi, H., Takehara, Y. & Endou, H. (1986) *Pflugers Arch.* **407**, 245-251.
63. Marples, D., Frokiaer, J., Dorup, J., Knepper, M. A. & Nielsen, S. (1996) *J. Clin. Invest.* **97**, 1960-1968.
64. Sands, J. M., Nonoguchi, H. & Knepper, M. A. (1987) *Am. J. Physiol.* **253**, F823-F832.
65. Galucci, E., Micelli, S. & Lippe, C. (1971) *Arch. Int. Physiol. Biochim.* **79**, 881-887.
66. Wall, S. M., Chou, C.-L. & Knepper, M. A. (1991) in *Vasopressin*, eds. Jard, S. & Jamison, R. (John Libbey Eurotext Ltd., pp. 483-491.
67. Karakashian, A., Timmer, R. T., Klein, J. D., Gunn, R. B., Sands, J. M. & Bagnasco, S. M. (1999) *J. Am. Soc. Nephrol.* **10**, 230-237.
68. Nielsen, S., Terris, J., Smith, C. P., Hediger, M. A., Ecelbarger, C. A. & Knepper, M. A. (1996) *Proc. Natl. Acad. Sci. USA* **93**, 5495-5500.
69. Shayakul, C., Steel, A. & Hediger, M. A. (1996) *J. Clin. Invest.* **98**, 2580-2587.
70. Smith, C. P., Potter, E. A., Fenton, R. A. & Stewart, G. S. (2004) *Am. J. Physiol.* **287**, C1087-C1093.
71. You, G., Smith, C. P., Kanai, Y., Lee, W. S., Stelzner, M. & Hediger, M. A. (1993) *Nature* **365**, 844-847.
72. Terris, J. M., Knepper, M. A. & Wade, J. M. (2001) *Am. J. Physiol.* **280**, F325-F332.
73. Sands, J. M. (2002) *J. Am. Soc. Nephrol.* **13**, 2795-2806.
74. Zhang, C., Sands, J. M. & Klein, J. D. (2002) *Am. J. Physiol.* **282**, F85-F90.
75. Blout, M. A., Mistry, A. C., Frohlich, O., Price, S. R., Chen, G., Sands, J. M. & Klein, J. D. (2008) *Am. J. of Physiol.* (In Press)
76. Klein, J. D., Frohlich, O., Blount, M., Martin, C., Smith, T. & Sands, J. M. (2006) *J. Am. Soc. Nephrol.* **17**, 2680-2686.
77. Blout, M. A., Klein, J. D., Martin, C. F., Tchapyjnikov, D. & Sands, J. M. (2007) *Am. J. Physiol.* **293**, 1308-1313.
78. Stewart, G. S., Fenton, R. A., Wang, W., Kwon, T.-H., White, S. J., Collins, V. M., Cooper, G., Nielsen, S. & Smith, C. P. (2004) *Am. J. Physiol.* **286**, F979-F987.
79. Kato, A. & Sands, J. M. (1999) *Am. J. Physiol.* **276**, F62-F71.
80. Sands, J. M., Flores, F. X., Kato, A., Baum, M. A., Brown, E. M., Ward, D. T., Hebert, S. C. & Harris, H. W. (1998) *Am. J. Physiol.* **274**, F978-F985.
81. Sands, J. M. & Kokko, J. P. (1990) *Kidney Int.* **38**, 695-699.
82. Stokes, J. B. (1990) *Kidney Int.* **38**, 679-686.
83. Preston, G. M., Carroll, T. P., Guggino, W. B. & Agre, P. (1992) *Science* **256**, 385-387.
84. Heymann, J. B. & Engel, A. (1999) *News Physiol. Sci.* **14**, 187-193.
85. Verkman, A. S. & Mitra, A. K. (2000) *Am. J. Physiol.* **278**, F13-F28.
86. Hatakeyama, S., Yoshida, Y., Tani, T., Koyama, Y., Nihei, K., Ohshiro, K., Kamiie, J., Yaoita, E., Suda, T., Hatakeyama, K. *et al.* (2001) *Biochem. Biophys. Res. Commun.* **287**, 814-819.
87. Gorelick, D. A., Praetorius, J., Tsunenari, T., Nielsen, S. & Agre, P. (2006) *BMC Biochemistry* **7**, 14.
88. Itoh, T., Rai, T., Kuwahara, M., Ko, S. B., Uchida, S., Sasaki, S. & Ishibashi, K. (2005) *Biochem. Biophys. Res. Commun.* **330**, 832-838.
89. Sasaki, S. & Noda, Y. (2007) *Curr. Opin. Nephrol. Hypertens.* **16**, 348-352.
90. Sohara, E., Rai, T., Yang, S.-S., Uchida, K., Nitta, K., Horita, S., Ohno, M., Harada, A., Sasaki, S. & Uchida, S. (2006) *Proc. Natl. Acad. Sci. USA* **103**, 14217-14222.
91. Deen, P. M. T., Verdijk, M. A. J., Knoers, N. V. A. M., Wieringa, B., Monnens, L. A. H., van Os, C. H. & van Oost, B. A. (1994) *Science* **264**, 92-95.

92. Rojek, A., Fuchtbauer, E.-M., Kwon, T.-H., Frokiaer, J. & Nielsen, S. (2006) *Proc. Natl. Acad. Sci. USA* **103**, 6037-6042.
93. Earm, J. H., Christensen, B. M., Frokiaer, J., Marples, D., Han, J. S., Knepper, M. A. & Nielsen, S. (1998) *J. Am. Soc. Nephrol.* **9**, 2181-2193.
94. Sands, J. M., Naruse, M., Baum, M., Jo, I., Hebert, S. C., Brown, E. M. & Harris, H. W. (1997) *J. Clin. Invest.* **99**, 1399-1405.
95. Wang, W., Li, C., Kwon, T.-H., Knepper, M. A., Frokiaer, J. & Nielsen, S. (2002) *Am. J. Physiol.* **283**, F1313-F1325.
96. Puliyanda, D. P., Ward, D. T., Baum, M. A., Hammond, T. G. & Harris, H. W. Jr. (2003) *Biochem. Biophys. Res. Commun.* **303**, 52-58.
97. Kwon, T.-H., Pushkin, A., Abuladze, N., Nielsen, S. & Kurtz, I. (2000) *Am. J. Physiol.* **278**, F327-F336.
98. Hager, H., Kwon, T.-H., Vinnikova, A. K., Masilamani, S., Brooks, H. L., Frokiaer, J., Knepper, M. A. & Nielsen, S. (2001) *Am. J. Physiol.* **280**, F1093-F1106.
99. Kim, Y.-H., Kim, J., Verkman, A. S. & Madsen, K. M. (2003) *Am. J. Physiol.* **285**, F550-F557.

Loss of Urinary Macromolecules in Mice Causes Interstitial and Intratubular Renal Calcification Dependent on the Underlying Conditions

Xue-Ru Wu[a], John C. Lieske[b], Andrew P. Evan[c], Andre J. Sommer[d], Lucy Liaw[e] and Lan Mo[a]

[a]*Departments of Urology and Pathology, New York University School of Medicine, New York, NY 10016; Veterans Affairs Medical Center in Manhattan, New York, NY 10010;*
[b]*Division of Nephrology and Hypertension, Mayo Clinic College of Medicine, Rochester, MN 55905;*
[c]*Department of Anatomy and Cell Biology, Indiana University School of Medicine, Indianapolis, IN 46220;*
[d]*Department of Chemistry and Biochemistry, Miami University, Oxford, OH 45056;*
[e]*Center for Molecular Medicine, Maine Medical Center Research Institute, Scarborough, ME 04074*

Abstract. Urinary protein macromolecules have long been thought to play a role in influencing the various phases of urolithiasis including nucleation, growth, aggregation of mineral crystals and their subsequent adhesion to the renal epithelial cells. However, compelling evidence regarding their precise role was lacking, due partly to the fact that most prior studies were done *in vitro* and results were highly variable depending on the experimental conditions. The advent of genetic engineering technology has made it possible to study urinary protein macromolecules within an *in vivo* biological system. Indeed, recent studies have begun to shed light on the net effects of loss of one or more macromolecules on the earliest steps of urolithiasis. This paper focuses on the *in vivo* consequences of inactivating Tamm-Horsfall protein and/or osteopontin, two major urinary glycoproteins, using the knockout approach. The renal phenotypes of both single and double knockout mice under spontaneous or hyperoxaluric conditions will be described. The functional significance of the urinary macromolecules as critical defense factors against renal calcification will also be discussed.

Keywords: urinary macromolecules, Tamm-Horsfall protein, osteopontin, knockout mice, urolithiasis, kidney stone
PACS: 01.30.Cc

URINARY PROTEIN MACROMOLECULES AND THEIR PROPOSED ROLES IN UROLITHIASIS

Urine of healthy people is often supersaturated with inorganic and organic substances. This state of super-saturation is intensified when the body is called upon to conserve water. However, crystallization usually does not occur, due to powerful defense mechanisms that effectively keep urinary solutes in a soluble state [1-5]. Indeed, normal urine is rich in substances that are capable of preventing mineral crystallization *in vitro*, although the precise importance of macromolecule inhibitors and the effects of their deficiency on lithogenic processes have been controversial.

CP1049, *Renal Stone Disease 2, 2nd International Urolithiasis Research Symposium,*
edited by A. P. Evan, J. E. Lingeman, J. A. McAteer, and J. C. Williams, Jr.

Despite the uncertainty, a diverse group of urinary proteins has become the center of attention, the most prominent of which are Tamm-Horsfall protein, osteopontin (or uropontin), members of the inter-alpha inhibitor family, and fragment 1 of urinary prothrombin [2,3,6-8]. Almost without exception, these proteins were initially identified as the organic components of human renal stones, and were later found to modulate crystal nucleation, growth, aggregation and attachment to renal epithelial cells *in vitro*. However, until recently little was known about the function(s) of these proteins in urinary stone formation *in vivo*. It is believed that renal crystallization results from an imbalance between urinary solutes and crystallization inhibitors [9-11]. Specifically, when the concentration of urinary solutes exceeds the metastable limit or when there are insufficient/ineffective inhibitors, or a combination of both, crystals will form in the urinary system. A critical test to these hypotheses has recently been provided by the creation of the knockout mice lacking one or more urinary macromolecules, particularly Tamm-Horsfall protein and/or osteopontin.

TAMM-HORSFALL PROTEIN AND ITS ABLATION IN MICE

Tamm-Horsfall protein (THP), also named uromodulin, is the most abundant protein in the urine of most mammals, with an excretion rate of up to 100 mg daily in humans [12]. Made by tubular cells in the thick ascending limb of Henle's loop of the kidney, THP is anchored to the apical membrane via glycophosphatidyl inositol (GPI) linkage and is released into the urine by the activity of either proteases or phospholipases [13-15]. Under physiological conditions, THP tends to self-aggregate via its juxtamembrane zona pellucida (ZP) domain, forming filament-like polymers [16]. Despite its abundance, interesting physicochemical properties and tissue specificity, the biological function(s) of THP have remained elusive [12,17]. The protein has been proposed to be a defender against type 1-fimbriated *E. coli*, a modulator of renal cytokine levels, a contributor to the water impermeability of the thick ascending limb of Henle's loop and a regulator of renal mineral crystallization.

Since the identification of THP as one of the major protein components in human renal stones, a number of *in vitro* studies have been carried out with purified THP, yielding conflicting results. Depending on the experimental conditions used, the methodology and the THP concentrations, THP was observed to act as a promoter or an inhibitor, or to have no effect on calcium oxalate crystallization [12,18-20]. Therefore, despite intense research, the role of THP in crystallization *in vivo* remained a mystery.

To better understand the role(s) of THP in renal physiology and diseases, two independent knockout mouse models were created that used the homologous recombination approach to ablate the THP gene in the mouse embryonic stem (ES) cells [21,22]. For the sake of brevity, work from only one of the knockout models (generated in the laboratory of the first author of this paper) will be described here [23]. Mice derived from the genetically engineered ES cells were completely viable, thrived, bred normally and exhibited no noticeable behavioral changes. Unlike the wild-type mice which strongly expressed THP, THP was completely absent in the kidney and urine of the THP KO mice, as evidenced by Northern blotting, RT-PCR, Western blotting and immunohistochemical staining. When subjected to von Kossa staining, kidneys of THP KO mice but not the wild-type controls contained micro-crystals, mainly in the renal papillary region [23]. The great majority of the crystals were located interstitially or in the basement membrane zone [24]. These crystals were distinctively light-reflective under polarizing light. By Fourier transform infrared microspectroscopy, these crystals were exclusively calcium phosphate [24]. Overall, 14-17% of the KO mice developed papillary calcinosis from two different cohorts [23,24]. Hemotoxylin/eosin-stained slides revealed no apparent inflammation surrounding the microcrystals. These data provide the first *in vivo* experimental evidence indicating that the loss of THP predisposes mice to spontaneous formation of microcrystals in the kidney.

Although the mechanism whereby THP deficiency leads to renal calcification is currently under study, it is possible that this pathological consequence results from multiple concurrent mechanisms. First, the loss of THP appears to increase the concentration of phosphorus and supersaturation for brushite (calcium phosphate) [24]. The reason for this is currently unclear but may be related to an increased food intake as a compensation for renal loss of sodium and chloride in the THP KO mice. Urinary supersaturation of phosphorus and calcium phosphate may directly result in crystallization, although the cellular steps leading to interstitial crystal deposition remain to be elucidated. Second, the lack of urinary THP may lead to increased crystal interaction with the renal epithelial cells. Indeed, when radiolabeled calcium oxalate monohydrate crystals were incubated with cultured MDCK cells in the presence of whole urines, there were significantly more crystals bound to the MDCK cells with urine from the KO mice than with urine from the wild-type mice [24].

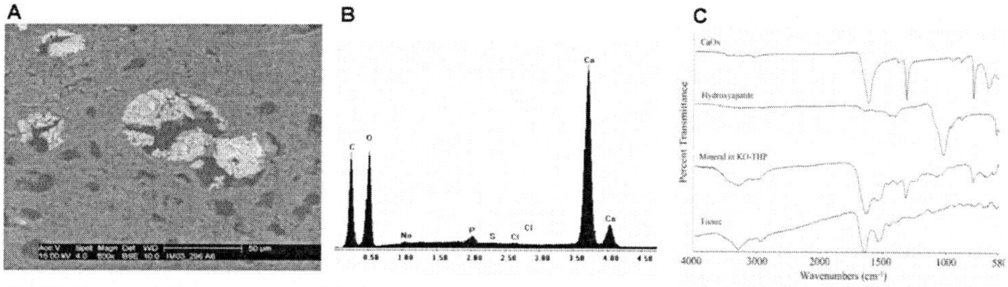

FIGURE 1. A kidney cross-section from a THP KO mouse treated with ethylene glycol was analyzed with scanning EM (**A**), X-ray elemental analysis (**B**) and infrared spectroscopy (**C**). **A**, several plugging intra-tubular crystals in white color. **B**, the crystals consisted of carbon, oxygen and calcium consistent with a calcium oxalate composition. **C**, top two panels represent standard spectra of calcium oxalate (CaOx) and hydroxyapatite; the third spectrum was obtained from crystals from THP KO mouse as in (**A**); the lower spectrum was obtained from a normal mouse kidney. Note that crystals in the KO mouse treated with ethylene glycol had a spectrum similar to CaOx standard.

Not only were the THP KO mice prone to developing spontaneous renal crystals, but they also were highly susceptible to chemically induced hyperoxaluric conditions. When mice were treated in the drinking water with 1% ethylene glycol (a precursor of oxalate) and 4 IU/ml vitamin D3 (which was intended to increase calcium absorption in the intestinal tract), 76% of the THP KO mice developed a large number of crystals in the kidney as revealed by von Kossa staining [23,24]. The crystals were widespread throughout the cross-sections of the kidney with outer medullary regions harboring the most crystals. The crystals were almost exclusively intra-tubular (Figure 1A). The renal epithelial damage and interstitial fibrosis were extensive. Electron microscopy with X-ray elemental analysis (Figure 1B) and infrared spectroscopy (Figure 1C) both showed that the crystals contained calcium oxalate. Wild-type mice were remarkably resistant to renal crystallization despite the fact they were as hyperoxaluric as the THP KO mice [23,24]. Taken together, our results established that THP is a potent inhibitor of both spontaneous and chemically induced renal calcium crystallization, and suggest that quantitative and qualitative defects of THP might be associated with an increased risk of urolithiasis in humans.

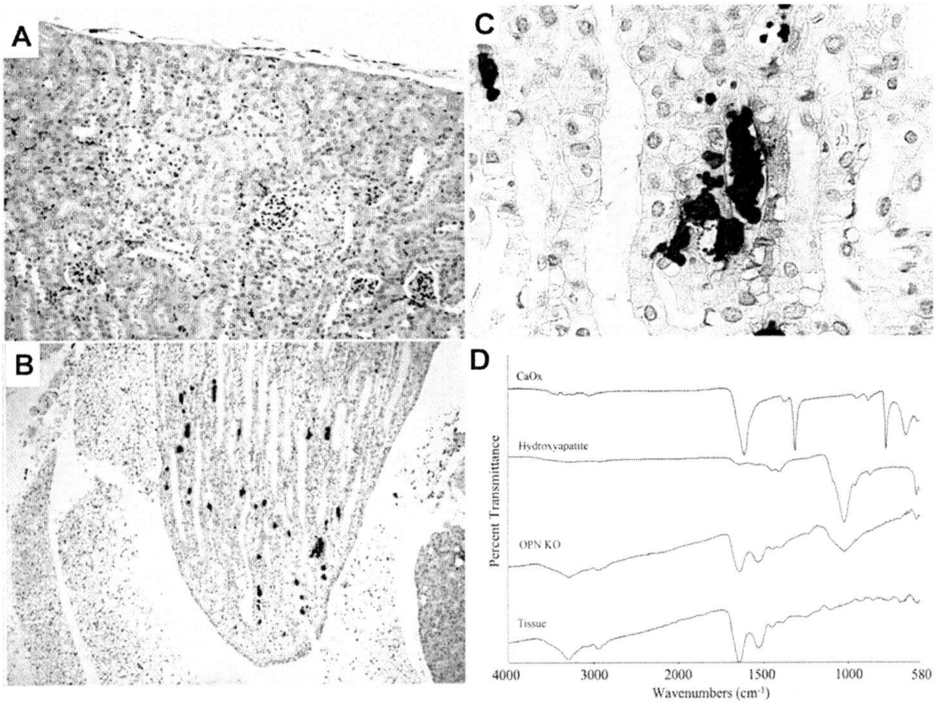

FIGURE 2. Spontaneous renal calcinosis in OPN KO mice. Cross-sections of an OPN KO mouse kidney were stained with a Yasue method (**A-C**) or analyzed with infrared spectroscopy (**D**). Note that the intra-renal crystals were absent in the cortex (**A**), but were abundant in the papilla (**B**) and were interstitial (**C**). Spectroscopy showed that the crystals of the OPN KO mouse consisted of hydroxyapatite.

OSTEOPONTIN AND ITS ABLATION IN MICE

Osteopontin (OPN) is an acidic phosphorylated glycoprotein that was initially isolated from bone matrix, and is believed to play a role in modulating mineralization by enhancing osteoclast activity and by suspending hydroxyapatite crystal growth [25]. Under normal conditions, OPN is also expressed by epithelial cells constituting the ascending limb of Henle's loop, although at a much lower level (4 mg/day) than THP [26]. Evidence supporting a role for OPN as an inhibitor of renal stone formation includes the observations that: OPN is a major component of human renal stones [27]; purified OPN inhibits the nucleation, growth and aggregation of calcium oxalate crystals and reduces binding of the crystals to renal epithelial cells *in vitro* [28]; OPN is up-regulated in renal tubules upon overexposure to calcium oxalate in experimental models [29]; and OPN-knockout mice develop experimentally induced renal stones after exposure to high levels of oxalate [30,31].

Naturally formed crystals had never before been noted within the kidneys of OPN KO mice until recently when we re-examined these mice carefully using von Kossa staining and observed microcrystals within the renal papillae of about 10% of OPN KO mice [24]. Like those in the THP KO mice, crystals in the OPN KO mice were mainly interstitial, were of calcium phosphate by FTIR analysis (Figure 2), and were not associated with any inflammation. The fact that renal papillae in mice are small in size and can be easily missed in cross-sections could explain why crystals were not observed in previous studies [31]. Similar to what Wesson and colleagues reported, the OPN mice also developed intra-tubular crystals under chemically induced hyperoxaluria, although crystallization was much less frequent and crystals were much smaller in size than those in the THP KO mice [24]. Based on these observations, it appears therefore that OPN is a less potent inhibitor of intrarenal calcification than THP. Interestingly, hyperphosphaturia was absent in the OPN KO mice, suggesting that under normal circumstances OPN utilizes different mechanisms to inhibit renal crystallization. Indeed, OPN appeared more potent for preventing calcium oxalate monohydrate crystals from adhering to the MDCK cells *in vitro* [24].

SYNERGY BETWEEN TAMM-HORSFALL PROTEIN AND OSTEOPONTIN

Several observations suggest that THP and OPN might act synergistically to prevent renal crystallization. Both THP and OPN KO mice developed spontaneous and chemically induced renal calcinosis. These two proteins appear to act on different steps in urolithiasis, and in the absence of THP hyperoxaluria triggered a dramatic, (possibly) compensatory induction of OPN [23]. To test this hypothesis, we recently generated mice lacking both THP and OPN [24]. Compared with THP or OPN single knockouts, which developed intra-renal crystals in 17% and 10% of the animals, 39% of the double KO mice formed intrarenal crystals spontaneously [24]. The crystals were also localized to within the papillary region and were largely interstitial. Under ethylene glycol treatment, 71% THP KO mice and 65% OPN KO mice developed renal calcinosis, respectively, whereas 95% double KO mice developed the lesion. After a relatively short (1-month) treatment with ethylene glycol, 18% of the THP/OPN-double null mice developed renal stones at the tip of renal papillae [24]. Some of these stones blocked the distal end of ducts of Bellini, leading to severe dilation of the proximal collecting ducts. Other stones were found in the renal pelvic cavity. Taken together, a recurring theme is emerging that spontaneously formed intra-renal crystals in THP, OPN and double KO mice are primarily interstitial and consist of calcium phosphate. In contrast, under hyperoxaluria the renal crystals are almost exclusively intra-tubular and made of calcium oxalate. Therefore, the location of intra-renal crystals during THP and/or OPN deficiency clearly depends on the underlying conditions. Finally, these data suggest that THP and OPN act synergistically in stone inhibition, and that deficiency of both proteins can render the host more vulnerable to hyperoxaluric conditions than deficiency in either one protein alone.

REDUNDANCY OF MACROMOLECULE INHIBITION

Since urine is often supersaturated, maintaining a crystal-free environment in the kidney requires a highly effective defense mechanism. Emerging evidence from knockout mice suggests that the potency of host urinary defenses may lie in the redundancy of the macromolecules. This was best illustrated by the incomplete penetrance of a crystal-forming phenotype in THP or OPN KO mice [23,24]. Rather, as discussed earlier, only a small percentage of the mice succumbed to renal crystal formation. Moreover, even inactivation of both THP and OPN did not lead to 100% penetrance of spontaneous renal calcinosis. This suggests that other macromolecules present in the urine can continue to function as inhibitors in the absence of THP and/or OPN, thereby compensating for the loss of these proteins. This type of redundancy may be built up gradually as a result of evolutionary pressure. It is worth noting that when overloaded with crystal-forming precursors, the compensatory effects were no longer sufficient for crystal inhibition in the absence of THP and/or OPN [24]. In this regard, it will be extremely interesting to find out whether deficiency of other known or unknown urinary macromolecules can also combine with THP and OPN inhibit renal calcification, and whether their loss can potentiate the effects of THP and OPN loss and significantly increase renal calcification further. The availability of additional KO mice will facilitate such studies. While human mutations affecting multiple genes encoding the urinary macromolecules are unlikely, it is entirely possible that under conditions that impair the renal tubular function the expression of multiple proteins could be affected simultaneously. It is under these conditions that urinary inhibition of crystals could be dramatically compromised and crystallization results. It is well established that human nephrolithiasis is closely associated with reduced renal function [32]. It will be important to determine whether generalized reduced renal function can contribute to stone formation in some of these patients.

ACKNOWLEDGMENTS

The authors acknowledge the grant support from National Institutes of Health (DK56903 and DK69688 to X.-R. Wu; and DK53399 and DK60707 to J.C. Lieske) and Veterans Administration (Merit Review Award). They thank Yasushi Nakagawa for urinalysis and Gerard Farell-Baril for technical assistance.

REFERENCES

1. F. L. Coe, A. Evan and E. Worcester, *J Clin Invest.* **115**, 2598-2608 (2005).
2. S. R. Khan and D. J. Kok, *Front Biosci.* **9**, 1450-1482 (2004).
3. J. R. Hoyer, L. Otvos, Jr. and L. Urge, *Ann N Y Acad Sci.* **760**, 257-265 (1995).
4. O. W. Moe, *Lancet.* **367**, 333-344 (2006).
5. V. Kumar and J. C. Lieske, *Curr Opin Nephrol Hypertens.* **15**, 374-380 (2006).
6. E. M. Worcester, *Semin Nephrol.* **16**, 474-486 (1996).
7. R. L. Ryall, *Pediatr Nephrol.* **10**, 656-666 (1996).
8. S. R. Marengo, M. I. Resnick, L. Yang and J. Y. Chung, *J Urol.* **159**, 1444-1450 (1998).
9. C. Barbas, A. Garcia, L. Saavedra and M. Muros, *J Chromatogr B Analyt Technol Biomed Life Sci.* **781**, 433-455. (2002).
10. M. Asselman and C. F. Verkoelen, *Curr Opin Urol.* **12**, 271-276 (2002).
11. S. R. Khan, *Urol Int.* **59**, 59-71 (1997).
12. F. Serafini-Cessi, N. Malagolini and D. Cavallone, *Am J Kidney Dis.* **42**, 658-676 (2003).
13. M. J. Rindler, S. S. Naik, N. Li, T. C. Hoops and M. N. Peraldi, *J Biol Chem.* **265**, 20784-20789 (1990).
14. D. Cavallone, N. Malagolini and F. Serafini-Cessi, *Biochem Biophys Res Commun.* **280**, 110-114 (2001).
15. S. Fukuoka and K. Kobayashi, *Biochem Biophys Res Commun.* **289**, 1044-1048. (2001).
16. L. Jovine, H. Qi, Z. Williams, E. Litscher and P. M. Wassarman, *Nat Cell Biol.* **4**, 457-461 (2002).
17. S. Kumar and A. Muchmore, *Kidney Int.* **37**, 1395-1401 (1990).
18. G. Bihl and A. Meyers, *Lancet.* **358**, 651-656. (2001).
19. B. Hess, *Urol Res.* **20**, 83-86 (1992).
20. E. M. Worcester, *J Am Soc Nephrol.* **5**, S46-53 (1994).
21. L. Mo, X. H. Zhu, H. Y. Huang, E. Shapiro, D. L. Hasty and X. R. Wu, *Am J Physiol Renal Physiol.* **286**, F795-802 (2004).
22. J. M. Bates, H. M. Raffi, K. Prasadan, R. Mascarenhas, Z. Laszik, N. Maeda, S. J. Hultgren and S. Kumar, *Kidney Int.* **65**, 791-797 (2004).
23. L. Mo, H. Y. Huang, X. H. Zhu, E. Shapiro, D. L. Hasty and X. R. Wu, *Kidney Int.* **66**, 1159-1166 (2004).
24. L. Mo, L. Liaw, A. P. Evan, A. J. Sommer, J. C. Lieske and X. R. Wu, *Am J Physiol Renal Physiol.* **293**, F1935-1943 (2007).
25. M. Mazzali, T. Kipari, V. Ophascharoensuk, J. A. Wesson, R. Johnson and J. Hughes, *Qjm.* **95**, 3-13 (2002).
26. W. Min, H. Shiraga, C. Chalko, S. Goldfarb, G. G. Krishna and J. R. Hoyer, *Kidney Int.* **53**, 189-193 (1998).
27. Y. Xie, M. Sakatsume, S. Nishi, I. Narita, M. Arakawa and F. Gejyo, *Kidney Int.* **60**, 1645-1657 (2001).
28. J. A. Wesson, E. M. Worcester, J. H. Wiessner, N. S. Mandel and J. G. Kleinman, *Kidney Int.* **53**, 952-957. (1998).
29. S. R. Khan, J. M. Johnson, A. B. Peck, J. G. Cornelius and P. A. Glenton, *J Urol.* **168**, 1173-1181 (2002).
30. L. Liaw, D. E. Birk, C. B. Ballas, J. S. Whitsitt, J. M. Davidson and B. L. Hogan, *J Clin Invest.* **101**, 1468-1478 (1998).
31. J. A. Wesson, R. J. Johnson, M. Mazzali, A. M. Beshensky, S. Stietz, C. Giachelli, L. Liaw, C. E. Alpers, W. G. Couser, J. G. Kleinman and J. Hughes, *J Am Soc Nephrol.* **14**, 139-147 (2003).
32. E. M. Worcester, J. H. Parks, A. P. Evan and F. L. Coe, *J Urol.* **176**, 600-603; discussion 603 (2006).

Molecular Basis of Urolithiasis: Role of Crystal Retention

Hari K. Koul and Sweaty Koul

Signal transduction and Molecular Urology Laboratory-Program in Urosciences, Division of Urology-Department of Surgery, School of Medicine, University of Colorado Denver, 4200 E. 9th Ave., Denver, Colorado 80262 USA

Abstract. Urolithiasis is a multifactorial disorder, and it is unlikely that a single cause is responsible for entire spectrum of this disorder. Nonetheless, increased concentrations of various urinary constituents (e.g., calcium and/or oxalate) have been associated with a majority of stone formers. Irrespective of the underlying metabolic conditions, crystal precipitation and crystal retention along the urinary tract are two essential pre-requisites for urinary tract stone formation. In this chapter we summarize underlying metabolic abnormalities associated with various sub-sets of stone formers. We will also present evidence in support of our hypothesis that crystal formation is a normal physiological process of eliminating toxic wastes as solid complexes, and that pathological events begin with crystal retention. In the end we present evidence supporting various mechanisms of crystal retention.

Keywords: crystal formation, crystal retention, tubular damage, Randall's Plaques, signaling events, inflammation
PACS: 87.15.nt

OVERVIEW AND UNDERLYING METABOLIC CONDITIONS

Nephrolithiasis is one of the oldest diseases afflicting mankind, with the earliest recorded example dating back to 324 BC. In the United States, the prevalence of renal calculi is estimated to be 2-3%, and the likelihood that a Caucasian male will develop stone disease by age 70 is about 1 in 8 [1,2]. Presently it is estimated that 720,000 Americans suffer from stone episodes yearly. Based on these estimates, 12 to 24 million Americans will develop stones in their lifetime. This disorder is predominant in 30-39 year old Caucasian males. Thus, the disease strikes during mid-adulthood, the most productive time of life. Human kidney stones are composed of crystals and organic material, up to 98% of the stone being crystalline. Approximately 80% of kidney stones are made of calcium oxalate. Despite the prevalence of this disorder, the exact mechanism for the initiation of renal stone formation is not fully understood. Idiopathic calcium oxalate nephrolithiasis is a multi- factorial disease [1] and it is unlikely that a single underlying condition will be responsible for the entire spectrum of this disease; however it appears that two important factors in its pathogenesis are abnormalities in calcium and oxalate metabolism. Hyperoxaluria and Hypercalciuria are the two most commonly associated risk factors for stone formation.

CP1049, *Renal Stone Disease 2, 2nd International Urolithiasis Research Symposium,*
edited by A. P. Evan, J. E. Lingeman, J. A. McAteer, and J. C. Williams, Jr.

With the advent of extracorporeal shock wave lithotripsy (ESWL) and refinements in percutaneous nephrolithotomy (PCNL), interventional approaches to treat renal stone disease have become less morbid. However, these interventions do not treat the underlying disease. Moreover, despite these advances in interventional approaches, the incidence of stone disease is on the rise in the US. Many of these procedures are also injurious to the kidney and are associated with increase recurrence rates. Progress in understanding the molecular basis of this multi-factorial disease has been slow.

Factors associated with urolithiasis can be broadly characterized as extrinsic and intrinsic categories (Figure 1). The extrinsic factors that influence stone disease are diet, environmental and geographic factors, seasonal and climatic factors and water intake. For instance, increased animal protein consumption, hot climates, foods rich in oxalate and low water intake, all increase the risk of urolithiasis. All these factors influence crystal formation in the kidney. The intrinsic factors include genetic background, age and sex, metabolic disorders, intestinal mal-absorption syndromes, renal tubular acidosis, and as yet uncharacterized renal dysfunction [3].

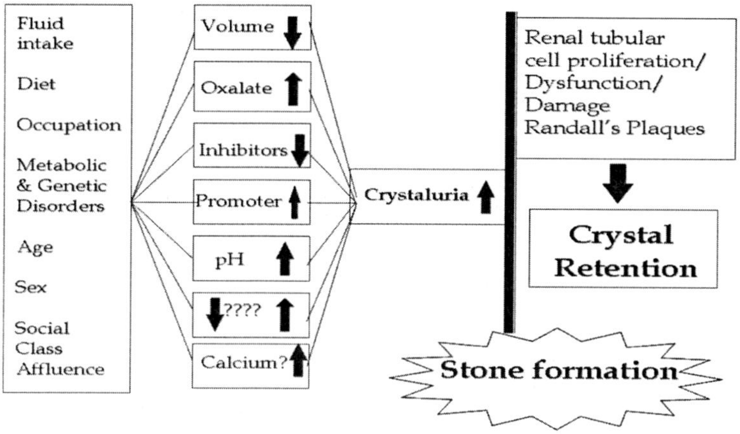

FIGURE 1. Extrinsic and Intrinsic factors and their influences on urinary constituents associated with crystal formation, and factors that promote crystal retention

The genetic background of an individual may play an important role in stone formation; for instance, the incidence of stone disease is lower in Blacks compared to Caucasians. Similarly, the age and sex of an individual may influence stone formation; the incidence of stone disease in males is three times that of females and peak incidence of stone disease occurs during third and fourth decade of life. Examples of rare hereditary disorders are primary hyperoxaluria, cystinuria, and xanthinuria. These conditions promote stone formation by directly increasing the concentrations of respective metabolites in the urine, and thus overwhelming the kidney. Metabolic disorders and intestinal malabsorption syndromes may also influence stone disease by increasing renal load of oxalate and or calcium resulting in excessive crystalline waste in the renal tubules. Renal Tubular Acidosis (RTA) is a clinical syndrome resulting from specific defects in renal tubular H^+ secretion and urinary acidification. RTA is classified as distal RTA (types I and III), proximal RTA (type II) and or diabetes-associated RTA (type IV). Up to 70% of adults with distal RTA have kidney stones, but the stones are mostly calcium phosphate. Type II RTA and type IV RTA are not known to increase the risk of stone formation.

From a simple physicochemical standpoint, for stones to form, urine has to be saturated with respect to the precipitating salts. Thus for calcium oxalate stones to form, the urinary concentrations of calcium and oxalate must rise above the solubility factor for these ions. Indeed, the distal tubular fluid in all individuals is supersaturated with respect to calcium and oxalate and these ions do nucleate to form calcium oxalate crystals. An increase in urinary constituent metabolites would promote increased crystal precipitation in the renal tubules. However, crystal formation is by no means equivalent to symptomatic stone disease, since most of the solid particles crystallizing within the urinary tract will be excreted freely [4,5]. In addition, crystaluria alone does not appear to distinguish stone formers from healthy people [4-8]. Finlayson calculated that given the most favorable conditions, it will take ~10h for a 1 mm calcium oxalate crystal to grow large enough to block the duct of Bellini, and become the nidus of a urinary stone [6]. Given the normal physiological parameters of urine flow and ionic concentrations, it is unlikely that single, free-standing crystals will be able to grow large enough in time to block the tubules in which they are formed. The crystals formed in the renal tubules are washed away with the free flowing urine.

Because of the short transit time from glomerulus to the renal pelvis, crystalline particles formed in urine flowing freely through the renal tubule cannot attain the dimensions required to block a collecting duct and form a urinary microlith. Thus for renal stone formation, crystals should be able to either grow large enough to block the renal tubules or alternately attach themselves to the lining of the renal tubules. Moreover, the normal lining of the renal tubules, the renal tubular epithelial cells, interact with the crystals in a dynamic fashion which remains poorly understood to date. The mechanism of stone formation is clearly more complex than a mere increase in the crystal formation. These considerations suggest the attachment of crystals to the renal epithelial cells and the cellular responses to crystal interaction are critical in understanding the pathogenesis of urolithiasis.

MOLECULAR MECHANISMS OF CRYSTAL RETENTION

Calcium oxalate crystal-cell interaction is a subject of active investigation in several laboratories [7-10]. Several proteins have been identified on renal cells that interact with crystals. We and others have shown that the interaction of calcium oxalate monohydrate (COM) crystals with renal epithelial cells results in a program of events, including alterations in gene expression, initiation of DNA synthesis, cell growth and death. Our studies have demonstrated that crystal cell interaction results in activation of p38 mitogen-activated protein kinase (p38 MAPK) signaling pathway, which plays an important role in modulating the response of renal epithelial cells to the COM crystals [11-12].

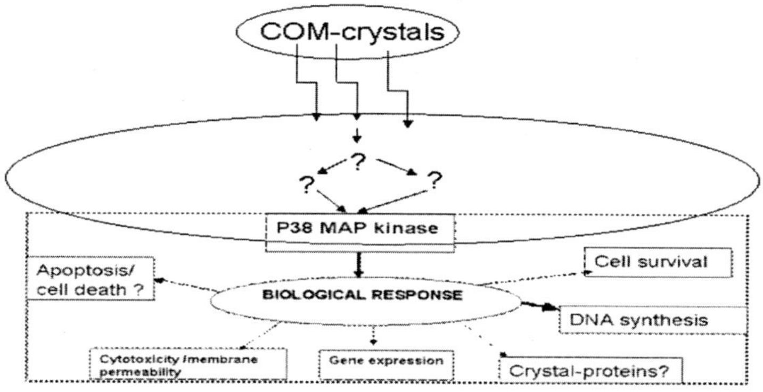

FIGURE 2. Schematic depiction of the role of p38 MAP kinase signal transduction pathway in mediating the effects of calcium-oxalate crystals (COM crystals) in renal epithelial cells: COM crystals interact with specific receptor sites on the cell membrane and activate p38 MAP kinase pathway by mechanisms that are not clearly understood. Inhibition of the p38 MAP kinase pathway resulted in modulation of several of the downstream targets that are activated by COM-crystals.

Based on these studies we hypothesis that the p38 MAPK signal transduction pathway plays a central role in mediating the effects of calcium-oxalate crystals and in modulating the cellular responses to calcium oxalate crystals (Figure 2). Although these exciting studies point to specific pathways, it is too early to define final and selective targets in stone disease. Additional studies in this direction are warranted. It is important to point out here that many of the conclusions drawn from studies to date are based on oxalate and crystal interactions in the renal cortical epithelial cells and little is known about these interactions in the papillary region, which is actual site of crystal retention.

In a series of excellent investigations, Evan et al. have demonstrated direct attachment of kidney stones with Randall's plaques in the papillary region, suggesting an important role for Randall's plaques in crystal retention [13]. However, the molecular events that lead to Randall's plaque formation remain unclear at present. In general, progress in our understanding of molecular events in the renal papillary region has been hampered by lack of human papillary epithelial cells. Recently we reported the establishment of primary cultures of epithelial cells (hIMCD cells: human Inner Medullary Collecting Duct cells) lining the papillary region [14]. The hIMCD cells grew in a monolayer. Cells showed the expression of epithelial specific markers, including cytokeratin, the tight-junction marker zonula occludens-1 and the cytoskeletal protein vimentin. They lacked expression of factor VIII, which is a glycoprotein synthesized by endothelial cells. To our knowledge we also noted for the first time uroplakin expression in collecting duct epithelial cells. This expression was maintained in primary culture. The hIMCD cells in culture were highly resistant to hypertonic solutions and they responded to hypertonicity by over-expression of cyclooxygenase-2. Moreover, these cells also survived prolonged periods of hypoxia. We have also established a continuous cell line by transfecting these cells with telomerase gene using an adenoviral vector system (unpublished work, Khandrika et al). Studies characterizing this cell line are currently underway in our laboratories. This cell line should provide an excellent tool for the investigation of the various molecular events that are associated with crystal attachment in the papillary region.

CRYSTAL RETENTION IS THE KEY TO UNDERSTANDING PATHOLOGICAL EVENTS ASSOCIATED WITH STONE FORMATION

We believe that crystal formation in the urinary tract is an efficient physiological process for conserving water and excreting toxic wastes as calcium complexes. The renal tubular epithelium is specially designed to handle crystalline waste. Crystal *retention* in the kidney is a pathological event, which is facilitated: a) when the load of urinary crystals overwhelms the defense mechanisms, and/or b) by tubular epithelial cell dysfunction. A hypothetical model describing the renal cell crystal handling is presented in Figure 3.

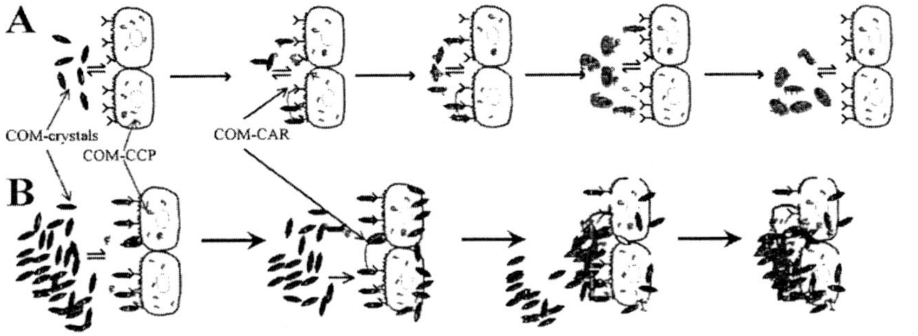

FIGURE 3. Hypothetical model system depicting crystal interactions with the renal cells. A) COM crystals interact with specific receptors on the renal epithelial cells. This crystal-cell interaction results in secretion of proteins that interact with the crystal surfaces and cover them. The coated crystals are not able to bind to the lining of the urinary tract and are eliminated harmlessly in the urine. B) When crystal load is in excess of what cells can handle or when the cells are dysfunctional—or when Randall's plaques are exposed to urinary milieu—crystals continue to bind in an uninterrupted fashion and eventually result in clinical stone disease.

Based on our model system, normal crystal interaction with the renal epithelial cells results in secretion and synthesis of proteins that cover the crystal surfaces. These coated crystals are harmlessly excreted in the urine (Figure 3A). On the other hand, when the calcium oxalate crystal load overwhelms the system, or if the cells are dysfunctional, or if Randall's Plaques are exposed to urinary milieu (Figure 3B), these crystal-coating mechanisms are inadequate and crystals continue to attach to the cells, initiating crystal retention. The underlying metabolic or genetic factors as well as dietary and other associated factors fit in this model system. For example, hyperoxaluria and other nephrotoxins that promote tubular damage will increase the incidence of crystal retention. Similarly hypercalciuria and other associated factors that may increase the incidence of calcium phosphate deposits in the kidney (e.g., Randall's plaques) will also promote crystal retention. Understanding the specific molecular events that are associated with crystal retention should help us develop strategies to inhibit the pathologic effects of calcium-oxalate and prevent crystal retention and renal stone formation. These mechanisms will be actively pursued in coming years.

ACKNOWLEDGMENTS

Financial support from NIH-NIDDK R01 DK54084 and Academic Enrichment funds from the University of Colorado Denver, School of Medicine and Department of Surgery are gratefully acknowledged.

REFERENCES

1. M. Menon and H. Koul. *J Clin Endocrinol Metab* 74(4):703-707, 1992.
2. J. Uribarri, M.S. Oh, and H.J. Carroll. *Ann Intern Med* 111(12):1006-1009, 1989.
3. F L. Coe, A. Evan, and E. Worcester. *J Clin Invest* 115(10):2598-2608, 2005.
4. B. Hess and D.J. Kok. Nucleation, growth, and aggregation of stone-forming crystals. In: *Kidney Stones: Medical and Surgical Management.* (Coe FL. Ed). Lippincott-Raven Publishers. Philadelphia, 1996.
5. J.S. Elliot and I.N. Rabinowitz. *J Urol* 123:324-327, 1980.
6. B. Finlayson and S. Reid. *Invest Urol* 15:442-448, 1978.
7. J.H. Wiessner, A.T. Hasegawa, L.Y. Hung, G.S. Mandel and N.S. Mandel. *Kidney Int* 59(2):637-44, 2001.
8. N.L. Miller, A.P. Evan and J.E. Lingeman. *Urol Clin North Am* 34(3):295-313, 2007.
9. S.R. Khan. *Urol Res* 34(2):86-91, 2006.
10. H.K. Koul, S. Koul, S. Fu, V. Santosham, A. Seikhon and M. Menon. *J Am Soc Nephrol* Suppl14:S417-21, 1999.
11. L.S. Chaturvedi, S. Koul, A. Sekhon, A. Bhandari, M. Menon and H.K. Koul. *J Biol Chem* 277(15):13321-30, 2002.
12. H. Koul, M. Menon, L.S. Chaturvedi, S. Koul, A. Sekhon, A. Bhandari and M. Huang. *J Biol Chem* 277(39):36845-52, 2002.
13. B.R. Matlaga, F.L. Coe, A.P. Evan and J.E. Lingeman. *J Urol* 177(1):31-8, 2007.
14. L. Khandrika, F.J. Kim, A. Campagna , S. Koul, R.B. Meacham and H.K. Koul. *J Urol* 179(5):2057-63, 2008.

Hyaluronan: A Matrix Component

Louise Rügheimer

Division of Integrative Physiology, Department of Medical Cell Biology, Biomedical Centre, PO Box 571, SE-751 23 Uppsala, Sweden
louise.rugheimer@mcb.uu.se

Abstract. The glucosaminoglycan hyaluronan is a key component of the extracellular matrix. It is a large, negatively charged molecule that can act as an ion exchange reservoir for positive ions. Hyaluronan is involved in renomedullary water handling through its water-binding capacity. In the renal medulla, the main source for hyaluronan production is the renomedullary interstitial cells. Hyaluronan synthases are found in the inner part of the plasma membrane and polymerize hyaluronan chains which are extruded into the extracellular space. Hyaluronidases are a family of enzymes involved in the degradation of hyaluronan. They have a wide range of properties, including differences in size, inhibitor sensitivities, catalytic mechanisms, substrate specificities and pH optima.

Keywords: Hyaluronan, renomedullary interstitial cells
PACS: 66.20.–d; 82.70.–y

HYALURONAN

Hyaluronan is a major structural component of the extracellular matrix and belongs to the family of glycosaminoglycans. Hyaluronan is a linear, high molecular weight polysaccharide composed of repeating disaccharide units of D-glucuronic acid (GlcUA) and N-acetyl-D-glucosamine (GlcNAc) (Figure 1).

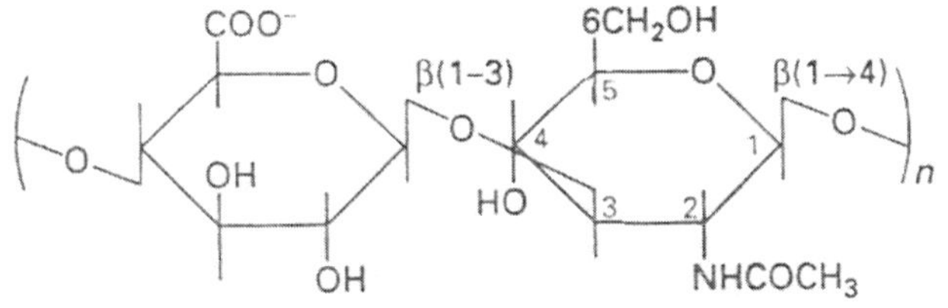

FIGURE 1. D-Glucuronic acid (left) and N-Acetyl-D-glucosamine (right), the two components that form the disaccharide that when repeated makes up the hyaluronan molecule.

If stretched end-to-end, one molecule would be 20 mm long, but individual segments of a hyaluronan molecule fold into a rod-like conformation because of the β linkages and extensive intrachain hydrogen bonding between adjacent sugar residues [1,2]. Hyaluronan is negatively charged due to ionization of the carboxyl groups of the glucuronic acid constituents at physiological pH [3]. The repulsion between the

CP1049, *Renal Stone Disease 2, 2nd International Urolithiasis Research Symposium,*
edited by A. P. Evan, J. E. Lingeman, J. A. McAteer, and J. C. Williams, Jr.

negatively charged carboxylate groups that protrude outward at regular intervals also contributes to the structure of the molecule [2]. Unlike other glycosaminoglycans, hyaluronan is neither sulfated nor does the primary structure contain peptide [3].

The negatively charged network attracts cations, for example Ca^{2+}, that give hyaluronan high osmotic activity and attract large amounts of water through osmosis. When hyaluronan in solution reaches a concentration of approximately 0.1 mg/ml, the molecule can form an entangled network: one gram of hyaluronan binds up to one liter of water. Given no constraints, a hyaluronan molecule will occupy a volume about 1000 times the space of the molecule itself. When placed in a confining space, such as in the extracellular matrix, the hyaluronan molecule will push outward, creating a turgor pressure that increases with the amount of water in the gel [2].

Hyaluronan is implicated in basic biological processes such as cell proliferation, differentiation, and migration. In pathological processes with enhanced extracellular matrix metabolism, such as rheumatoid arthritis and cancer, hyaluronan is recognized as one of key participants [4].

HYALURONAN RECEPTORS

Hyaluronan interacts with cell surface receptors [5]. Several hyaluronan receptors have been identified: CD44, RHAMM (receptor for hyaluronan mediated motility), LEC (liver endothelial cell clearance receptor), HARE (hyaluronan receptor for endocytosis), layilin and LYVE-1 (hyaluronan receptor in the lymphatic vessel endothelium) [6-8].

CD44 is the best studied and most common hyaluronan receptor found in a variety of cells [9-11]. The CD44 receptor is a transmembrane glycoprotein and consists of four functional domains. The receptor is known to participate in matrix-cell signaling, cell migration, cell-cell aggregation and receptor mediated internalization/degradation of hyaluronan [12,13].

Hyaluronan binds not only to these surface receptors but also to aggrecans, which are peptide cores associated with glycosaminoglycans, and other proteins in the extracellular matrix. The binding is reinforced by small link proteins that aggregate onto the hyaluronan chain. Binding to these proteins is considered important, for the arrangement and modulation of the extracellular matrix.

TURNOVER OF HYALURONAN—SYNTHESIS

There are three homologous mammalian hyaluronan synthases known as HAS 1, 2 and 3 [14-16]. They have impressive catalytic activity and can polymerize about 100 monosaccharide/sec *in vitro* [17]. HAS 1 and HAS 2 polymerize hyaluronan chains of similar lengths between $2x10^5$–$2x10^6$ Da, whereas HAS 3 polymerizes shorter hyaluronan chains, in the range of $<2x10^5$ Da to $3x10^5$ Da (Figure 2).

Hyaluronan chains of different lengths have different effects on cell behavior. Short hyaluronan chains stimulate cell proliferation and initiate signaling cascades; they may be involved in angiogenesis and inflammatory responses. High-molecular-weight hyaluronan chains are antiangiogenic and have the opposite effect of inhibiting cell proliferation [3,18-22].

Hyaluronan synthases are found in the inner part of the plasma membrane and newly synthesized hyaluronan is extruded into the extracellular space [23,24]. Renomedullary interstitial cells are major producers of hyaluronan and the level of hyaluronan in the supernatant of renomedullary interstitial cells in culture changes according to the osmotic power of the culture media [25,26].

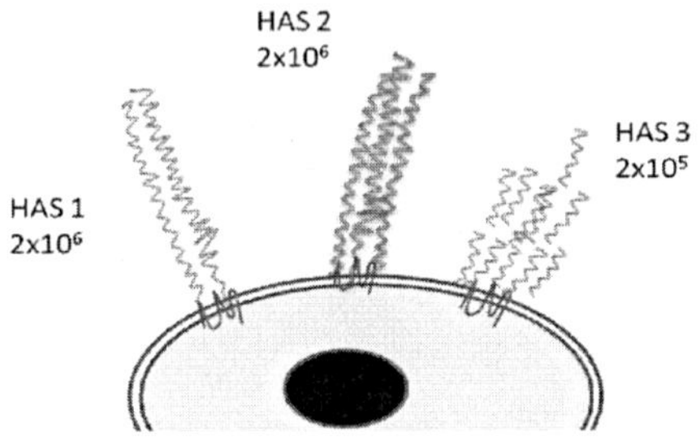

FIGURE 2. A schematic picture of a cell synthesizing hyaluronan. Hyaluronan synthase (HAS) 1 produces small amounts of high-molecular-weight hyaluronan. HAS 2 produces more high-molecular-weight hyaluronan. HAS 3 is the most active of the hyaluronan synthases, yet produces low molecular weight hyaluronan chains.

TURNOVER OF HYALURONAN—CATABOLISM

Hyaluronidases (HYAL) are a family of enzymes involved in the degradation of hyaluronan [1]. They have a wide range of properties, including differences in size, inhibitor sensitivities, catalytic mechanisms, substrate specificities and pH optima [27-29]. There are six known human isoforms of hyaluronidase; HYAL 1-6 [27,29-31].

Normal turnover of plasma hyaluronan is about 15-35% a minute [32] and tissue half-life of hyaluronan ranges from 0.5 to 3 days. When reaching the blood stream, 85-90% of hyaluronan is eliminated in the liver by receptor-facilitated uptake. The kidney extracts about 10% but excretes only 1-2% in the urine. The lymph nodes also have a capacity for extraction and catabolism of hyaluronan. The lymphatic system is only present in the renal cortex (not in the medulla), where it can drain the interstitium of larger molecules, such as hyaluronan.

The levels and/or expression of hyaluronidases are changed in the tissues, sera, or urine in cases of disease, such as cancer and diabetes [33-38]. The connections of these changes to the pathogenesis of these diseases are not clear.

The CD44 receptor is involved in the turnover of hyaluronan through uptake and intracellular breakdown by acid hydrolysis in lysosomes, as has been shown for macrophages, cultured fibroblasts and chondrocytes [12,13]. The process involves hyaluronan being tethered to the cell surface by CD44 in caveolin-enriched invaginations. It is cleaved to 20 kDa fragments by HYAL 2 on the plasma membrane, endocytosed, and ultimately delivered to low pH intracellular organelles/lysosomes, where it is further digested by HYAL 1 [39].

Many biological systems are under negative control. Stimulation of synthesis does not usually occur when quick responses are required; instead, there is a release from negative control. Inhibition of catabolism by hyaluronidase inhibitors may be responsible for the release from negative control and quick rate of hyaluronan increase. Little is known about hyaluronidase inhibitors, but levels of hyaluronidase inhibitors are elevated in the serum of cancer patients and in liver disease [40,41].

THE ROLE OF HYALURONAN IN THE KIDNEY

Hyaluronan is found predominantly in the renal inner medulla (papilla), whereas, in the renal cortex, hyaluronan content is low and only about 1-3% of that in the renal medulla [42-45] (Figure 3). This heterogeneous distribution is important for the ability to produce concentrated or dilute urine during normal physiological conditions. Hyaluronan plays an important role in water homeostasis through the distribution and movement of water [1], and together with vasopressin regulated aquaporins to determine water reabsorption in the medullary structures.

Hyaluronan and water form gel-like structures at low hyaluronan concentrations (about 0.1 mg/ml), which in turn create a swelling of the extracellular matrix. The gels formed have different pore sizes and charge density; they are selective and can regulate the traffic of molecules and cells according to their size and/or charge (steric exclusion) [46]. The renomedullary content of hyaluronan in the rat during baseline conditions has been calculated to about 0.6 mg/ml [44]; i.e., the medullary interstitium behaves as a gel. The antagonism of water reabsorption by interstitial hyaluronan may involve changes in the interstitial hydrostatic pressure. Elevations in hyaluronan decreases water transport and an intraperitoneal injection of hyaluronan decreases peritoneal fluid absorption [47,48]. In the interstitium, hyaluronan diminishes the water permeability of the membrane [49,50].

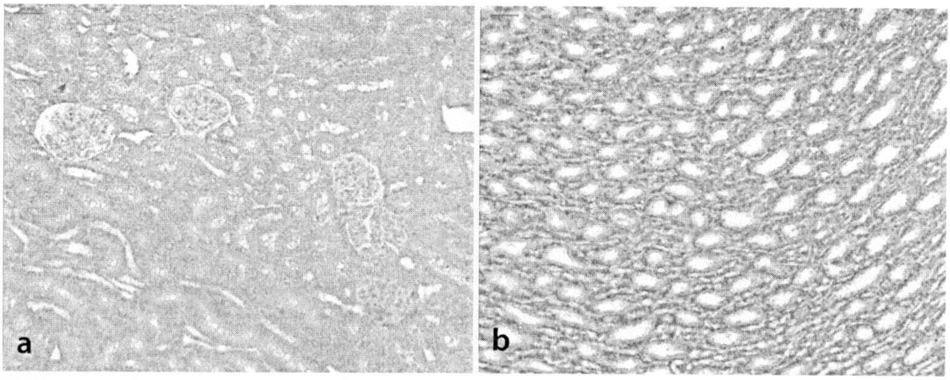

FIGURE 3. Histochemical staining for interstitial hyaluronan in sections of renal cortex and medulla from rats. The renal cortex (a) is virtually devoid of hyaluronan and contains only a few percent of that in the medulla (b). The interstitial hyaluronan is seen as dark-purple staining. Bar represents 50 μm

When urine is formed, the pelvic wall contracts in order to force the urine out of the kidney and down along the ureter. This force compresses the hyaluronan gel structure in the medullary interstitium and can theoretically give rise to two types of effects for inner medullary concentration. One is the lowering of osmolality in the surrounding interstitial fluid and the other is to use the stored mechanical energy to drive water absorption from the tubule. Hyaluronan may in this respect function as a mechano-osmotic transducer [32]. The contractions are shown in hamster papillae which are very long and thin [51]. The effects are if any smaller in the rat or human papilla that is wider and thicker.

Hyaluronan is involved in water homeostasis, during acute hydration medullary hyaluronan increases [44,45,52], which can reduce water reabsorption across the interstitium. In contrast, medullary hyaluronan content decreases during water deprivation/dehydration leading to increased water reabsorption across the interstitium. This implies that the mechanisms by which hyaluronan regulates renal water handling are different to that of vasopressin, as the latter increases during water deprivations leading to increased insertion of aquaporins and water permeability. A tubular system with large amounts of vasopressin regulated aquaporins situated in an interstitial environment with reduced hyaluronan content should allow excessive water reabsorption. In 1958, Ginetzinsky found that the amount of hyaluronidase excreted in the urine increases during dehydration and drops to zero after hydration [53]. This suggests that elevated hyaluronidase activity during dehydration reduces interstitial hyaluronan, and vice versa.

Under pathological conditions, hyaluronan is inappropriately regulated. During renal ischemia-reperfusion injury, tubulointerstitial inflammation and renal transplant rejection renal cortical levels of hyaluronan increase heavily, whereas renal papillary levels are largely unaltered, which may contribute to the pathophysiology of the disease process [42,54-56].

RENOMEDULLARY INTERSTITIAL CELLS (RMIC)

Renomedullary interstitial cells are fibroblasts and the major contributors of hyaluronan in the renal medulla. Renomedullary interstitial cells in culture produce less hyaluronan during hyperosmotic conditions than during iso- and hypoosmotic conditions, supporting the *in vivo* observations that hyaluronan content decreases during dehydration and increases during hydration [25,26]. Furthermore, CD44 expression on medullary interstitial cells increases during hyperosmotic conditions and decreases during hypo-osmotic conditions [26] and can provide a mechanism to increase/decrease the intracellular breakdown of hyaluronan, leading to changes in interstitial hyaluronan during dehydration and hydration. The vasopressin receptor V_1 is present on renomedullary interstitial cells [8]. Vasopressin increases prostaglandin (PGE_2) production in renomedullary interstitial cells, and prostaglandin (PGE_2) increases hyaluronan production [57,58]. The angiotensin receptors AT_1 and AT_2 are found on medullary interstitial cells as well as many other receptors for vasoactive peptides [59].

REFERENCES

1. J. R. Fraser, T. C. Laurent and U. B. Laurent, J Intern Med **242** (1), 27-33 (1997).
2. H. Lodish, Berk, A., Zipursky, L., Matsudaira, P., Baltimore, D., Darnell, J. , *Molecular cell biology*, 4 ed. (W.H. Freeman and Company, New York, 2002).
3. T. C. Laurent and J. R. Fraser, Faseb J **6** (7), 2397-2404 (1992).
4. B. P. Toole, Q. Yu and C. B. Underhill, Methods Mol Biol **171**, 479-485 (2001).
5. B. P. Toole, J Clin Invest **106** (3), 335-336 (2000).
6. D. G. Jackson, Trends Cardiovasc Med **13** (1), 1-7 (2003).
7. P. Bono, K. Rubin, J. M. Higgins and R. O. Hynes, Mol Biol Cell **12** (4), 891-900 (2001).
8. J. L. Zhuo, Clin Exp Pharmacol Physiol **27** (7), 465-473 (2000).
9. B. P. Toole, Curr Opin Cell Biol **2** (5), 839-844 (1990).
10. C. Underhill, J Cell Sci **103 (Pt 2)**, 293-298 (1992).
11. P. Lesavre, G. Choukroun, A. Francois, L. H. Noel, L. Mecarelli and D. Droz, Adv Nephrol Necker Hosp **26**, 317-339 (1997).
12. M. Culty, H. A. Nguyen and C. B. Underhill, J Cell Biol **116** (4), 1055-1062 (1992).
13. Q. Hua, C. B. Knudson and W. Knudson, J Cell Sci **106 (Pt 1)**, 365-375 (1993).
14. A. P. Spicer, M. L. Augustine and J. A. McDonald, J Biol Chem **271** (38), 23400-23406 (1996).
15. P. H. Weigel, V. C. Hascall and M. Tammi, J Biol Chem **272** (22), 13997-14000 (1997).
16. P. L. DeAngelis, Cell Mol Life Sci **56** (7-8), 670-682 (1999).
17. Varki, *Essential Glycobiology*, 1 ed. (The consortium of glycobiology Editors, Los Angeles, 1999).
18. W. D. Comper and T. C. Laurent, Physiol Rev **58** (1), 255-315 (1978).
19. R. Deed, P. Rooney, P. Kumar, J. D. Norton, J. Smith, A. J. Freemont and S. Kumar, Int J Cancer **71** (2), 251-256 (1997).
20. D. C. West, I. N. Hampson, F. Arnold and S. Kumar, Science **228** (4705), 1324-1326 (1985).
21. M. Slevin, J. Krupinski, S. Kumar and J. Gaffney, Lab Invest **78** (8), 987-1003 (1998).
22. V. B. Lokeshwar and M. G. Selzer, J Biol Chem **275** (36), 27641-27649 (2000).
23. P. Prehm, Biochem J **220** (2), 597-600 (1984).
24. L. H. Philipson and N. B. Schwartz, J Biol Chem **259** (8), 5017-5023 (1984).
25. P. Hansell, C. Maric, D. Alcorn, V. Goransson, C. Johnsson and R. Hallgren, Acta Physiol Scand **165** (1), 115-116 (1999).
26. V. Goransson, P. Hansell, S. Moss, D. Alcorn, C. Johnsson, R. Hallgren and C. Maric, Matrix Biol **20** (2), 129-136 (2001).
27. G. Kreil, Protein Sci **4** (9), 1666-1669 (1995).
28. G. I. Frost, Csoka, T., Stern, R., Trends in glycoscience and glycotechnology **8** (44), 419-434 (1996).
29. A. B. Csoka, G. I. Frost and R. Stern, Matrix Biol **20** (8), 499-508 (2001).
30. A. J. Bollet, W. M. Bonner, Jr. and J. L. Nance, J Biol Chem **238**, 3522-3527 (1963).
31. L. Sun, E. Feusi, A. Sibalic, B. Beck-Schimmer and R. P. Wuthrich, Kidney Blood Press Res **21** (6), 413-418 (1998).
32. M. A. Knepper, G. M. Saidel, V. C. Hascall and T. Dwyer, Am J Physiol Renal Physiol **284** (3), F433-446 (2003).
33. V. B. Lokeshwar, B. L. Lokeshwar, H. T. Pham and N. L. Block, Cancer Res **56** (3), 651-657 (1996).
34. V. B. Lokeshwar, M. J. Young, G. Goudarzi, N. Iida, A. I. Yudin, G. N. Cherr and M. G. Selzer, Cancer Res **59** (17), 4464-4470 (1999).
35. A. Laudat, J. Guechot, K. Lecourbe, R. Damade and A. M. Palluel, Clin Chim Acta **301** (1-2), 159-167 (2000).
36. P. Bertrand, N. Girard, C. Duval, J. d'Anjou, C. Chauzy, J. F. Menard and B. Delpech, Int J Cancer **73** (3), 327-331 (1997).
37. K. Tamakoshi, F. Kikkawa, O. Maeda, N. Suganuma, S. Yamagata, T. Yamagata and Y. Tomoda, Br J Cancer **75** (12), 1807-1811 (1997).
38. M. Ikegami-Kawai, R. Okuda, T. Nemoto, N. Inada and T. Takahashi, Glycobiology **14** (1), 65-72 (2004).
39. B. Formby and R. Stern, Biochem Biophys Res Commun **305** (1), 203-208 (2003).
40. R. Stern, Eur J Cell Biol **83** (7), 317-325 (2004).
41. K. Mio and R. Stern, Matrix Biol **21** (1), 31-37 (2002).
42. C. Johnsson, G. Tufveson, J. Wahlberg and R. Hallgren, Kidney Int **50** (4), 1224-1229 (1996).
43. A. F. Wells, E. Larsson, A. Tengblad, B. Fellstrom, G. Tufveson, L. Klareskog and T. C. Laurent, Transplantation **50** (2), 240-243 (1990).
44. P. Hansell, V. Goransson, C. Odlind, B. Gerdin and R. Hallgren, Kidney Int **58** (5), 2061-2068 (2000).
45. V. Goransson, C. Johnsson, O. Nylander and P. Hansell, J Physiol **542** (Pt 1), 315-322 (2002).

46. Alberts, *Molecular biology of the cell*, 4 ed. (Garland Science, New York, 2002).
47. T. Wang, H. H. Cheng, O. Heimburger, C. Chen, J. Waniewski, J. Bergstrom and B. Lindholm, Kidney Int **55** (2), 667-673 (1999).
48. T. Wang, H. H. Cheng, O. Heimburger, J. Waniewski, J. Bergstrom and B. Lindholm, Kidney Int **53** (2), 496-502 (1998).
49. S. J. Lai-Fook and L. V. Brown, J Appl Physiol **70** (5), 1928-1932 (1991).
50. D. C. Zawieja, C. Garcia and H. J. Granger, Am J Physiol **262** (1 Pt 2), H136-143 (1992).
51. M. E. Pruitt, M. A. Knepper, B. Graves and B. Schmidt-Nielsen, Am J Physiol Renal Physiol **290**(4), F892-896 (2006).
52. L. Rugheimer, C. Johnsson, C. Maric and P. Hansell, Acta Physiol (Oxf) **193** (2), 191-198 (2008).
53. A. G. Ginetzinsky, Nature **182** (4644), 1218-1219 (1958).
54. V. Goransson, C. Johnsson, A. Jacobson, P. Heldin, R. Hallgren and P. Hansell, Nephrol Dial Transplant **19** (4), 823-830 (2004).
55. A. B. Nilsson, C. Johnsson, P. Friberg and P. Hansell, Acta Physiol Scand **173** (3), 343-350 (2001).
56. J. Melin, O. Hellberg, K. Funa, R. Hallgren, E. Larsson and B. C. Fellstrom, Nephron Exp Nephrol **103** (3), e86-94 (2006).
57. P. Mahadevan, R. G. Larkins, J. R. Fraser, A. J. Fosang and M. E. Dunlop, Diabetologia **38** (3), 298-305 (1995).
58. T. R. Beck, A. Hassid and M. J. Dunn, J Pharmacol Exp Ther **215** (1), 15-19 (1980).
59. C. Maric, G. P. Aldred, P. J. Harris and D. Alcorn, Kidney Int **53** (1), 92-99 (1998).

Hyaluronan and Stone Disease

Marino Asselman

Department of Urology, Erasmus Medical Center Rotterdam,
Room H1098, P.O. Box 2040, 3000 CA Rotterdam, The Netherlands

Abstract. Kidney stones cannot be formed as long as crystals are passed in the urine. However, when crystals are retained it becomes possible for them to aggregate and form a stone. Crystals are expected to be formed not earlier than the distal tubules and collecting ducts. Studies both *in vitro* and *in vivo* demonstrate that calcium oxalate monohydrate crystals do not adhere to intact distal epithelium, but only when the epithelium is proliferating or regenerating, so that it possesses dedifferentiated cells expressing hyaluronan, osteopontin (OPN) and their mutual receptor CD44 at the apical cell membrane. The polysaccharide hyaluronan is an excellent crystal binding molecule because of its negative ionic charge. We hypothesized that the risk for crystal retention in the human kidney would be increased when tubular cells express hyaluronan at their apical cell membrane. Two different patient categories in which nephrocalcinosis frequently occurs were studied to test this hypothesis (preterm neonates and kidney transplant patients). Hyaluronan (and OPN) expression at the luminal membrane of tubular cells indeed was observed, which preceded subsequent retention of crystals in the distal tubules. Tubular nephrocalcinosis has been reported to be associated with decline of renal function and thus further studies to extend our knowledge of the mechanisms of retention and accumulation of crystals in the kidney are warranted. Ultimately, this may allow the design of new strategies for the prevention and treatment of both nephrocalcinosis and nephrolithiasis in patients.

Keywords: Kidney stones, tubular nephrocalcinosis, hyaluronan, osteopontin, renal tubular epithelial cells
PACS: 01.30.Cc; 87.19.X–; 87.18.Ed; 87.15.hg.

INTRODUCTION

Calcium salts (and other poorly soluble waste salts) often form crystals in the urine as the concentration of urine increases along the nephron. Stone formers differ from non-stone formers in the fact that these crystals are retained and accumulate in their kidneys (a condition we will call 'crystal retention') to ultimately become cemented together with organic material into a kidney stone [1]. Almost 30 years ago leading investigators in the stone field emphasized that crystal retention is a crucial requisite for kidney stone formation, and they postulated that this process could take place inside the tubular lumen, perhaps when crystals are retained at the luminal membrane of epithelial cells lining the renal tubules [2]. This concept inspired researchers worldwide to search for so-called "crystal binding molecules." These molecules would be expressed by tubular epithelial cells and have affinity for binding crystals, and thus could play a role in the retention of crystals in the kidney [3,4]. A corollary of this

CP1049, *Renal Stone Disease 2, 2nd International Urolithiasis Research Symposium,*
edited by A. P. Evan, J. E. Lingeman, J. A. McAteer, and J. C. Williams, Jr.

concept was that these molecules could be expressed by tubular cells of stone formers, but less so in non-stone formers.

Previous Work

Dr. Carl Verkoelen and his co-workers from the department of Urology of the Erasmus Medical Center Rotterdam started to work on the subject of crystal-cell interaction over ten years ago [5]. They carried out *in vitro* studies with MDCK-I cells [6-9], a cell line very like that of the epithelium of the renal distal tubules/collecting ducts [10-13]. Cells were cultured on porous supports to mimic the *in vivo* situation; it has been shown the use of these permeable supports allows cells to develop with higher levels of differentiation compared to cells cultured on solid supports [7,14]. Using the permeable supports, the MDCK-I cells form a tight layer of columnar cells with short microvilli on their luminal membrane [7,14,15].

Crystal-cell interaction studies were done using these MDCK-I cells; because the formation of crystals along the nephron would be expected not earlier than the distal nephron—unless oxalate plasma concentrations are raised to very high levels, such as in unusual situations such as poisoning with ethylene glycol or primary hyperoxaluria [16]—the use of a distal cell line such as MDCK-I is appropriate. It was found that calcium oxalate monohydrate (COM) crystals did not adhere to well differentiated cells (those populating confluent monolayers with high transepithelial electrical resistance). In contrast, crystals adhered to cells in developing, subconfluent cultures and to migrating cells at the border of cell groups in cultures with low transepithelial electrical resistance [6]. It was later shown that the difference between the crystal-binding phenotype of confluent cultures and subconfluent (or scrape-damaged) cultures could be explained by the expression of hyaluronan at the apical membrane of proliferating and regenerating cells, where hyaluronan could serve as a crystal binding molecule, whereas fully differentiated cells which do not express hyaluronan, would thus not be able to bind crystals [8]. Hyaluronan is an excellent binding molecule for crystals because it is negatively charged with its many carboxyl groups [17], while the crystals are positively charged because of calcium ions protruding from the crystal lattice. We found that the pericellular matrices (PCMs) containing hyaluronan extended several microns from the cell surface in subconfluent cells, but these PCMs disappeared when cultures reached confluence [18].

PRIMARY CULTURES OF HUMAN RENAL TUBULAR CELLS

Similar *in vitro* studies were repeated using primary cultures of human proximal and distal tubular/collecting duct cells. Again, cells were found to be susceptible to crystal binding during the first days of growth, but they lost this affinity when cultures developed into confluent monolayers with functional tight junctions. The transmembrane receptor CD44—and its ligands, osteopontin (OPN) [19] and hyaluronan [20]—were expressed at the apical membrane of proliferating human epithelial cells, but when confluence was reached, CD44 was expressed on the basolateral membrane, and OPN and hyaluronan were no longer detectable in the cultures [21]. As with the MDCK-I cultures, proliferating cells of human renal tubular origin were found to be surrounded by hyaluronan-rich PCMs. Disintegration of these PCMs with hyaluronidase significantly decreased the cell affinity for crystals. These studies confirmed the results with MDCK-I cells and suggested that (1) intact, fully differentiated distal tubular epithelium of the human kidney does not bind crystals, and that (2) crystal retention in the human kidney may depend on the expression of CD44 at the luminal membrane of damaged cells, with the associated PCMs rich in OPN and hyaluronan [21].

We hypothesized from these results that the risk for crystal retention in the human nephron is increased when tubular cells express hyaluronan at their apical cell membrane [4,8,22]. The next step was to investigate this hypothesis *in vivo*, looking at crystal retention in cases of renal tubular injury and hyaluronan expression.

CRYSTAL RETENTION IN INJURED RAT KIDNEYS

Hyaluronan in the healthy kidney is hardly detectable in the cortex but is abundantly present as the main component of the renal inner medullary interstitium [23]. Hyaluronan in the kidney is upregulated during some inflammatory disease states [24-28]. In the healthy kidney, OPN is confined to the distal potions of only some nephrons. During inflammation, however, OPN can be dramatically upregulated in most segments of the nephron [26,27,29-31]. CD44 is also upregulated in the kidney during inflammation [26,27].

Rats were treated with ethylene glycol to induce renal tubular cell damage and calcium oxalate crystalluria. It was found that there was no crystal retention in the absence of tubular injury/regeneration, but that crystals were retained as soon as renal tubules were injured or regenerating. Crystals were found adherent to the apical surface of cells expressing hyaluronan, OPN and CD44. These *in vivo* results support the concept that crystal retention is associated with hyaluronan expressed at the surface of injured/regenerating cells [32]. The next step was to investigate this concept in nephrocalcinosis, a condition in which patients retain crystals inside their renal tubules.

CRYSTAL RETENTION IN HUMAN RENAL TISSUE

We selected two populations of patients that commonly develop nephrocalcinosis: preterm neonates and kidney transplant patients. Fetal kidneys contain proliferating and/or regenerating tubular cells, because the formation of new nephrons is not completed until 36 weeks of gestation. In renal transplants, ischemia and nephrotoxic immunosuppressive drugs may lead to injury and subsequent repair. In renal tissue from preterm neonates, the expression of hyaluronan and OPN was studied along with tubular crystal localization and colocalization with luminal OPN and hyaluronan. Tubular crystal localization and colocalization with luminal OPN and hyaluronan was also studied in kidney biopsies after transplantation [33].

Hyaluronan and OPN were found to be expressed at the luminal cell membrane of nephrons during nephrogenesis and at the luminal surface of distal tubules in post-transplantation biopsies. The expression of hyaluronan and OPN occurred before the retention of crystals in both groups [33]. From these results we proposed that this crystal binding phenotype may play an important role in the development of nephrocalcinosis.

In summary, our studies suggest that normal epithelium in the distal nephron has no affinity for crystals, so that under normal conditions crystal retention should not occur inside the renal tubules. However, the luminal membranes of proliferating cells during development as well as regenerating/(re)differentiating cells during injury and repair show a high affinity for calcium oxalate crystals. The difference is explained by expression of molecules at the apical cell membrane, and hyaluronan seems to be an important crystal binding molecule, perhaps because of its formation of PCMs. Luminal hyaluronan is found during nephrogenesis and during tubular regeneration in epithelial repair. It is thought to play a key role in (re)establishment of the epithelial barrier integrity and restoration of renal function, but as a negative side-effect it turns a non-crystal binding epithelium into a crystal-binding one due to its crystal binding properties [3,6,8,18,21,22,32-34].

CRYSTAL RETENTION IN THE RENAL TUBULES

From these studies, the question arises as to whether crystals binding to hyaluronan-expressing tubular cells are found in the kidneys of stone formers; that is, if the old hypothesis is true that crystal binding in the tubular lumen is crucial for initiating kidney stones, and if the hyaluronan-mediated binding of crystals is a viable mechanism, then one would expect to find such binding happening in the kidneys of stone formers. In 2003, Evan and Lingeman and their colleagues published the first of a series of studies utilizing high-resolution endoscopic mapping of the kidneys of stone formers during percutaneous nephrolithotomy, and also collecting biopsies of renal tissue from these patients [35]. This first study was on idiopathic, calcium oxalate stone formers; surprisingly, no tubular injury—and no intratubular crystals—were observed. These patients had interstitial apatite crystal deposits (Randall's plaques) beginning in the basement membranes of the thin limbs of the loops of Henle extending into the interstitium surrounding the collecting ducts and downwards towards the papillae just beneath the papillary epithelium [36,37]. Thus, there seems to be no evidence of crystal-binding to tubular cells in this type of stone former. Rather, retention of urinary crystals can be attributed to the present of the Randall's plaques. However, more recent work by the same group has shown that both intratubular crystals and hyaluronan staining *are* seen in biopsies from the kidneys of patients who had hyperoxaluria as the result of intestinal bypass surgery for obesity [93]. Thus, although binding of crystals to the luminal membranes of tubular cells may not occur in the common, idiopathic stone formers, such a mechanism does appear to be important in at least some other forms of stone disease.

NEPHROLITHIASIS AND NEPHROCALCINOSIS

Nephrolithiasis indicates the presence of kidney stones, and as such is a term understood by all; in contrast the definition of nephrocalcinosis is less clear. Nephrocalcinosis can refer to *diffuse renal parenchymal calcification demonstrable by radiology imaging techniques* [40], and as such seems to be a condition rather dependent on the method used for its detection. For example, during ultrasonography of the kidney, diffuse scattering of small, hyperechogenic lesions in either the cortex or medulla can be called nephrocalcinosis [41], and diverse conditions show this ultrasound image pattern [42]. However, neither x-ray or ultrasonic imaging methods show whether the deposits in the kidney are intratubular or interstitial, and these methods are probably not sensitive enough to detect the early stages of nephrocalcinosis. Nephrocalcinosis should be subdivided on the basis of the location of calcium deposits at the microscopic level, separating interstitial nephrocalcinosis (deposition of crystals in the renal medullary interstitium) and tubular nephrocalcinosis (retention of crystals in the renal tubules) [38].

The incidence of interstitial nephrocalcinosis is known to rise with age [43]. This form of nephrocalcinosis is probably relatively benign until it erodes through the epithelium of the renal papilla to become an exposed Randall's plaque. These plaques certainly could be the nidus for stone attachment in at least a subset of kidney stones, since calcium oxalate stones have been found attached these plaques [44,94]. Randall's plaques are more common in idiopathic calcium oxalate stone patients than in non-stone formers, and this suggests an alteration in the solubility of calcium phosphate in the renal interstitium of stone formers [44]. In theory, the concentration of calcium phosphate in the interstitium could be increased in stone formers compared to normal individuals, or the interstitial inhibitors of crystallization could be less effective.

Tubular nephrocalcinosis is defined as calcium deposits inside the renal tubules and occurs if crystals are retained inside the nephron [22]. As described above, our studies have contributed significantly to the understanding that crystals are retained when renal tubular cells are triggered to express hyaluronan at their luminal membrane [33]. Besides in preterm neonates [45] and kidney transplants [46], tubular nephrocalcinosis also occurs in sarcoidosis [47], primary hyperoxaluria [48], Dent's disease [49,50], distal renal tubular acidosis [51-53], carbonic anhydrase deficiency [54], Bartter's syndrome [55,56], cystic fibrosis [57,58], Sjögren's syndrome [59], intestinal bypass surgery patients [60,93], Crohn's disease [44,61], acute phosphate nephropathy [62], and brushite stone formers [4,22,39,63].

The molecular/cellular bases for intratubular crystals has not been studied in most of these conditions. For each of these conditions, it would be valuable to have renal biopsies stained for hyaluronan and examined for the presence of intratubular crystals. A recent study by Vervaet *et al.* has shown that indeed in Dent's disease, sarcoidosis, primary hyperoxaluria and acute phosphate nephropathy the same association of crystals with hyaluronan expressing tubular epithelial cells was observed [64]. The commonality of hyaluronan expression with tubular nephrocalcinosis in these diverse conditions suggests that hyaluronan may be foundational in the formation of tubular nephrocalcinosis.

CLINICAL RELEVANCE

Tubular nephrocalcinosis does not usually lead to acute renal failure, except in extreme cases, such as in ethylene glycol poisoning [65]. However, the long-term effects of calcium deposits in the tubules are largely unstudied. The first report of nephrocalcinosis in preterm infants was only 26 years ago [66]. The intratubular deposits in these patients were found to be predominantly calcium oxalate, but calcium phosphate crystals were also observed in the neonatal kidneys [67]. The incidence of tubular nephrocalcinosis has been reported to be as high as 83% in very premature infants (gestation between 24 and 28 weeks) [68]. This form of nephrocalcinosis is thought to disappear later in life, but Schell-Feith *et al.* showed in their large group of 83 patients with nephrocalcinosis that it persisted in 15% of these patients after 30 months follow-up [45,69]. 15% of preterm infants who had nephrocalcinosis showed mild chronic renal insufficiency (15%) at a mean follow-up age of 7.5 years, in contrast to similar preterm infants who did not have nephrocalcinosis (6%) [70]. Prematurity *per se* was associated with high blood pressure and distal tubular dysfunction (low plasma bicarbonate and early-morning urine osmolality) but nephrocalcinosis seemed to confer an additional risk on compromising renal function later in life [70]. This poor prognosis can easily be attributed to crystal retention, which could lead to irreversible damage of nephrons as a result of crystal aggregates obstructing the tubular lumen. Our results with preterm neonates—showing that hyaluronan and OPN is expressed at the luminal membrane of proliferating distal tubular cells during nephrogenesis—is in agreement with the important role that has been attributed to these molecules during kidney development [71,72]. In preterm neonates, supersaturation of calcium salts is increased because of a calcium- and vitamin D-rich diet, low urinary citrate and long-term furosemide treatment, all of which contribute to crystalluria [33,73,74]. We have shown that hyaluronan and OPN expressed at the luminal membrane of proliferating distal tubular cells precedes nephrocalcinosis in these infants, which strongly suggests that this increased crystal binding phenotype played a role in crystal retention [33]. The subsequent decline of kidney function in 15% of preterm infants with persistent nephrocalcinosis after 30 months follow-up described by Schell-Feith *et al.* therefore could easily be the result of crystal retention [69,70].

Another condition in which nephrocalcinosis unmistakably plays a role is chronic allograft nephropathy in kidney transplants. It has recently been shown that in these patients nephrocalcinosis occurs and is associated with long-term graft failure [4,33,46,75,76]. Merneo *et al.* examined 40 allograft nephrectomies in patients with transplant kidney failure between 2 days and 11 years after transplantation who had neither primary nor secondary hyperoxaluria as the cause of initial end-stage renal disease, or a history of kidney stones. These authors showed that calcium oxalate crystal retention in the renal tubules was frequently observed in failing renal grafts, because in 88% of allograft nephrectomies birefringent crystals were observed mainly on the distal tubular epithelium [75]. Serum oxalate concentrations increase during chronic renal failure and accumulate in the body during dialysis. Within the first few days after transplantation oxalate is mobilized and excreted with the urine, and therefore it was proposed that the recipient's chronic renal failure was related to early calcium oxalate deposition in the renal tubules [75]. In another study, nephrocalcinosis in allograft biopsies was found in 76% of patients with post-transplantation acute tubular necrosis (ATN), whereas nephrocalcinosis was not observed in patients with normal renal function after transplantation [77].

In 213 patients with 586 protocol biopsies obtained 6 weeks, 3 and 6 months after transplantation, nephrocalcinosis increased from 6 to 18%. Although three months after transplantation some crystals were found in the interstitium, the majority were located inside the renal tubules [78]. Our study of protocol renal allograft biopsies taken 3 and 6 months post-transplantation showed an increase in nephrocalcinosis from 20% to 60% [33]. In general, biopsies obtained from dysfunctional renal allografts more often contain crystals in the renal tubules than those from functional allografts. It should be noticed, however, that this does not establish the cause and effect relationship between poor renal graft function and nephrocalcinosis. Pinheiro *et al.* performed percutaneous renal transplant biopsies in 97 patients within three months post-transplantation and reanalyzed them after ten years. An overall incidence of calcium oxalate deposits of 53% was observed from which 86% of the patients the calcium oxalate deposits were already found in the first biopsy, which was higher than expected. The calcium oxalate deposits were observed only in the tubular lumen [76]. Chronic allograft nephropathy is the result of cumulative and incremental damage to nephrons as a result of ischemic injury and chronic stress by nephrotoxic immunosuppressive agents in which impaired tubular repair/regeneration eventually leads to fibrosis and loss of function [46], Pinheiro et al. not only found a higher incidence of calcium oxalate deposits in patients with tubular dysfunction and ATN in early post-transplantation biopsies but there was also an independent association between calcium oxalate deposition and a poorer allograft survival, because ATN-free patients with nephrocalcinosis poorer graft survival than ATN-free patients without nephrocalcinosis [76]. The observation that patients with early nephrocalcinosis had a four-fold higher risk of losing the graft than those without nephrocalcinosis again indicates that renal dysfunction is the consequence rather than the cause of nephrocalcinosis. The authors themselves concluded that a high incidence of post-transplantation nephrocalcinosis may have a negative impact on graft survival [76].

It should be emphasized that all of the above mentioned studies were performed with renal tissue specimens prepared for routine histology. We [38] and others [79] have demonstrated, however, that a substantial part of crystals in renal tubules are lost during routine tissue preparation. It is therefore not unlikely that the incidence and severity of nephrocalcinosis could even be underestimated.

We have shown in transplant kidneys that expression of hyaluronan and OPN is upregulated, which probably occurs in response to ischemic/reperfusion renal damage, cyclosporine toxicity and chronic allograft rejection. Subsequent biopsies of transplant kidneys showed an increase in crystal retention in time, which again suggests that this increased crystal binding phenotype played a role in crystal retention [33]. These results also indicate that crystals themselves were not injurious to tubular cells because tubular injury preceded crystal retention. These *in vivo* results are in correspondence with cell culture studies, which showed that calcium oxalate crystals are not injurious to distal tubular/collecting duct cells [80]. We propose that calcium oxalate crystals are not the primary cause of decline of renal function in kidney transplants of patients with nephrocalcinosis but crystal retention could eventually lead to irreversible damage to nephrons as a result of large crystal aggregates obstructing the lumen.

Nephrocalcinosis also occurs in primary hyperoxaluria type 1, a genetic metabolic disorder of oxalate metabolism. This rare autosomal recessive inborn error of glyoxylate metabolism is characterized by a functional defect of the liver specific enzyme alanine glyoxylate aminotransferase (AGT) leading to hyperoxaluria and hyperglycolic aciduria [48]. In 57 primary hyperoxaluria type 1 patients in the Netherlands progression to renal insufficiency was statistically associated with the presence of nephrocalcinosis, detected by ultrasound and response to pyridoxine therapy also predicted outcome of renal function but progression to renal insufficiency was not associated with the level of urinary oxalate or with AGT activity [81]. In another paper it was shown that all patients with cortical nephrocalcinosis in primary hyperoxaluria developed end-stage renal disease [82].

TREATMENT STRATEGIES

Tubular nephrocalcinosis is the result of the combination of crystal formation and crystal retention. The risk of crystal formation is significantly higher when concentrations of citrate in the urine is low and concentrations of calcium and/or oxalate are high [83]. Efforts should therefore be made to keep urinary calcium and oxalate levels low and citrate concentrations high. Hyperoxaluria was found in 35% of kidney transplant recipients and hypocitraturia in 69% [84]. High urinary oxalate probably results from the release of oxalate that was accumulated during the dialysis period in body stores like bone and tissue [85]. Renal tubular acidosis (RTA) is common in preterm infants [73] and renal transplant patients [86]. RTA leads to hypercalciuria and hypocitraturia [87]. To avoid crystal formation, these patients should be treated with potassium citrate. Potassium citrate treatment increases urinary pH to the physiological range which prevents further release of calcium from the bone and it leads to increased urinary citrate that binds calcium and thereby prevents calcium crystal formation. Crystal formation can also be influenced by adjustments in the diet. To avoid crystal formation as much as possible, it is recommended that the patients maintain an ideal body weight, drink at least 2 L water/day, limit sodium chloride intake, limit protein intake, consume normal amounts of dairy products (30 mmol calcium per day) and consume fruits and vegetables, except spinach and rhubarb [74,88].

It is more difficult to prevent crystal retention by influencing the crystal binding phenotype of the distal tubular epithelium. Previously, it was found that prostaglandin

E_2 (PGE_2) increases hyaluronan synthesis in renal glomerular cells and that this could be inhibited by the cyclooxygenase (COX) inhibitor (NSAID) indomethacin [89]. This prompted us to study the effect of NSAIDs on hyaluronan-mediated crystal binding to regenerating MDCK-I cells (data not yet published). These *in vitro* studies showed that hyaluronan-dependent calcium oxalate crystal binding to regenerating dedifferentiating tubular cells is COX-2 mediated and can be modulated by NSAIDs which suggests that COX inhibitors could be used to reduce the risk for nephrocalcinosis in patients. This does not mean, however, that we generally propose the use of NSAIDs for the prevention of nephrocalcinosis, because NSAIDs have important adverse effects on the function of the kidney due to the role of COX-2 in renin release, regulation of sodium excretion, and maintenance of renal blood flow [90]. The most important conclusion is that it is possible to lower the expression of hyaluronan at the surface of renal tubular cells temporarily, and thereby reduce the risk for nephrocalcinosis, but strategies should be developed that are safe to the kidney.

FUTURE STUDIES AND PERSPECTIVES

It is interesting to look again at earlier reports and interpret data following the line of thoughts that tubular crystal retention is the result from increased expression of hyaluronan at the luminal membrane of distal tubular epithelial cells during injury/regeneration. In *The Lancet* in 1994, for example, extracorporeal shock-wave lithotripsy (ESWL) treatment of a calyceal stone in a reported case of a twenty-six years old patient with primary hyperoxaluria resulted in fatal renal failure within one month [91]. Since the age of three this patient had recurrent nephrolithiasis. One month after treatment hemodialysis was necessary and within three months symptoms of oxalosis became apparent: peripheral neuritis and cardiac rhythm abnormalities as a result of systemic deposition of calcium oxalate. Within two years a kidney transplant failed due to oxalosis of the transplanted kidney and rejection, and the patient died of sepsis after a cerebrovascular accident. The authors emphasized the fact that ESWL treatment causes renal damage in most cases, along with an immediate decline in total effective renal plasma flow [91,92]. Apparently the combination of hyperoxaluria and renal damage led to this catastrophic series of events resulting in renal failure, but the authors did not recognize the fact that renal damage might have caused an increased risk of crystal retention. In this patient subsequent kidney transplantation again failed as a result of widespread deposition of calcium oxalate crystals (oxalosis). It is plausible that injury in the transplant kidney due to ischemia/reperfusion and nephrotoxic drugs in combination with oxalate crystalluria resulted in obstructive tubulopathy and graft failure in this patient.

The concept that crystal retention in the kidney leads to renal calcification disorders is indisputable. Interstitial nephrocalcinosis (Randall's plaques) result from the deposition of crystals in the renomedullary interstitium and there are strong indications that hyaluronan in the inner medullary interstitium plays a role in this process [22]. Tubular nephrocalcinosis is caused by the attachment of crystals to renal tubular cells.

Each form of tubular nephrocalcinosis probably has its own specific mitogen/stress conditions leading to the expression of regenerating crystal binding cells in the renal tubules. The initial site of crystal retention in idiopathic stone formers remains an open question. Studying the mechanisms of retention of crystals inside the lumen of the renal tubules is needed because it is obvious that prevention of kidney stone disease is better than only treating symptomatic kidney stone disease. Another particularly relevant reason to extend these studies is the fact that tubular nephrocalcinosis could eventually lead to irreversible damage of nephrons since nephrocalcinosis has been found to be associated with decline of renal function in preterm neonates and patients with kidney transplants.

To explore these concepts future studies should include histological studies of snap frozen human renal tissue specimens of different kidney stone formers, and of other specific patient groups associated with nephrocalcinosis like Dent's disease and primary hyperoxaluria. Human renal tissue specimens are difficult to obtain whereas urine samples are not. Therefore, urine samples of well-defined patient populations should be collected and determined whether molecules can be detected in the urine which could have a relation with hyaluronan biosynthesis by renal tubular epithelial cells. The concentration of hyaluronan itself and its molecular size, for example, can be detected in the urine and quantified with an ELISA. The aim of such studies is to reveal whether there are urinary markers that can identify patients with tubular injury/regeneration and an increased risk for crystal retention. Urine samples of patients before and after ESWL-treatment for example could be used, since ESWL is known to temporarily cause renal damage. More interesting are urine samples during follow-up of post-transplantation patients, preterm neonates and primary hyperoxaluria patients. *In vitro* studies of renal distal tubular epithelial cells in culture should be extended in order to determine which hyaluronan-binding proteins are involved in PCM formation and degradation, because identification of such proteins could eventually give reason to test their presence in urine of patients and evaluate whether or not they could also be used as urinary markers of tubular injury/regeneration. The aim of such studies is to extend our knowledge of the mechanisms of retention and accumulation of crystals in the kidney, in order to ultimately design new strategies for the prevention and treatment of both nephrocalcinosis and nephrolithiasis in patients.

ACKNOWLEDGMENTS

I want to thank Carl Verkoelen for the time that I had the pleasure to work with him. He was the driving force of the kidney stone research group of our department at the Erasmus Medical Center Rotterdam and he is greatly missed by the international kidney stone research community after his unfortunate death last year. The studies that have been performed and are discussed here were the result of a close collaboration between our stone research group (M. Asselman, C. Bangma, E. van Ballegooijen, M. Schepers-Kok and C. Verkoelen) and a renal research unit at the department of nephrology at the university of Antwerp, Belgium (A. Verhulst, P. D'Haese, M. Helbert, V.Persy, B. Vervaet and M. de Broe).

This work was supported by the Oxalosis and Hyperoxaluria Foundation (Grant. No. 2749036).

REFERENCES

1. N. Mandel, Semin Nephrol **16**(5), 364 (1996).
2. B. Finlayson and F. Reid, Invest Urol **15**(6), 442 (1978).
3. M. Asselman and C. F. Verkoelen, Curr Opin Urol **12**(4), 271 (2002).
4. C. F. Verkoelen and A. Verhulst, Kidney Int **72**(1), 13 (2007).
5. C. F. Verkoelen, J. C. Romijn, W.C. De Bruijn et al., Kidney Int **48**(1), 129 (1995).
6. C. F. Verkoelen, B. G. van der Boom, A. B. Houtsmuller et al., Am J Physiol **274**(5 Pt 2), F958 (1998).
7. C. F. Verkoelen, B. G. van der Boom, D. J. Kok et al., Kidney Int **55**(4), 1426 (1999).
8. C. F. Verkoelen, B. G. Van Der Boom, and J. C. Romijn, Kidney Int **58**(3), 1045 (2000).
9. C. R. Gaush, W. L. Hard, and T. F. Smith, Proc Soc Exp Biol Med **122**(3), 931 (1966).
10. J. C. Richardson, V. Scalera, and N. L. Simmons, Biochim Biophys Acta **673**(1), 26 (1981).
11. O. Devuyst, R. Beauwens, J. F. Denef et al., Cell Tissue Res **277**(2), 231 (1994).
12. M. Gekle, S. Wunsch, H. Oberleithner et al., Pflugers Arch **428**(2), 157 (1994).
13. W. Pfaller, G. Gstraunthaler, U. Kersting et al., Ren Physiol Biochem **12**(5-6), 328 (1989).
14. G. C. Hansson, K. Simons, and G. van Meer, Embo J **5**(3), 483 (1986).
15. K. Svennevig, K. Prydz, and S. O. Kolset, Biochem J **311**(Pt 3), 881 (1995).
16. D. J. Kok, Endocrinol Metab Clin North Am **31**(4), 855 (2002).
17. B. P. Toole, Glycoforum website 'The Science of Hyaluronan Today' Chaper 8, 1 (1998).
18. M. S. Schepers, M. Asselman, R. A. Duim et al., Nephron Exp Nephrol **94**(3), e103 (2003).
19. G. F. Weber, S. Ashkar, M. J. Glimcher et al., Science **271**(5248), 509 (1996).
20. A. Aruffo, I. Stamenkovic, M. Melnick et al., Cell **61**(7), 1303 (1990).
21. A. Verhulst, M. Asselman, V. P. Persy et al., J Am Soc Nephrol **14**(1), 107 (2003).
22. C. F. Verkoelen, J Am Soc Nephrol **17**(6), 1673 (2006).
23. M. A. Knepper, G. M. Saidel, V. C. Hascall et al., Am J Physiol Renal Physiol **284**(3), F433 (2003).
24. E. Feusi, L. Sun, A. Sibalic et al., Nephron **83**(1), 66 (1999).
25. C. Johnsson, G. Tufveson, J. Wahlberg et al., Kidney Int **50**(4), 1224 (1996).
26. A. J. Lewington, B. J. Padanilam, D. R. Martin et al., Am J Physiol Regul Integr Comp Physiol **278**(1), R247 (2000).
27. V. Sibalic, X. Fan, J. Loffing et al., Nephrol Dial Transplant **12**(7), 1344 (1997).
28. A. Wells, E. Larsson, E. Hanas et al., Transplantation **55**(6), 1346 (1993).
29. V. P. Persy, W. A. Verstrepen, D. K. Ysebaert et al., Kidney Int **56**(2), 601 (1999).
30. Y. Xie, S. Nishi, S. Iguchi et al., Kidney Int **59**(3), 959 (2001).
31. Y. Xie, M. Sakatsume, S. Nishi et al., Kidney Int **60**(5), 1645 (2001).
32. M. Asselman, A. Verhulst, M. E. De Broe et al., J Am Soc Nephrol **14**(12), 3155 (2003).
33. A. Verhulst, M. Asselman, S. De Naeyer et al., Kidney Int **68**(4), 1643 (2005).
34. M. Asselman, A. Verhulst, E. S. Van Ballegooijen et al., Kidney Int **68**(1), 71 (2005).
35. A. P. Evan, J. E. Lingeman, F. L. Coe et al., J Clin Invest **111**(5), 607 (2003).
36. D. A. Bushinsky, J Clin Invest **111**(5), 607 (2003).
37. A. Randall, Ann Surg **105**, 1009 (1937).
38. M. T. Kummeling, B. W. de Jong, C. Laffeber et al., J Urol **178**(3):1097 (2007).
39. J. A. Sayer, G. Carr, and N. L. Simmons, Clin Sci (Lond) **106**(6), 549 (2004).
40. D. Schepens, G. Verswijvel, D. Kuypers et al., Nephrol Dial Transplant **15**(7), 1080 (2000).
41. P. T. Dick, B. M. Shuckett, B. Tang et al., Pediatr Radiol **29**(1), 68 (1999).
42. U. S. Alon, Curr Opin Pediatr **9**(2), 160 (1997).
43. E. Beer, J Path and Bact **9**, 225 (1904).
44. A. P. Evan, F. L. Coe, J. E. Lingeman et al., Urol Res **33**(5), 383 (2005).
45. E. A. Schell-Feith, J. E. Kist-van Holthe, N. Conneman et al., Kidney Int **58**(5), 2102 (2000).
46. B. J. Nankivell, R. J. Borrows, C. L. Fung et al., N Engl J Med **349**(24), 2326 (2003).
47. U. Gobel, R. Kettritz, W. Schneider et al., J Am Soc Nephrol **12**(3), 616 (2001).
48. D. S. Milliner, D. M. Wilson, and L. H. Smith, Kidney Int **59**(1), 31 (2001).
49. V. Cebotaru, S. Kaul, O. Devuyst et al., Kidney Int **68**(2), 642 (2005).

50. Y. K. Wong, K. T. Tang, J. C. Wu et al., J Cell Biochem **82**(1), 58 (2001).
51. T. Boettger, C. A. Hubner, H. Maier et al., Nature **416**(6883), 874 (2002).
52. L. J. Bruce, D. L. Cope, G. K. Jones et al., J Clin Invest **100**(7), 1693 (1997).
53. J. A. Nicoletta and G. J. Schwartz, Curr Opin Pediatr **16**(2), 194 (2004).
54. K. J. Borthwick, N. Kandemir, R. Topaloglu et al., J Med Genet **40**(2), 115 (2003).
55. J. A. Sayer and S. H. Pearce, Ann Clin Biochem **38**(Pt 5), 459 (2001).
56. A. J. Shaer, Am J Med Sci **322**(6), 316 (2001).
57. S. M. Katz, L. J. Krueger, and B. Falkner, N Engl J Med **319**(5), 263 (1988).
58. M. Soleimani and C. E. Burnham, Kidney Int **57**(2), 371 (2000).
59. H. M. Moutsopoulos, J. Cledes, F. N. Skopouli et al., J Intern Med **230**(2), 187 (1991).
60. D. R. Mole, C. R. Tomson, N. Mortensen et al., Qjm **94**(2), 69 (2001).
61. E. M. Worcester, M. Chuang, B. Laven et al., Urol Res **33**(5), 380 (2005).
62. D. Markovich and P.S. Aronson, Annu Rev Physiol **69**, 361 (2007).
63. A. P. Evan, J. E. Lingeman, F. L. Coe et al., Kidney Int **67**(2), 576 (2005).
64. B. A. Vervaet, A. Verhulst, G.S. Markowitz et al., European Urology Meetings **2**(3) (2007).
65. R.W. Schrier, In: Diseases of the Kidney and Urinary Tract, pp 1316 (2001).
66. K.G. Hufnagle, S.N. Khan, D. Penn et al., Pediatrics **70**, 360(1982).
67. F.C. McCormick, K. Brady, and C.E. Keen, Pediatr Pathol Lab Med **16**, 479(1996).
68. D.J. Cranefield, D.E. Odd, J.E. Harding et al., Pediatr Radiol **34**(2), 138 (2004).
69. E. A. Schell-Feith, J. E. Kist-van Holthe, P. H. Van Zwieten et al., Pediatr Nephrol **18**(11), 1102 (2003).
70. J. E. Kist-van Holthe, P. H. van Zwieten, E. A. Schell-Feith et al., Pediatrics **119**(3), 468 (2007).
71. M. Pohl, H. Sakurai, R.O. Stuart et al., Develop Biol **224**, 312 (2000).
72. S.A. Rogers, B. J. Padanilam, and K.A. Hruska, Am J Physiol **272**, F469 (1997).
73. P. Sikora, B. Roth, and A. Kribs, Kidney Int **63**, 2194 (2003).
74. L. Borghi, T. Schianchi, T. Meschi et al., N Engl J Med 346(2), **77** (2002).
75. L. Memeo, I. Pecorella, A. Ciarda et al., Transplant Proc **33**(1-2), 1262 (2001).
76. H.S. Pinheiro, N.O. Camara, K.S. Osaki et al., Am J Transplant **5**(2), 323 (2005).
77. S. Olsen, J. F. Burdick, P. A. Keown et al., Medicine (Baltimore) **68**(3), 173 (1989).
78. W. Gwinner, S. Suppa, M. Mengel et al., Am J Transplant **5**(8), 1934 (2005).
79. S. R. Marengo, D. H. Chen, A. P. Evan et al., Urol Res **34**(3), 200 (2006).
80. M. S. Schepers, E. S. van Ballegooijen, C. H. Bangma et al., Kidney Int **68**(4), 1543 (2005).
81. C. S. van Woerden, J. W. Groothoff, R. J. Wanders et al., Nephrol Dial Transplant **18**(2), 273 (2003).
82. O. Diallo, F. Janssens, M. Hall et al., AJR Am J Roentgenol **183**(6), 1767 (2004).
83. C. Y. Pak, Am J Kidney Dis **18**(6), 624 (1991).
84. L. Stapenhorst, R. Sassen, B. Beck et al., Pediatr Nephrol **20**(5), 652 (2005).
85. B. Hoppe, M. J. Kemper, A. Bokenkamp et al., Kidney Int **56**(1), 268 (1999).
86. C. Schwarz, T. Benesch, K. Kodras et al., Nephrol Dial Transplant **21**(9), 2615 (2006).
87. R. J. Alpern, Kidney Int **47**(4), 1205 (1995).
88. L. Borghi, T. Meschi, U. Maggiore et al., Nutr Rev **64**(7 Pt 1), 301 (2006).
89. P. Mahadevan, R. G. Larkins, J. R. Fraser et al., Diabetes **45**(1), 44 (1996).
90. R. C. Harris and M. D. Breyer, Clin J Am Soc Nephrol **1**(2), 236 (2006).
91. I. L. Tan, H. M. Zonderland, and E. R. Boeve, Lancet **344**(8924), 757 (1994).
92. B. R. Baumgartner, K. W. Dickey, S. S. Ambrose et al., Radiology **163**(2), 531 (1987).
93. A.P. Evan, F.L. Coe, D. Gillen, et al., Anat Rec **291**(3), 325 (2008).
94. A.P. Evan, F.L. Coe, J.E. Lingeman, et al. Anat Rec **290**(10), 1315 (2007).

III. URETERAL STENTS AND PHYSIOLOGY

Implications of Biofilm Formation on Urological Devices

Peter A. Cadieux[a-c], Geoffrey R. Wignall[a], Rupp Carriveau[d], and John D. Denstedt[a,c]

[a]Department of Surgery, Division of Urology and [b]Department of Microbiology and Immunology, University of Western Ontario, 1151 Richmond St. Suite 2, London, Ontario, Canada, N6A5B8
[c]Lawson Health Research Institute, 268 Grosvenor St., London, Ontario, Canada, N5A4V2
[d]Department of Civil and Environmental Engineering, University of Windsor, 401 Sunset Avenue, Windsor, Ontario, Canada N9B3P4

Abstract. Despite millions of dollars and several decades of research targeted at their prevention and eradication, biofilm-associated infections remain the major cause of urological device failure. Numerous strategies have been aimed at improving device design, biomaterial composition, surface properties and drug delivery, but have been largely circumvented by microbes and their plethora of attachment, host evasion, antimicrobial resistance, and dissemination strategies. This is not entirely surprising since natural biofilm formation has been going on for millions of years and remains a major part of microorganism survival and evolution. Thus, the fact that biofilms develop on and in the biomaterials and tissues of humans is really an extension of this natural tendency and greatly explains why they are so difficult for us to combat. Firstly, biofilm structure and composition inherently provide a protective environment for microorganisms, shielding them from the shear stress of urine flow, immune cell attack and some antimicrobials. Secondly, many biofilm organisms enter a metabolically dormant state that renders them tolerant to those antibiotics and host factors able to penetrate the biofilm matrix. Lastly, the majority of organisms that cause biofilm-associated urinary tract infections originate from our own oral cavity, skin, gastrointestinal and urogenital tracts and therefore have already adapted to many of our host defenses. Ultimately, while biofilms continue to hold an advantage with respect to recurrent infections and biomaterial usage within the urinary tract, significant progress has been made in understanding these dynamic microbial communities and novel approaches offer promise for their prevention and eradication. These include novel device designs, antimicrobials, anti-adhesive coatings, biodegradable polymers and biofilm-disrupting compounds and therapies.

Keywords: ureteral stent, uropathogen, conditioning film, biofilm, adhesion, persister, antibiotic resistance
PACS: 87.18.Fx; 87.19.xb

BIOFILMS: WHAT, WHERE AND WHY?

A biofilm can be defined as a community of microorganisms (bacterial, fungal, algal) attached to a liquid-surface interface and enveloped within a matrix of exopolysaccharides and other biological constituents [1,2]. In general, their main purpose is to enable a microbial population to remain within an environment that they

CP1049, *Renal Stone Disease 2, 2nd International Urolithiasis Research Symposium,* edited by A. P. Evan, J. E. Lingeman, J. A. McAteer, and J. C. Williams, Jr.

find favorable to both survival and reproduction. Thus, on a very basic level, a urinary biofilm on a ureteral stent is no different from those found on an infected heart valve, at a deep sea hydrothermal vent or in the piping of a water intake system [3,4]. In addition to their adherence role, biofilms provide a degree of protection for a microbial population. Although microorganisms can survive and multiply quite effectively as planktonic (free swimming) cells within a liquid milieu (such as uropathogens in urine), they are largely exposed to any unfavorable environmental conditions that might arise and may be swept away from an advantageous environment via shear forces within the surrounding fluid (such as during urine voiding). Thus, if a planktonic population is exposed to a sudden lethal change in temperature or high concentration of a toxic compound, all cells in the population may be killed. The structure and makeup of a biofilm protects many cells within the population by physically shielding them from the surrounding environment and inducing changes in gene expression that result in metabolic dormancy and/or increased resistance to many inhibitory substances [5]. Although biofilms are far more complex in reality than described here, it is obvious that they improve microorganism survival, growth and reproduction through multiple mechanisms. It is therefore not surprising that biofilms are relatively ubiquitous throughout nature, or more relevant here, urinary tract devices. Clearly, biofilms are the greatest challenge faced by medicine in terms of treating wounds, using biomaterials and designing compounds for the prevention and treatment of infection.

Biofilm Development and Structure

When studying biofilms on a macroscopic level, most appear fairly simple in structure, as uncomplicated layers of organisms attached to a surface. However, upon closer examination, it becomes clear that in the majority of cases this is quite the contrary. Most biofilms, especially those occurring in nutrient-limiting environments, are highly complex structures designed to maximize survival and spread. This complexity has largely been shown to be a planned behavior and not simply a matter of architecture. As such, every organism within a biofilm appears to have a purpose, each contributing to the overall population. For instance, some organisms within biofilms undergo a type of suicide akin to "apoptosis" under certain conditions to reduce the nutrient requirements of the population, directly supply nutrients to the remaining organisms and/or contribute DNA and other compounds to the biofilm matrix [6,7]. Furthermore, another portion of cells (termed persisters) will often enter a state of metabolic dormancy that renders them more tolerant to lethal factors such as antibiotics or host nitric oxide [8]. In this sense, a biofilm may be described as a distinct entity, a multicellular organism comprised of diversely differentiated cells throughout, all with a common goal [9]. This complexity and adaptability are largely driven by the rapid environmental changes that microorganisms face on a continual basis, whether in nature or in association with human tissues and biomaterials, and offers some explanation as to why medical biofilms are virtually impossible to eradicate once formed. Biofilms can be homogeneous, consisting of only one organism type or heterogeneous, comprised of two or more different organisms. In urology, as in nature, both types are commonly found and the type that will occur in any specific situation depends upon multiple factors, including the surface and organism type, the surrounding environment and organism inter-relationships.

All biofilms start with an organism's attachment to a surface (Figure 1). This can be a single cell, group of cells or a matrix-enclosed cluster sloughed off a previous biofilm. The success of this initial attachment will depend upon multiple factors, some of bacterial origin and others environmental and/or host-derived. Surface molecule expression and cell viability are the most critical bacterial determinants and as such they express numerous appendages, receptor ligands and polysaccharides involved in adherence including pili, lipopolysaccharides, exopolysaccharides, adhesins and flagella [1]. Importantly, the presence and expression of these factors can vary significantly between different bacteria, even down to the strain level. As the organism approaches the surface, one or several factors will contact the surface and a reversible attachment will take place. The success of this interaction is dependent not only on the initial attachment but also the environmental properties of the surface and surrounding fluid (i.e., surface hydrophobicity, energy and charge, fluid shear stress, temperature, osmolarity, etc.). This attachment allows time for additional factors to adhere and stimulates changes in bacterial gene expression that drive polysaccharide production and other events that lead to irreversible adherence [9,10]. In the case of a biomaterial, once this irreversible attachment has taken place and a biofilm begins to form, at present it is virtually impossible to eradicate.

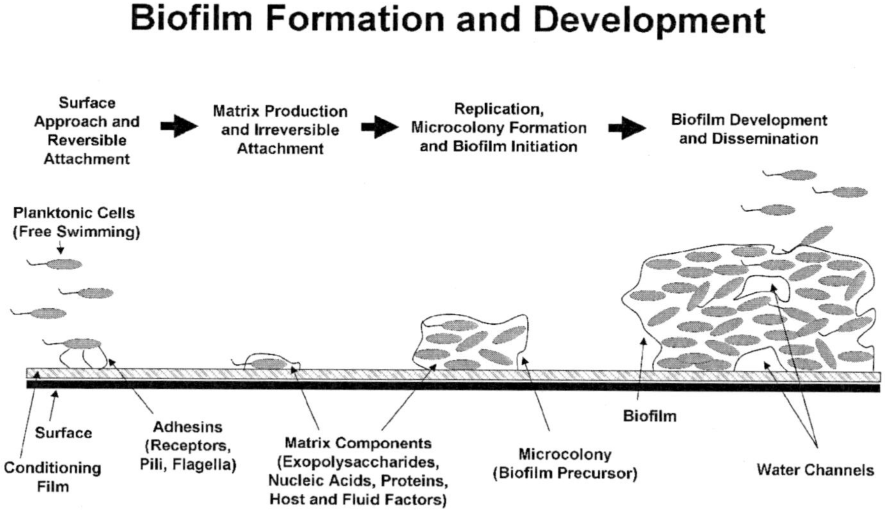

FIGURE 1. Schematic representation of the process of biofilm formation and development.

Within the urinary tract, biomaterial colonization is further complicated by the presence of biological constituents within the surrounding urine (and sometimes blood) that also adhere to the biomaterial and form what is termed a "conditioning film" (Figures 1 and 2) [2]. This film assists the attaching microbe in three critical ways: Firstly, it masks the intended surface properties of the device and may block the release of an impregnated compound (e.g., an antimicrobial). Secondly, it provides additional molecules for the organism to attach to, which increases its ability to make and maintain contact with the surface. Finally, it provides a source of nutrients for the organism immediately where attachment and biofilm formation occur. Ultimately, it is two key aspects of the bacterium-biomaterial interaction—namely multiple attachment strategies and the constant deposition of a urinary conditioning film—that make it increasingly difficult to produce biofilm-resistant prostheses for urology.

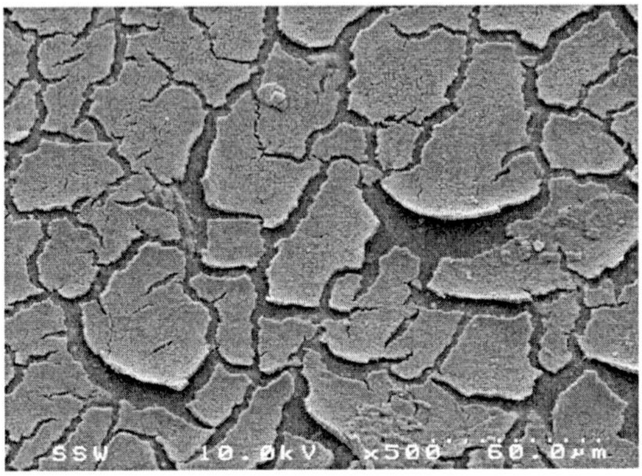

FIGURE 2. A ureteral stent with a sterile conditioning film formed over 48 hours incubation in artificial urine. The cracked appearance is due to drying in preparation for scanning electron microscopy (SEM), revealing the relative thickness of the film to be in the micrometer range.

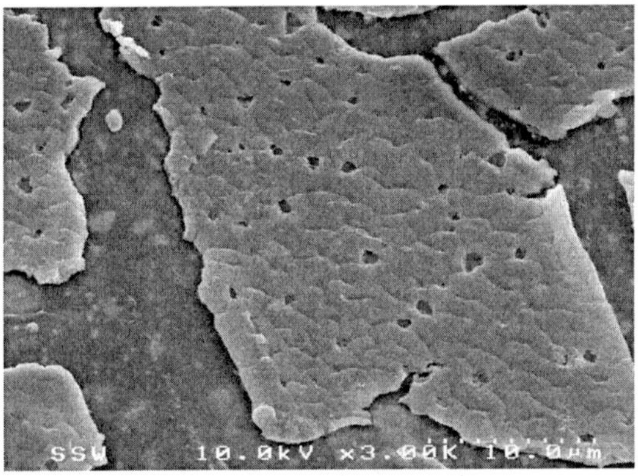

FIGURE 3. A *K. pneumoniae* biofilm formed in artificial urine over 48 hours, showing water channels (visible holes) throughout the film for nutrient uptake and waste removal.

As described, biofilm configuration and development highly depend upon the local growth conditions. Thus, there is no one standard biofilm structure and a multitude of arrangements can exist (e.g., towers, mushrooms, streamers), often with fluid-filled channels (Figure 3) and spatial variations ranging from nanometers to millimeters [1,2]. Furthermore, it is not uncommon to find that the same organism produces biofilms of varying structure and density dependent upon environmental conditions

[11]. In general, relatively flat and unstructured biofilms tend to develop in nutrient-rich habitats while more highly structured, complex films form when nutrients are restricted [1]. This is likely due, at least in part, to the fact that when nutrients are scarce, elaborate structures maximizing surface area and fluid flow will be required while those with ample nutrients in the surrounding fluid and buried within the matrix will not. In considering the local environmental conditions of the urinary tract, the above findings would suggest that relatively flat films possessing high effective diffusion rates would tend to develop on urinary prostheses, as ample nutrient levels and low flow velocities generally exist immediately around them. Studies investigating ureteral stents inserted up to 128 days support this, finding that biofilms formed in the absence of encrustation did not induce blockage of any of the devices, even in patients whose biofilms developed over several months [12,13]. Furthermore, when the devices were examined using scanning electron microscopy they revealed relatively flat biofilms with depths in the micrometer range. Thus, in the majority of cases, it would appear that the major clinical difficulties associated with urinary biofilms are not due to device failure but more to their associated infections. However, this would not be the case for biofilms associated with urease-producing organisms (e.g., *Proteus mirabilis*), since the rapid alkalinization of the urine they induce would lead to rapid encrustation and subsequent blockage of the device due to more crystalline biofilms with higher densities [14,15].

Communication within Biofilms

The success of microorganism survival in general is largely owed to their ability to sense even minute environmental changes and make rapid adjustments. To achieve this, they have developed a multitude of ligand-receptor and sensor-response regulator systems for assessing their local conditions and eliciting a response [16]. These triggers can work alone or in combination and may result in the organism altering a number of biological processes including growth rate, movement, membrane permeability, efflux rates, exopolysaccharide production and cell lysis. It is therefore understandable that cells within biofilms would also constantly assess their own population dynamics and adjust their phenotypes accordingly. The best characterized example of cell-cell communication is that of quorum-sensing in the marine bacterium *Vibrio fischeri*, in which the buildup of a secreted factor (inducer) due to cell density (quorum) leads to the activation of bioluminescence. These inducer-receptor systems have since been found in virtually all microorganisms tested and have been shown to regulate a multitude of biological processes [17,18]. Typical quorum-sensing compounds for Gram-negative and -positive bacteria are acylated homoserine lactones and processed oligo-peptides, respectively [17,19]. Multiple studies have further argued that quorum-sensing systems may be used specifically by biofilm organisms to mobilize to more amenable locations within the film, modify the local environment and attract and detach organisms to and from the biofilm, respectively [20-22].

BIOFILM-ASSOCIATED INFECTION AND COMPLICATIONS

Hydrodynamics of the Urinary Tract

Urine flow from the kidney to the bladder is largely peristaltic, although many of the details of this process remain unresolved [23,24]. A second component of the flow is driven purely by a pressure gradient developed between the renal pelvis and the bladder. This second flow component can be problematic should pressures in the bladder exceed those at the renal pelvis. Furthermore, computational analysis has demonstrated that the normal initiation of peristalsis can itself momentarily reverse the flow in segments of the ureter nearest its upstream entrance [24]. Since the placement of a ureteral stent relaxes the annular muscles at the stent-ureter interface, subsequently disabling the peristaltic urine transport, it can further encourage this backward flow. Under these conditions urine flow, through and around the stent, become completely driven by the pelvis-bladder pressure differential. This reduced and at times retrograde flow enhances the ability of biofilms to migrate along the device or actively detach from it and flow toward the kidneys, potentially leading to pyelonephritis [25]. Mathematical modeling has shown that the perforating holes common to most stents act to reduce this potential for reflux [25], being generally inactive during normal flow but becoming stimulated once there is a blockage [26].

In general, urethral urine flow has received little theoretical attention, although recent work on surgically-separated canine urethras has suggested that it is most likely laminar [27]. However, it should be noted that flow may briefly or sporadically transition to a non-laminar state in humans [28]. Common flow rates in the human urethra typically vary between 10-20 mL/s. With the placement of a catheter, however, the characteristics of lower urinary tract flow change substantially. By extending into the bladder the catheter effectively holds the internal sphincter open so as to create a constant drip flow through the catheter to a collection device. This sort of low energy flow has negative consequences for the patient as the higher shear rates associated with normal urination are no longer present. High flow velocities in normal urinary flow are due to the driving pressure built up in the bladder by a closed, internal sphincter. The higher shear rates connected with these flows are often successful at flushing out many of the potentially detrimental resident bacteria. A further catheter complication stems from the balloons attached to maintain catheter position. Often the balloon and catheter orientation can lead to the formation of a urine sump at the bottom of the bladder leading to an accumulation of bacteria and deposits. In an attempt to regain some of the advantages the healthy urine flushing regimen, some research has focused on the development of an electronic catheter valve. The valve can be opened on a programmable time release basis or manually by the patient. Clinical trials of this device are due to finish around 2009 [29]. Clearly, this is an area where substantial gains can be made for patient comfort with innovative solutions that tap microbiologic, urologic, and engineering expertise.

Urethral Catheters and Ureteral Stents

In North America alone more than 100 million urethral catheters and ureteral stents are inserted annually, translating into millions of device-associated infections and billions of dollars in additional health care expenditures [30]. The major problem associated with their usage is that they present novel, non-host surfaces on which bacteria can colonize and form biofilms. The most common use for urethral catheters is during surgery to monitor urinary output and in the majority of cases these patients do not develop a clinical infection due to a sufficiently short indwelling time. That being said, there are a growing number of patients who require long-term catheterization and most will eventually suffer from chronic recurrent bladder infections. It has been estimated that the risk of bacteriuria increases by roughly 10% for each day that a urethral catheter is in place and that virtually all catheterized patients will develop a urinary tract infection when the catheter remains beyond 28 days [31]. At the root of the problem is the simple fact that a urethral catheter directly connects the urinary tract with the outside environment. Since a patient's own skin is enveloped in microorganisms, as well as the close proximity of the urinary tract to the gastrointestinal tract and numerous other environmental and patient factors (e.g., decreased immunity, hospitalization, hygiene), it is easy to understand how most long-term catheterized patients eventually become infected [32]. The more opportunity a device has to become colonized, the higher the risk for biofilm development, migration to the bladder and development of infection. As alluded to previously, not only can the colonization of a urinary catheter lead to urinary tract infections but it may also affect the functioning of the catheter through obstruction with encrustation, especially in the case of urease-producing organisms [31].

Ureteral stents are likewise subject to biofilm development, infection and encrustation, although rates of occurrence are greatly reduced. For instance, one study examining urine culture and stent colonization in ~150 patients found colonization rates of 0, 33, 50 and 54% when stent indwelling times were < 2 weeks, < 4 weeks, 4-6 weeks and > 6 weeks [33]. The major reason for this decreased rate compared to catheters is the fact that a ureteral stent is placed entirely within the body. Thus, aside from contamination during placement or the presence of an existing infection, bacteriuria or other medical condition allowing organisms into the tract, the device is not subjected to microbes on a continual basis like that of a urethral catheter. For instance, at one extreme, forgotten stents have remained in patients for several years before retrieval and never developed an infection or microbial biofilm (although they commonly severely encrust) [34]. Thus, if a ureteral stent goes into a sterile urinary tract without surgical contamination, how does it still become colonized as indwelling time increases? This is due at least is part to the fact that the urinary tract is not a completely sterile environment all of the time. Transient bacteriuria is hypothesized to occur within the general population (especially in women and the elderly), though goes unnoticed in the majority of cases [35,36]. When a ureteral stent is present, those transient visitors have the opportunity to attach to its surface before the subject's urinary tract and immune system flush them out. This can then develop into recurrent bacteriuria or infection. A final point of interest from the aforementioned stent colonization study was that a positive urine culture only corroborated actual device colonization in 69% of cases [33]. This highlights the fact that not all biofilm organisms can be cultivated directly off of urinary tract devices [37]. This can develop into a very dangerous clinical situation, especially if the patient continues to provide negative cultures and the infected device continues to indwell. This is one of the major reasons prophylactic antibiotics are commonly prescribed by clinicians upon stent placement, even for short term indwelling [33].

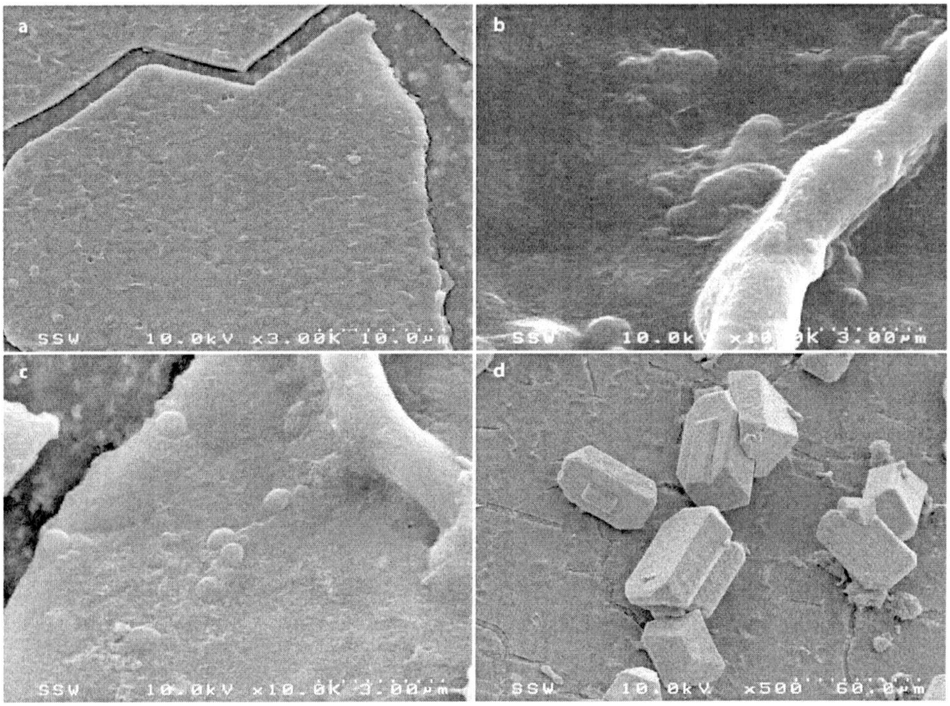

FIGURE 4. Bacterial biofilms formed on ureteral stents in artificial urine after 48 hour challenge, specifically *E. coli* (a), *K. pneumoniae* 280 (b), *S. aureus* Newman (c) and *P. mirabilis* 296 (d).

The major bacterial species involved in catheter and stent infections are Escherichia coli, Proteus mirabilis, Klebsiella pneumoniae, Pseudomonas aeruginosa, Staphylococcus spp. (mainly S. epidermidis, S. aureus, S. saprophyticus) and Enterococcus spp. (mainly E. faecalis, E. faecium). Several of these are shown in Figure 4. In addition, there are countless opportunistic pathogens that can form biofilms on urinary devices and cause infection depending upon the patient's health and immune status, as well as microbial exposure. Management of patients with long-term catheterization and stenting remains a challenge. In most situations, only patients at risk for sepsis or those with symptomatic infections should be actively treated while those with isolated bacteriuria may be observed. Routine device changes may help reduce bacterial load and allow for more effective antibiotic therapy when required as mature biofilms may be more difficult to treat than those less established [38].

Biofilm Shedding and Migration

Detachment and dispersal of biofilm cells into the environment is the least known aspect of biofilm formation but is critical to bacterial spread and thus to overall population survival [1,10,39]. In terms of biomaterial use, this shedding can lead to biofilm and infection spread, sepsis, the reappearance of infection following antimicrobial treatment (often leading to chronic infection) and the growth of the original biofilm. For example, bacterial cells released from a ureteral stent biofilm have the potential to: **1**) Travel down to the bladder and instigate or regenerate a previously-cleared cystitis; **2**) Travel up the device itself (e.g., *Proteus mirabilis* swarming, biofilm migration) [40,41] or via urine reflux induced by the device to the kidney, causing pyelonephritis [25,42,43]; **3**) Adhere again to the device and/or existing biofilm increasing its surface area and density; **4**) Adhere to a potential calculus within the tract, creating a further nidus of infection and potentially inhibiting stone treatment options; **5**) Promote the formation of calculi if the organism expresses urease [31] and **6**) Enter the underlying layers of the urinary tract epithelia and even the bloodstream if local damage has been induced by the device or infection, or the organism possesses the ability to do so on its own [44]. All of these scenarios enhance the ability of the organism to remain in the tract following device removal and/or replacement, and can greatly increase the severity of infection. Previous work by our group compared a standard ureteral stent placed in conjunction with pre- and post-operative antibiotics to one impregnated with the antimicrobial triclosan in chronically-stented patients [13]. We observed that every stent placed in a patient with a positive urine culture during instillation had adherent, viable biofilms upon removal at three months, despite the fact that they all went through multiple courses of antimicrobial therapy during the indwelling period. Furthermore, biofilm organisms from every one of these devices matched the original urinary isolate as well as any organisms recovered from their previous stent(s). This strongly suggests that ureteral stents placed within an infected urinary environment will become infected, regardless of the device type or antimicrobial therapy regimen used and highlights the ability of biofilms to induce chronic infections. Shedding is one of the most clinically-relevant biofilm aspects as it provides organisms that enhance, spread and prolong infections.

Biofilm Resistance to Antibiotics

The fact that biofilms are inherently resistant to antibiotics has been well documented and is the greatest obstacle in treating chronic infections, especially those associated with prostheses. As a consequence, infections associated with biofilms are rarely resolved using antibiotic therapy alone, even in patients with fully functioning immune defenses. Studies have shown that some organisms within biofilms can survive antibiotic concentrations >1000 fold higher than those required to kill their planktonic counterparts [45,46]. This resistance is multi-factorial, dependent upon the organism challenged and agent utilized, the structure and makeup of the biofilm matrix, local environmental factors and the presence of persister cells.

It was originally hypothesized that the EPS matrix of biofilms was the primary factor involved in their resistance to antimicrobials, strictly due to the inability of the antimicrobial agent to reach cells buried within the biofilm. While the matrix can inhibit the transfer of particular compounds (including antibiotics) through it via chelation, destruction and direct blockage, it is largely agent- and microbe-dependent [47-49]. Ultimately, these impediments may result in only sub-lethal concentrations of the antibiotic reaching cells within the biofilm or delay the buildup of the compound to cidal levels, allowing resistance mechanisms to be activated or acquired. Examples of this include strains expressing beta-lactamase (destroys most penicillin and cephalosporin class antibiotics) [45], and the chelation of aminoglycoside antibiotics by negatively charged particles within the biofilm matrix of *P. aeruginosa* [48].

Another proposed mechanism is the development of various microenvironments within the biofilm that may be anaerobic, have altered pH and/or vary highly in solute and waste product levels. These changes may result in antibiotic destruction in that region or induce phenotypic changes in some cells that result in a low-dividing state or reduced membrane permeability. This idea is supported by studies showing reduced susceptibility in membrane porin mutants [50], loss of activity of some antibiotics under anaerobic conditions [51] and the fact that several classes of antibiotics are only effective on rapidly-dividing cells.

A third mechanism of escape from treatment is the production of persister cells, a sub-population of metabolically dormant cells within biofilms that are akin to bacterial spores [8]. These cells are highly tolerant to antimicrobials and appear to be produced maximally during stationary phase growth, suspected to be the phase of growth in which most biofilm cells reside. They do not apparently need to possess any particular resistance mechanisms to survive and can resume growth once the concentration of antibiotic drops to sub-lethal concentration. Although planktonic persisters can be mopped up by immune cells following antimicrobial therapy that kills the majority of the remaining population, cells buried within a biofilm are protected from immune clearance. This explains how persisters can be formed during both planktonic and biofilm infections but only become a clinical problem with respect to biofilms.

BIOFILM PREVENTION AND TREATMENT STRATEGIES

The prevention and treatment of biofilms in urology, especially those on prostheses, has involved multiple research and clinically-based approaches. Most strategies have concerned modifications to the biomaterial [52-54] or the development and application of surface coatings [55,56] in attempts to prevent bacterial attachment by rendering the surface less attractive to microbes. This line of investigation has evolved further to include the use of adherent, impregnated and oral antimicrobials to kill or inhibit the growth of organisms that are ultimately successful in surface adherence [57-59]. Although no single approach has proven entirely successful, several have demonstrated some clinical benefit in reducing infections and many have shown superior efficacy during *in vitro* and/or animal studies. Although there currently exists no biofilm-resistant biomaterial or device in urology, there are several major avenues of research aimed at developing one.

Antimicrobials

Silver

The most studied and arguably successful surface-based strategy to date for preventing device-related infections in urology is that of silver-coated urethral catheters, which have been in use for over 20 years. The broad-spectrum antimicrobial effects of silver have been known since ancient times, and studies have revealed that it acts by blocking multiple enzymatic processes via interaction with electron donors (especially sulfhydryl groups) [60] and through membrane destabilization [61]. Several meta-analyses comparing over 20 studies have made a case that silver alloy (but not silver oxide) coated devices are effective in reducing overall catheter-associated urinary tract infection (CAUTI) rates by up to 45% [60,62]. However, it is important to note that many of those studies could not show significance statistically, and wide variations in overall efficacy were observed [30,62]. In addition, the higher cost of these devices over standard catheters further clouds the issue. Ultimately, despite intense research and over two decades of use, it remains unclear as to whether silver coated catheters are the best clinical tool for significantly decreasing CAUTI .

Antimicrobial Hydrogels

Maeyama et al. [63] developed a novel surface based on a biodegradable polymer consisting of an antimicrobial catechin found in green tea extracts. The surface erodible polymer, Epigalocatechin-3-gallate (EGCg), showed dose-dependent effects in inhibiting *E. coli* biofilm formation while enhancing destruction. The target of EGCg was found to be DNA gyrase, the enzyme also targeted by the quinolone antibiotics [64]. This novel, hydrophilic surface treatment swells in the presence of a physiological fluid and releases EGCg to the bulk phase. Over time, surface erosion proceeds and more EGCg is released, resulting in high local concentrations near the surface. Such concentrations contribute to the destruction of the three-dimensional biofilm interface as well as the biofilm/substrate interface. Direct consequences of these effects are the subsequent detachment, removal, or washout of the biofilm. Further studies are required to determine clinical potential.

Numerous other antimicrobials have been coated onto urological devices for biofilm prevention and treatment including multiple antibiotics (gentamicin, cefazolin and several quinolones) [57,65,66], as well as innate immune factors such as nitric oxide [58]. In addition, certain hydrogels have been developed that release stored antimicrobials only upon the application of ultrasonic waves to allow for tight regulation of compound release [67]. Overall, these studies widely vary in their results which range from no perceived effect to complete biofilm prevention and tend to be antimicrobial and strain specific. These largely conflicting results, combined with generally short elution periods observed with these types of coatings and the growing trend of antimicrobial resistance and tolerance have prevented this line of research from being deemed a clinical success.

Triclosan

Triclosan is a broad-spectrum antimicrobial that has been in use for over forty years and is currently found in numerous consumer and medical products including surgical scrubs and vicryl suture [68]. At sub-lethal concentrations it acts by inhibiting the bacterial enoyl-acyl carrier protein (ACP) reductase (FabI), a critical enzyme in fatty acid biosynthesis, while at bactericidal concentrations is believed to act through multiple, non-specific mechanisms including membrane destabilization [69]. Two urological approaches have been recently applied to investigate its ability to prevent device-associated biofilm-formation and infection: 1) elution from a ureteral stent impregnated with triclosan (Triumph®, Boston Scientific Corp. Inc.) and 2) elution from catheter balloons impregnated with the antimicrobial [13,70]. Triclosan-eluting stents demonstrated significant antimicrobial and infection clearance effects during preliminary *in vitro* and *in vivo* studies, as well as anti-inflammatory effects in cell culture [71-73]. However, a clinical trial involving chronically-stented patients showed no improvement in device colonization or urine culturing despite a significant reduction in antibiotic usage compared to controls [13]. Thus, at least within this complicated patient population, the elution of triclosan alone from the device was unable to prevent colonization and biofilm formation. Jones et al. conducted preliminary *in vitro* experiments involving catheters whose retention balloons were filled with triclosan [70]. Their results were encouraging as biofilm formation was completely prevented for several major uropathogens (including *E. coli* and *P. mirabilis*) and greatly inhibited for others such as *E. faecalis*, which possess moderate TCN resistance. As expected, no biofilm inhibition was observed for *P. aeruginosa*, which exhibits high level resistance to the agent via membrane impermeability and efflux pump expression [72, 74].

Biofilm Disrupting Agents

We have already discussed cell-cell communication within biofilms as a means for microorganisms to control their biofilm development and spread. However, these factors also offer a potential opportunity to influence biofilm development on medical devices either through surface coating or exogenous application [75]. Studies have already examined several of these quorum-sensing factors on *P. aeruginosa* biofilms and shown them to inhibit biofilm formation and promote biofilm dissolution [76,77]. In addition, ureteral stents coated with the quorum-sensing inhibitor RNA III inhibiting peptide from *S. aureus* were found to resist biofilms of that organism *in vitro* and in a rat model of device infection, especially when combined with the antibiotic teicoplanin [78,79]. Although still in its infancy, this line of research may prove to be fruitful as it specifically targets biofilm organisms by using their own naturally-evolved signaling factors against them. Furthermore, these factors can be combined with other agents such as antimicrobials to either kill or inhibit the growth of organisms released from the biofilms before they can adhere again.

Novel Anti-fouling Coatings

Following many uses in industrial applications, diamond-like coatings (DLC) are being adapted for biomedical applications. These amorphous carbon coatings are known for their superior tribologic properties and their biocompatibility. Laube et al. developed a low temperature, low pressure, plasma-enhanced chemical vapor deposition technique for coating polymeric medical implants with DLC [80]. The coating was assessed for its ability to decrease the extent of crystalline biofilm formation, as well as the potential stent side effects and patient comfort. Results indicated *in vivo* biofilm formation and encrustation was effectively reduced. Subsequently, patients were more tolerant of replacement of the low-friction devices. While the precise reasons for the positive performance characteristics of DLC are still not clear, results certainly warrant additional research.

Previous work involving hydrogels containing poly(ethylene glycol) (PEG) have shown considerable success as antifouling agents due to PEG's hydrophilic nature, high degree of mobility, and steric hindrance in its chemical structure. The polyether structure of PEG allows it to couple large numbers of water molecules, reducing its coefficient of friction and driving it to behave more like a fluid. Importantly, PEG has shown considerable success in resisting not only bacterial attachment, but that of proteins and mammalian cells as well, suggesting that it may be able to resist conditioning film development. To date, the main concerns with using PEG have been the inability to anchor enough of the molecules to generate a robust, high-density coating and prevent its thermal, oxidative or hydrolytic degradation during this process. A novel approach for attaching PEG and other molecules to device surfaces is derived from nature, employing peptide mimics based upon the adhesive proteins involved in the mussel adherence to underwater surfaces. *In vitro* and *in vivo* studies involving surfaces coated with PEG conjugated to one of these biological glues, namely 3,4-dihydroxyphenylalanine (DOPA) demonstrated the inhibition of both conditioning and biofilm formation, as well as a significant reduction in UPEC adherence within a rabbit model of cystitis [81,82]. Future studies are underway to address its true clinical potential.

Novel Stent Designs

While urinary stenting has been in medicine for over 2000 years [80], modern stents have changed very little in terms of overall design. Recent investigations have brought to light an apparent lack of clear design rationale for some aspects of common stents—in particular, the number, size, and orientation of the pass-through holes in the stent [26]. Some researchers have even questioned the efficacy and necessity of the central bore associated with a typical stent. A novel stent designed for biliary drainage was developed with a winged cross section [83]. Numerical modeling confirmed that this design offered a larger surface area for flow, higher flow velocity, and an increased flow rate compared to that of a conventional tubular stent. In addition, the lack of a central bore eliminates the potential for luminal occlusion. Though originally designed for biliary drainage, such a novel design may be adapted for urology.

Responding to high stenting failure rates in patients with extrinsic ureteral obstruction, some minor modifications have been made to the traditional stent with limited results [84,85]. Representing a more radical departure, some have attempted the simultaneous insertion of two ipsilateral stents, yielding better flow rates with time [86]. Unfortunately, the logistical challenges associated with installation and removal may outweigh the benefits of the configuration. In light of this, monolithic double "barreled" or double-lumen stents were developed by ACMI and Cook Urological. Hafron et al. evaluated these dual-lumen stents in *ex vivo* porcine kidney models with extrinsic ureteral obstruction [87]. The prototype double stents provided excellent flow that rivaled that of two stents juxtaposed. While these stents were assessed under conditions of extrinsic obstruction, it could be rationally postulated that the built-in redundancy of the design may increase their efficacy during intrinsic blockage.

CONCLUSIONS

The development of biofilms by microorganisms is both a natural and vital part of their biological imperative, namely survival. The fact that these organisms also form biofilms on and within the human body can be rationalized as a simple extension of this natural tendency, not necessarily a distinct phenomenon. Biofilms pose an enormous challenge in medicine as they can form rapidly on almost any surface and once formed, are virtually impossible to remove. This is understandable since microorganisms use multiple strategies to form biofilms and can rapidly adjust to changing environmental conditions including resistance to host immunity and antimicrobials. Most strategies to date for inhibiting biofilms deal with the use of antimicrobials but generally only work to reduce the planktonic organisms shed from them. It is interesting to note that the human immune system is largely successful against infectious microorganisms that enter the body through the concerted efforts of a wealth of innate and acquired immune strategies. Thus, it may simply be that one or two strategies employed at a time are not sufficient to prevent or rid biofilms and their related infections. Perhaps a multi-faceted approach to device development employing eluting antimicrobials with surface bound silver and biofilm-disrupting agents may be more successful. This strategy has the potential to attack the pathogen in multiple ways simultaneously while also allowing the host's natural immune system to play a role. In addition, the use of antibiotics prior to device placement or between device changes is critical for preventing certain infections.

Biofilm prevention and eradication have been at the forefront of both clinical and industrial research on urological devices for several decades, and countless studies have looked into developing biofilm-resistant materials, surface coatings, signaling molecules, antimicrobials and physical treatments with proven clinical benefit. Although many of these studies have shown powerful *in vitro* and *in vivo* evidence of biofilm inhibition, nothing has ultimately led to a device or treatment modality that would be considered a clinical triumph in the field. This is not entirely surprising as biofilm-associated device infections are multi-factorial and depend upon not only bacterial aspects, but the host and environment as well. Exhaustive studies have revealed that the vast majority of biofilms cannot be eradicated by antimicrobials once formed, and that their repeated use in these situations may instead promote resistance. That being said, their ability to at least slow biofilm formation and clear planktonic organisms is of critical clinical importance and their use toward this end must be continued until better therapeutic options are available. Novel device designs and coatings are constantly under development in attempts to build upon previous failures and achieve a resistant device. Currently, the most promising molecules are those involved in bacterial communication as they can target biofilm organisms specifically and may be able to break down existing biofilms. Their application thus far appears to be optimal when utilized in conjunction with antimicrobials, as planktonic organisms and those released from existing biofilms can be killed. Ultimately, success in biofilms and their related infections may not come in the form of complete prevention or clearance, but more in clinically-relevant control.

ACKNOWLEDGMENTS

Peter Cadieux is an American Urological Association Foundation Research Scholar. Scanning electron micrographs were imaged by Ross Davidson and Wayne Chang at Surface Science Western at the University of Western Ontario (www.uwo.ca/ssw). Work involving triclosan was supported through grants from Boston Scientific (Natick, MA, USA) and the Lawson Health Research Institute, while that involving PEG-DOPA based anti-fouling coatings was funded by Nerites Corporation Limited (Madison, WI, USA).

REFERENCES

1. J W Costerton, *The Biofilm Primer*. (Springer, New York, 2007).
2. Surman S Jass J, Walker J T, in *Medical Biofilms: Detection, Prevention and Control*, edited by Surman S Jass J, Walker J T (John Wiley and Sons, Hoboken, 2003), pp. 1.
3. P. Saravanan, Y. V. Nancharaiah, V. P. Venugopalan et al., *Biofouling* **22** (5-6), 371 (2006).
4. S. L. Stramer and M. J. Starzyk, *Microbios* **23** (93-94), 193 (1978).
5. R. M. Donlan and J. W. Costerton, *Clin Microbiol Rev* **15** (2), 167 (2002).
6. M. Allesen-Holm, K. B. Barken, L. Yang et al., *Mol Microbiol* **59** (4), 1114 (2006)
7. C. B. Whitchurch, T. Tolker-Nielsen, P. C. Ragas et al., *Science* **295** (5559), 1487 (2002).
8. K. Lewis, *Nat Rev Microbiol* **5** (1), 48 (2007).
9. K. Sauer, A. K. Camper, G. D. Ehrlich et al., *J Bacteriol* **184** (4), 1140 (2002).
10. P. Stoodley, K. Sauer, D. G. Davies et al., *Annu Rev Microbiol* **56**, 187 (2002).
11. G. Jackson, H. Beyenal, W. M. Rees et al., *J Microbiol Methods* **47** (1), 1 (2001).
12. G. Reid, J. D. Denstedt, Y. S. Kang et al., *J Urol* **148** (5), 1592 (1992).
13. P. A. Cadieux, B. H. Chew, L. Nott et al., *J Endourology* (submitted) (2008).
14. N. S. Morris, D. J. Stickler, and R. J. McLean, *World J Urol* **17** (6), 345 (1999)
15. D. Stickler, N. Morris, M. C. Moreno et al., *Eur J Clin Microbiol Infect Dis* **17** (9), 649 (1998).
16. A. Khorchid and M. Ikura, *Int J Biochem Cell Biol* **38** (3), 307 (2006).
17. D. L. Erickson, R. Endersby, A. Kirkham et al., *Infect Immun* **70** (4), 1783 (2002).
18. T. S. Murray, M. Egan, and B. I. Kazmierczak, *Curr Opin Pediatr* **19** (1), 83 (2007).

19. W. R. Abraham, *Curr Med Chem* **13** (13), 1509 (2006).
20. D. G. Allison and P. Gilbert, *J Ind Microbiol* **15** (4), 311 (1995).
21. M. C. Hansen, R. J. Palmer, and D. C. White, *J Microbiol Methods* **40** (3), 233 (2000).
22. P. Stoodley, S. Wilson, L. Hall-Stoodley et al., *Appl Environ Microbiol* **67** (12), 5608 (2001).
23. S. Boyarsky, C. W. Gottschalk, E. A. Tanagho et al., *Hydrodynamics of the Ureter and Renal Pelvis*. (Academic Press, New York - London, 1971).
24. B. Vahidi and N. Fatouraee, in *Proc29th Ann Intl Conf IEEE EMBS Cite Intl* (IEEE, Lyon, France, 2007).
25. L. J. Cummings, S. L. Waters, J. A. D. Wattis et al., *J Math Biol* **49** (1), 26 (2004).
26. J. C. K. Tong, E. M. Sparrow, and J. P. Abraham, *J Biomech Eng* **129**, 6 (2007).
27. A. A. Bykova and S. A. Regirer, *Fluid Dyn* **40** (1), 19 (2005).
28. H. S. Lecamwasam, M. P. Sullivan, S. V. Yalla et al., *Neurol and Urodyn* **18** (5), 21 (1999).
29. C. Evans-Pughe, *Instit Elec Eng (IEE) Rev* **51** (2), 40 (2005).
30. S. M. Jacobsen, D. J. Stickler, H. L. Mobley et al., *Clin Microbiol Rev* **21** (1), 26 (2008).
31. D. Stickler, *Biofouling* **94**, 293 (1996).
32. K. B. Waites, K. C. Canupp, and M. J. DeVivo, *J Spinal Cord Med* **27** (5), 448 (2004).
33. B. Lojanapiwat, *World J Urol* **24** (6), 681 (2006).
34. K. Park, S. S. Jeon, H. Park et al., *Urol Res* **32** (6), 416 (2004).
35. F. J. Meijman, *Ned Tijdschr Geneeskd* **145** (15), 716 (2001).
36. G. Rahav, E. Pinco, G. Bachrach et al., *Age Ageing* **32** (6), 670 (2003).
37. D. A. Lifshitz, H. Z. Winkler, M. Gross et al., *J Endourol* **13** (10), 735 (1999).
38. H. Anwar, M. Dasgupta, K. Lam et al., *J Antimicrob Chemother* **24** (5), 647 (1989).
39. J. W. Costerton, K. J. Cheng, G. G. Geesey et al., *Annu Rev Microbiol* **41**, 435 (1987).
40. B. Purvedorj, J. W. Costerton, and P. Stoodley, *Appl Environ Microbiol* **68** (9), 8 (2002).
41. D. Stickler, *Curr Opin Microbiol* **2** (3), 270 (1999).
42. C. Choisy, A. Herard, V. Vernet-Garnier et al., *Bull Acad Natl Med* **182** (8), 1709 (1998).
43. S. Choong and H. Whitfield, *BJU Int* **86** (8), 935 (2000).
44. D. A. Rosen, T. M. Hooton, W. E. Stamm et al., *PLoS Med* **4** (12), e329 (2007).
45. J. N. Anderl, M. J. Franklin, and P. S. Stewart, *Antimicrob Agents Chemother* **44** (7), 1818 (2000).
46. P. S. Stewart and J. W. Costerton, *Lancet* **358**, 3 (2001).
47. R. A. Brady, J. G. Leid, A. K. Camper et al., *Infect Immun* **74** (6), 3415 (2006).
48. R. Ramphal, M. Lhermitte, M. Filliat et al., *J Antimicrob Chemother* **22** (4), 483 (1988).
49. W. W. Nichols, S. M. Dorrington, M. P. Slack et al., *Antimicrob Agents Chemother* **32** (4), 518 (1988).
50. K. Otto and M. Hermansson, *J Bacteriol* **186** (1), 226 (2004).
51. K. J. Tack and L. D. Sabath, *Chemotherapy* **31** (3), 204 (1985).
52. G. Legeay, F. Poncin-Epaillard, and C. R. Arciola, *Int J Artif Organs* **29** (4), 453 (2006).
53. P. Petrini, C. R. Arciola, I. Pezzali et al., *Int J Artif Organs* **29** (4), 434 (2006).
54. J. M. Schierholz, J. Beuth, A. Rump et al., *J Chemother* **13 Spec No 1** (1), 239 (2001).
55. S. Hou, E. A. Burton, K. A. Simon et al., *Appl Environ Microbiol* **73** (13), 4300 (2007).
56. M. Vigeant, S. N. Rothstein, and J. J. Cacciatore, in *AIChE Ann Meeting, Conf Proc* (American Institute of Chemical Engineers Cincinnati, Ohio, USA, 2005).
57. V. DiTizio, G. W. Ferguson, M. W. Mittelman et al., *Biomaterials* **19** (20), 1877 (1998).
58. B. J. Nablo, H. L. Prichard, R. D. Butler et al., *Biomaterials* **26** (34), 6984 (2005).
59. G. Reid, M. Habash, D. Vachon et al., *Int J Antimicrob Agents* **17** (4), 317 (2001).
60. R. M. Slawson, M. I. Van Dyke, H. Lee et al., *Plasmid* **27** (1), 72 (1992).
61. P. Dibrov, J. Dzioba, K. K. Gosink et al., *Antimicrob Agents Chemother* **46** (8), 2668 (2002).
62. K. Davenport and F. X. Keeley, *J Hosp Infect* **60** (4), 298 (2005).
63. R. Maeyama, I. Kwon, Y. Mizunoe et al., *J Biomed Mater Res Part A* **75A** (1), 146 (2005).
64. H. Gradisar, P. Pristovsek, A. Plaper et al., *J Med Chem* **50** (2), 264 (2007).
65. T. John, A. Rajpurkar, G. Smith et al., *J Endourol* **21** (10), 1211 (2007).
66. J. L. Pugach, V. DiTizio, M. W. Mittelman et al., *J Urol* **162** (3 Pt 1), 883 (1999).
67. P. Norris, M. Noble, I. Francolini et al., *Antimicrob Agents Chemother* **49** (10), 4272 (2005).

68. H. N. Bhargava and P. A. Leonard, *Am J Infect Control* **24** (3), 209 (1996).
69. R. J. Heath, Y. T. Yu, M. A. Shapiro et al., *J Biol Chem* **273** (46), 30316 (1998).
70. G. L. Jones, C. T. Muller, M. O'Reilly et al., *J Antimicrob Chemother* **57** (2), 266 (2006).
71. P. A. Cadieux, B. H. Chew, B. E. Knudsen et al., *J Urol* **175** (6), 2331 (2006).
72. C. N. Elwood, B. H. Chew, S. Seney et al., *J Endourol* **21** (10), 1217 (2007).
73. B. H. Chew, P. A. Cadieux, G. Reid et al., *J Endourol* **20** (11), 949 (2006).
74. R. Chuanchuen, K. Beinlich, T. T. Hoang et al., *Antimicrob Agents Chemother* **45** (2), 428 (2001).
75. T. B. Rasmussen and M. Givskov, *Int J Med Microbiol* **296** (2-3), 149 (2006).
76. M. Hentzer, K. Riedel, T. B. Rasmussen et al., *Microbiology* **148** (Pt 1), 87 (2002).
77. D. C. Laux, J. M. Corson, M. Givskov et al., *Microbiology* **148** (Pt 6), 1709 (2002).
78. N. Balaban, P. Stoodley, C. A. Fux et al., *Clin Orthop Relat Res* (437), 48 (2005).
79. O. Cirioni, R. Ghiselli, D. Minardi et al., *Antimicrob Agents Chemother* **51** (12), 4518 (2007).
80. N. Laube, L. Kleinen, J. Bradenahl et al., *J Urol* **177**, 1923 (2007).
81. R. Ko, P. A. Cadieux, J. L. Dalsin et al., *J Endourol* (2008).
82. A. Pechey, C. N. Elwood, G. R. Wignall et al., *J Urol* (Submitted) (2008).
83. G. Raju, R. Sud, A. Elfert et al., *Gastroint Endoscopy* **63** (2), 317 (2006).
84. R. Shick, E. M. Seidal, T. Kalem et al., *J Endourol* **12**, 37 (1998).
85. M. Tliguri, M. Nouri, R. You et al., *Progres en Urologie* **10**, 92 (2000).
86. P. Rotariu, P. Yohannes, M. Alexianu et al., *J Endourol* **15**, 979 (2001).
87. J. Hafron, M. Ost, B. Tan et al., *Urology* **68** (4), 911 (2006).

Biodegradable Ureteral Stents

Ben H. Chew, Boris A. Hadaschik, Ryan F. Paterson and Dirk Lange

Department of Urologic Sciences, University of British Columbia, Vancouver, BC, Canada

Abstract. Ureteral stents have been associated with painful symptoms and require a secondary procedure for removal if the suture tether is removed. Biodegradable stents have been attempted in the past, but are no longer used since they resulted in histological inflammation or unpredictable variability in degradation time. This article reviews past degradable materials used in both the prostatic urethra and ureter as well as identifies a new degradable ureteral stent that lasts between 2 to 4 weeks in a porcine model.

Keywords: Ureter, stent, degradable
PACS: 01.30.Cc

INTRODUCTION

Ureteral stents are commonly used in urology today. The quest continues for the ideal stent which would be radiopaque, comfortable, easily manufactured, and resists encrustation and infection. Various coatings and materials have been utilized in an attempt to improve ureteral stent properties and minimize such stent-related problems as infection, encrustation, and bothersome symptoms. The exact cause of ureteral stent-related pain and symptoms is unknown. If a suture tether is not used, the stent must be removed via a secondary cystoscopic procedure resulting in costs, surgeon time, and discomfort. In an effort to make ureteral stent removal easier, efforts such as a magnet on the bladder curl and a urethral catheter with the opposing magnet has been used to facilitate removal [1].

Stent symptoms occur in more than 80% of stented patients and may consist of hematuria, flank pain, dysuria, and infection [2]. Furthermore, 58% of patients studied were unable to continue working normally or experienced negative economic impact [2]. Softer stents have been designed in an attempt to reduce ureteral stent symptoms. A randomized trial of soft versus firm polymers utilizing the validated Ureteral Stent Symptom Questionnaire revealed no difference in stent symptoms at one and four weeks post-stent insertion [3]. The exact mechanism of stent symptoms is unknown and although softer materials did not reduce stent symptoms, the amount of stent curl in the bladder did significantly increase symptoms. Rane et al. examined the amount of stent protruding into the bladder and found that ureteral stents that crossed the midline of the bladder resulted in significantly more bothersome symptoms [4].

Ureteral stents require a secondary procedure for removal if the suture tether is removed. Many physicians remove this tether as they can be a cause of early stent extrusion and some patients object to a suture protruding from their urethra. Even

CP1049, *Renal Stone Disease 2, 2nd International Urolithiasis Research Symposium,*
edited by A. P. Evan, J. E. Lingeman, J. A. McAteer, and J. C. Williams, Jr.

worse, some patients are unaware that a stent has been placed and may lead to a "forgotten stent" that remains in for years. Such forgotten stents become severely encrusted (Figure 1) and take, on average, three operations for complete removal utilizing techniques such as percutaneous nephrolithotomy, shockwave lithotripsy, and ureteroscopy [5]. Severely encrusted stents can also result in renal failure and potentially even death [6].

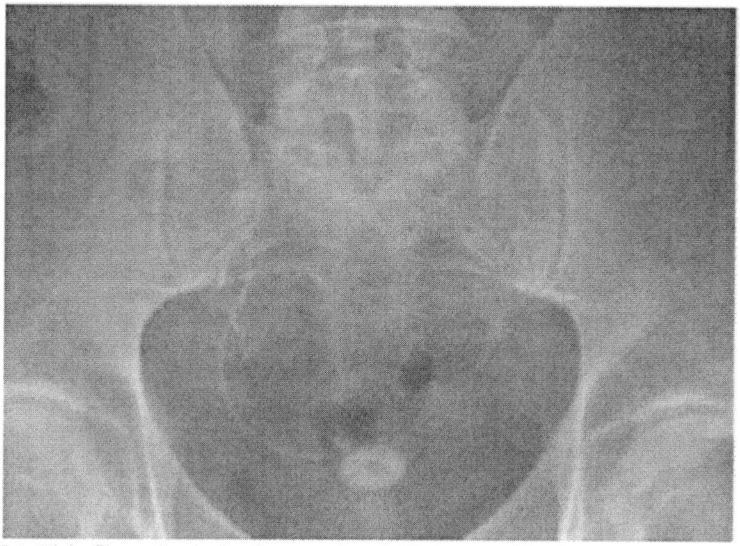

FIGURE 1. Plain film radiograph of a severely calcified stent with a large calcified bladder curl.

BIODEGRADABLE STENTS

Biodegradable stents are designed to degrade over time while providing upper tract urinary drainage. The design of a biodegradable stent must take into consideration the biocompatibility properties of the material, as well as the degree of expansion and degradation rates, and most importantly it must be able to fulfill the basic requirement of a stent in that it must be able to guarantee urinary flow from the renal pelvis through the ureter and into the bladder for the desired period of time. One of the challenges involved in designing a biodegradable stent is the control of the rate of degradation. Schlick and Planz [7,8] designed a stent composed of plastics, the degradation of which was dependent upon the urine pH. *In vitro* experiments with artificial urine showed that the stents were stable at urine pH less than 7.0 for at least 30 days, while they dissolved completely within 48 hours at pH greater or equal to 7.0. The principle behind this stent is that it will remain stable at physiological urine pH of 5-6, and can be triggered to dissolve by medically altering urinary pH. Although very promising, this technology remains at an experimental stage and awaits animal trials. An additional factor that may need to be taken into consideration is the influence of encrustation as it can form a platform for bacterial adherence and infection. In addition to this, stent encrustation and bacterial adherence may also influence urine pH. Uropathogens in general are known to increase urine pH, and may have an effect *in vivo*. In addition to this, medically increasing the urinary pH may introduce an additional risk for infection as more alkaline pH favors bacterial survival and some increased stone formation (calcium phosphate and magnesium ammonium phosphate (struvite) stones which precipitate at higher pH). In addition, encrustation of the stent may also prevent exposure of the stent to its environment and the altered pH, thus limiting its rate of decomposition.

Other biodegradable ureteral stents have been designed and attempted previously, but are no longer used due to biocompatibility issues in porcine ureters or because they dissolved in an inhomogeneous, premature, or delayed fashion. Lingeman et al. tested the Temporary Ureteral Drainage Stent (TUDS, Boston Scientific) in phase I and phase II trials [10,11]. In the Phase II trial, 88 patients were stented with the TUDS and followed to assess time to degradation. The primary objective was to achieve urinary drainage for at least 48 hours. Seventy (81%) of 87 patients retained the stent for the first 48 hours with 17 stents undergoing early extrusion. Three of these 17 patients with early stent extrusion required intervention: 1 required cystoscopy to reposition a retrogradely migrated stent and the other 2 required intravenous narcotics to relieve discomfort and obstructing symptoms. The median time to eliminate the stent was 15 days. By 30 days, only 14 of the 88 patients had any stent pieces visible on radiography. At 90 days, 3 of the patients had retained fragments and 2 of these underwent shockwave lithotripsy with subsequent passage of the fragments. The remaining patient underwent ureteroscopy followed by shockwave lithotripsy to eliminate the stent fragments. It appears that because of the 3 patients who had retained fragments at 3 months, this stent was no longer available on the market. Several other important points have arose from this study, however. It does provide some evidence that a stent does not need to be *in situ* for very long following ureteroscopy—17 of the patients extruded the stent and only 2 of them had some discomfort. Furthermore, this stent provided good drainage for the vast majority of patients in the study with significantly less discomfort than regular stents (vis-à-vis a questionnaire performed by patients in the study who previously had experienced a ureteral stent). Although the TUDS biodegradable stent was discontinued, the search for a stent that was more comfortable and does not require removal continues today.

The authors are testing a new stent made from a variation of biodegradable co-polymers similar to polymers used in absorbable sutures (Figure 2; Uriprene^{TM}, Poly-Med Inc, Greenfield, SC, marketed by Indevus Pharmaceuticals, Lexington, MA). While the hydrophobic mesh of the coating of this new stent dissolves rapidly, the inner coil dissolves later and provides the necessary structure to facilitate urinary drainage. The stent is a combination of L-glycolic acid, polyethylene glycol, and barium sulfate. Animal studies have been performed to assess time to degradation and the physiological responses elicited in a porcine model as compared to standard ethylene vinyl acetate and polyurethane stents. Two versions of the stent have been tested. The first version of the stent consisted of a single pigtail curl in the renal portion and took between 7 to 10 weeks to fully dissolve.[9] It was fully biocompatible and elicited only mild inflammatory changes which were indistinguishable from that caused by non-degradable control stents. Furthermore, there was significantly less hydronephrosis in the degradable stent group than in controls (Figure 3).

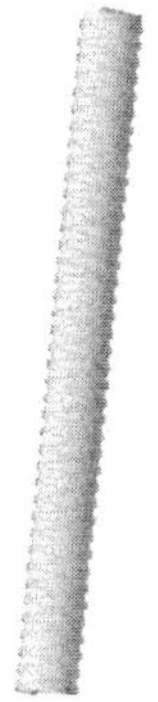

FIGURE 2. The novel degradable ureteral stent (Uriprene™, Poly-Med Inc., Greenville, SC, marketed by Indevus Pharmaceuticals, Cranbury, NJ)

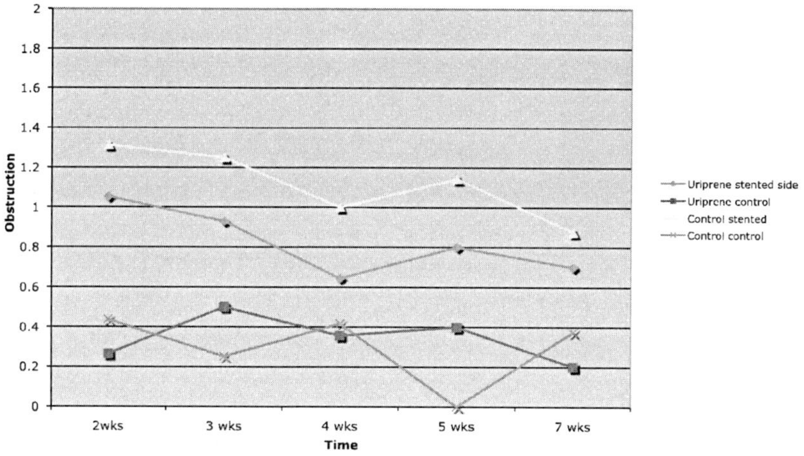

FIGURE 3. Degree of kidney obstruction (hydronephrosis) as seen following intravenous injection of radiographic contrast (intravenous pyelogram or IVP). The control stent (yellow line) produced consistently more dilation than the Uriprene (blue) which was not statistically significant from the control unstented ureters. Obstruction level 0=normal time to see contrast and no delayed imaging of contrast from renal collecting system, Level 1=minimal delay in time to see contrast in the kidney and minimal delay in excretion from kidney. Level 2= moderate delay in time to see contrast and moderate delay in excretion of contrast from kidney or moderate degree of distention in the renal collecting system. Level 3=severely obstructed kidney where it takes >20 minutes for contrast to be seen in the kidney and the renal collecting system is very dilated with possible dilation of the ureters on IVP.

A pathologist blinded to the treatment groups found no difference in the level of inflammation in the kidneys, ureters, and bladder. In fact, there was significantly less ureteral dilation in the Uriprene stented group in the proximal (Figure 4, P=0.045) and distal ureters (Figure 5, P=0.0006) than control stented kidneys. The Uriprene stented ureters were not significantly more dilated than the control (unstented) ureters from both groups).

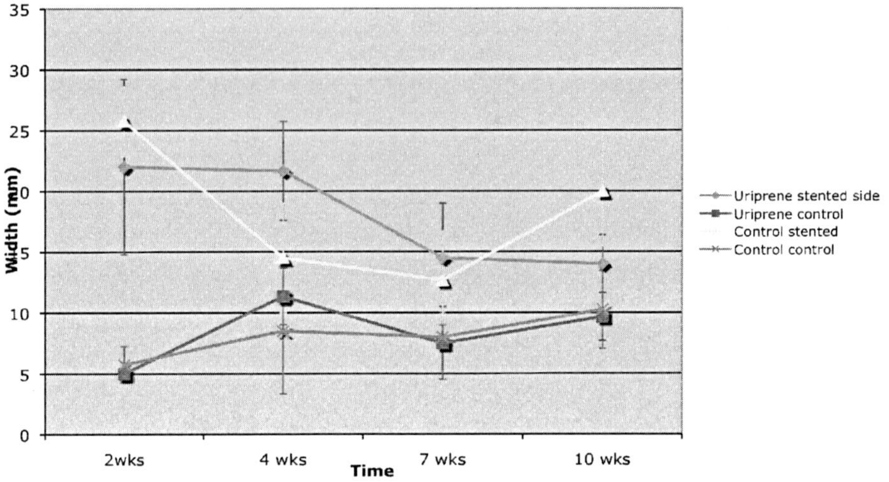

FIGURE 4. Measured widths of the lumen of the upper ureter at the time of necropsy. At the end of 10 weeks, the upper ureters were significantly more dilated in the control group as compared to the Uriprene group.

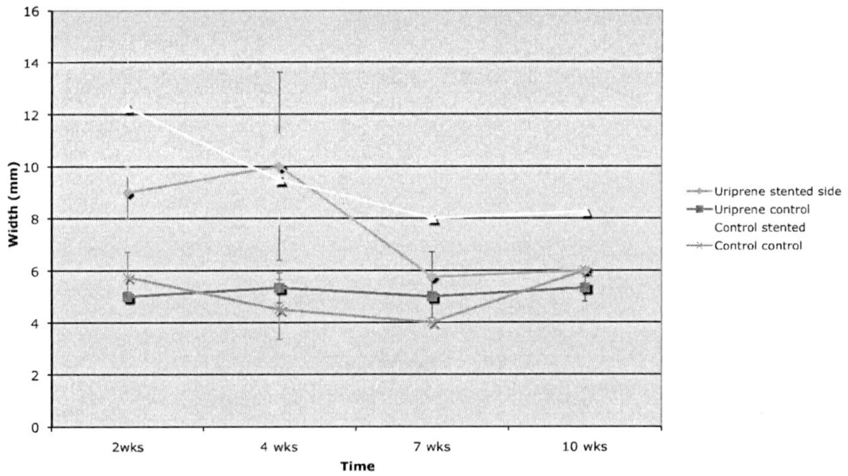

FIGURE 5. Measured widths of the lumen of the distal ureter at the time of necropsy. At the end of 10 weeks, the distal ureters were significantly more dilated in the control group compared to the Uriprene group.

DEGRADATION TIME

Degradation times for the initial version of the stent are outlined in Figure 6. All stents began to partially degrade at week 3 and 60% of all stents were completely degraded by week 7 and 100% by week 10. The stents degraded in an even fashion without causing "stent-strasse". There is more degradable coating on the proximal renal curl than the distal end, thus causing the stent to degrade from the bottom to the top, and thus avoiding distal ureteral obstruction.

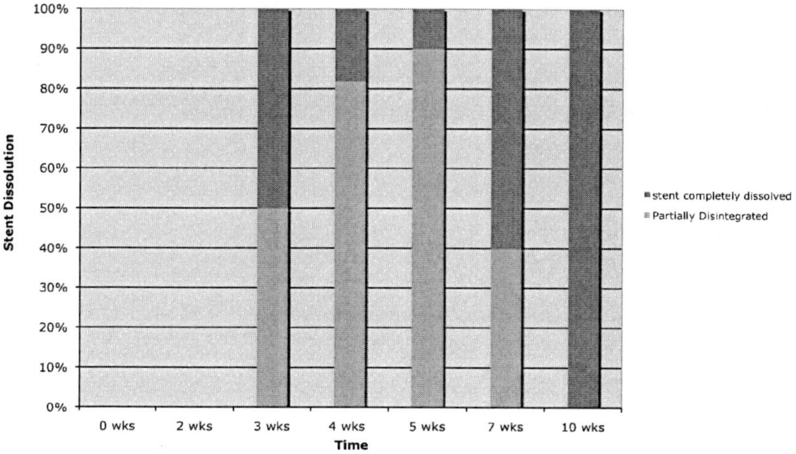

FIGURE 6. Degradation time of the Uriprene degradable stent. All stents began to dissolve (at least partially) by 3 weeks and were all degraded between 7 and 10 weeks after placement.

Seven to 10 weeks for the stent to degrade was decidedly too long as most urologists remove stents between 48 hours to 30 days. Therefore, the polymer was adjusted to dissolve more quickly. Secondly, a second curl was added to the bladder portion so that it resembled other current "double-J" designs. The number of coils per inch was increased to 36 to facilitate easier stent placement and reinforce the stent in the axial plane. This second generation stent was tested in another 32 pigs (16 control polyurethane stents and 16 Uriprene stents) who were all implanted cystoscopically and euthanized after 10 weeks to analyze histological inflammation. Intravenous pyelograms (IVPs) and renal ultrasounds were performed at 0, 2, 4, 7, and 10 weeks following implantation. The results showed that 80% of the stents degraded between 4 and 7 weeks with the remaining 20% degrading between 7 and 10 weeks (Figure 7).

Similar to the first generation stents, the second generation stents degraded in a uniform fashion in small microparticles that did not result in renal obstruction. The histopathology and inflammation was minor and did not differ between Uriprene and Control groups. The degree of hydronephrosis, however, was less in the Uriprene group (Figure 8).

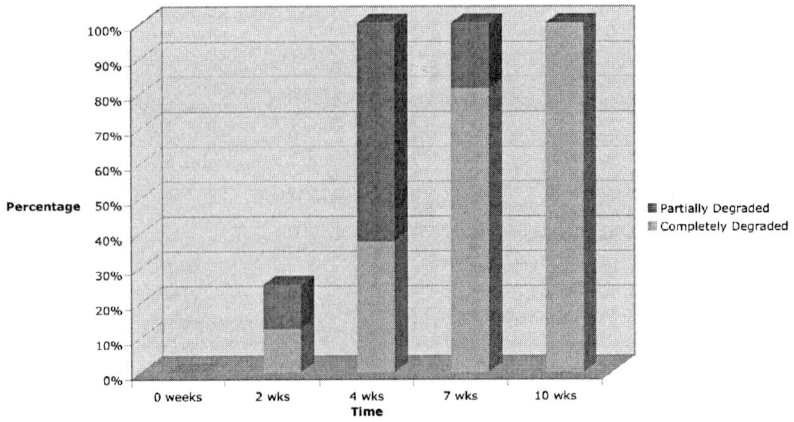

FIGURE 7. Degradation time of 2nd generation Uriprene stent in a 10 week pig study. Stents degraded faster than the first generation stents which degraded between 7 and 10 weeks. The majority of the 2nd generation stents degraded between 4 and 7 weeks.

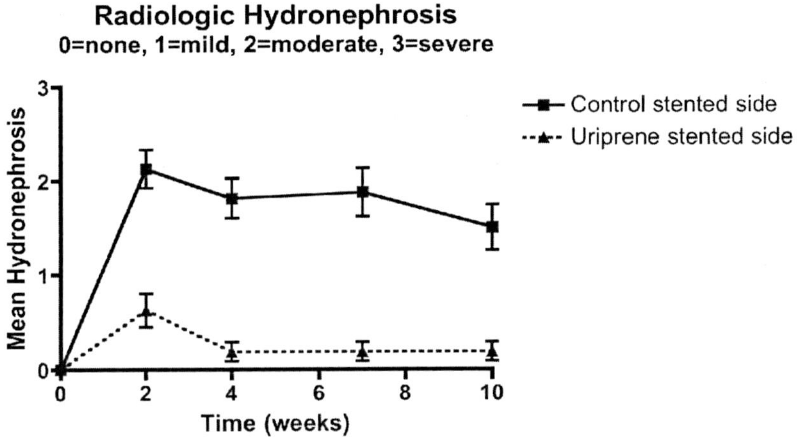

FIGURE 8. Radiologic hydronephrosis of Uriprene stented kidneys versus control stented kidneys as assessed by renal ultrasound. The control stents resulted in significantly more hydronephrosis than the Uriprene group at all time points after 0 weeks (P=0.04)

THIRD GENERATION DEGRADABLE URETERAL STENTS

The second generation Uriprene stent degraded between 4 and 7 weeks which was still longer than typically used in clinical situations. Also, it was implantable over a PTFE guidewire, but it was still preferable to insert over a hydrophilic wire. Therefore, a third generation stent was designed to degrade faster and to be easily implantable over a PTFE guidewire. Indeed, this final (third generation) version of the stent degraded between 3 and 4 weeks after implantation (Figure 9) and was easily implantable over a PTFE guidewire. The outer coating was altered to degrade faster and degraded in a very predictable fashion from the distal to proximal end without any obstruction as observed by ultrasound and IVP.

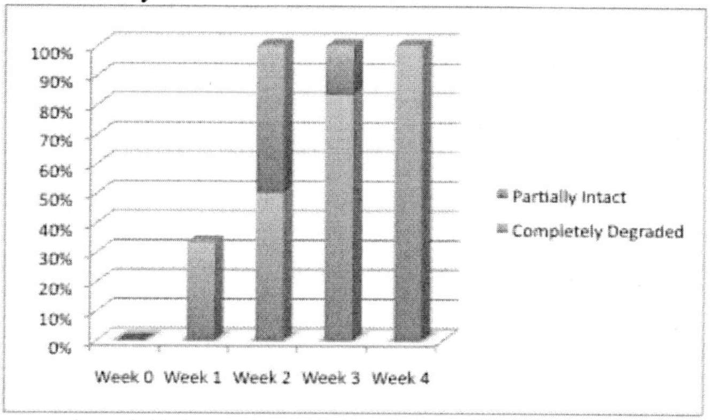

FIGURE 9. Degeneration of third generation Uriprene ureteral stents in a porcine model. All stents were at least partially degraded by 2 weeks and all stents degraded between 3 and 4 weeks.

The combination of the increased density of coils and altered coating allowed increased lubricity for easy insertion of this third generation of ureteral stent over the PTFE guidewire.

FUTURE OF DEGRADABLE STENTS

This third generation of degradable Uriprene ureteral stent that degrades within 3 to 4 weeks will be used in a clinical trial to assess its ability to provide urinary drainage post uncomplicated ureteroscopy. Secondary endpoints will include the time to degradation and patient comfort as compared to a control polyurethane ureteral stent. Its ability to be inserted into humans and provide adequate urinary drainage will be assessed in this clinical trial.

Biodegradable ureteral stents are also the perfect medium to incorporate drug-eluting technology. As the stent material degrades, drug that is loaded directly into the bulk stent material is then released to exert its effects on the local tissues. This may be helpful for stent comfort, combating urinary tract infection, preventing stent encrustation, and potentially for treatments of such conditions as upper urinary tract urothelial cell carcinoma, interstitial cystitis or chronic prostatitis.

SUMMARY

Biodegradable ureteral stents have been attempted in the past and were fairly successful except in a few patients who required either early (less than 48 hours) or late (greater than 3 month) intervention related to the stents. The Uriprene degradable ureteral stent has been tested and refined in its third generation of animal studies and is about to begin clinical trials. The future of ureteral stents will be to improve patient comfort and reduce encrustation and infection.

ACKNOWLEDGEMENTS

The authors wish to thank Dr. Ladan Fazli (pathologist, The Prostate Centre at Vancouver General Hospital) and Estelle Li for their work regarding the pathology of the porcine subjects. Dr. Shalaby Shalaby and Mr. Kenneth Clinkscales from Poly-Med Inc. (Greenville, SC) produce and manufacture the Uriprene stent. Ian Dobson (medical student) assisted with the weekly x-rays of the animals. The UBC and Jack Bell Animal Care Facilities provided excellent care of the animals. Funding for this project was provided by Valera Pharmaceuticals and Indevus Pharmaceuticals. Dr. Boris Hadaschik is a post-doctoral Urology Fellow who was funded by the Deutsche Forschungsgemeinschaft (German Research Foundation). Dr. Ben Chew received funding from Vancouver Costal Health Research Institute, Department of Urologic Sciences-UBC, the Canadian Urological Association Scholarship Foundation and is a Michael Smith Foundation Scholar.

REFERENCES

1. W. N. Taylor & Mcdougall, I. T. (2002) Minimally invasive ureteral stent retrieval. *J Urol,* 168, 2020-3.
2. H. B. Joshi, Newns, N., Stainthorpe, A., Macdonagh, R. P., Keeley, F. X., Jr. & Timoney, A. G. (2003) Ureteral stent symptom questionnaire: development and validation of a multidimensional quality of life measure. *J Urol,* 169, 1060-4.
3. H. B. Joshi, Chitale, S. V., Nagarajan, M., Irving, S. O., Browning, A. J., Biyani, C. S. & Burgess, N. A. (2005) A prospective randomized single-blind comparison of ureteral stents composed of firm and soft polymer. *J Urol,* 174, 2303-6.
4. A. Rane, Saleemi, A., Cahill, D., Sriprasad, S., Shrotri, N. & Tiptaft, R. (2001) Have stent-related symptoms anything to do with placement technique? *J Endourol,* 15, 741-5.
5. G. Haleblian, Kijvikai, K., De La Rosette, J. & Preminger, G. (2008) Ureteral stenting and urinary stone management: a systematic review. *J Urol,* 179, 424-30.
6. V. Singh, Srinivastava, A., Kapoor, R. & Kumar, A. (2005) Can the complicated forgotten indwelling ureteric stents be lethal? *Int Urol Nephrol,* 37, 541-6.
7. R. W. Schlick & Planz, K. (1997) Potentially useful materials for biodegradable ureteric stents. *Br J Urol,* 80, 908-10.
8. R. W. Schlick & Planz, K. (1998) In vitro results with special plastics for biodegradable endoureteral stents. *J Endourol,* 12, 451-5.
9. B. A. Hadaschik, Paterson, R. F., Fazli, F., Clinkscales, K. W., Shalaby, S. W. & Chew, B. H. (2008) Investigation of a novel degradable ureteral stent in a porcine model. *J Urol,* 180.
10. J. E. Lingeman, D. A. Schulsinger, D. A., & Kuo, R. L. (2003) Phase I trial of a temporary ureteral drainage stent. *J Endourol* 17(3): 169-171.
11. J. E. Lingeman, Preminger, G. M., Berger, Y., Denstedt, J. D., Goldstone, L., Segura, J. W., Auge B. K., Watterson, J. D., & Kuo, R. L. (2003) Use of a temporary ureteral drainage stent after uncomplicated ureteroscopy: results from a phase II clinical trial. *J Urol.* 169(5):1682-8.

Ureteral Stents. New Materials and Designs

Manoj Monga

Department of Urologic Surgery, University of Minnesota, 420 Delaware St SE (MMC 394), Minneapolis MN 55455. endourol@yahoo.com

Abstract. Issues of stent migration and challenges of stent placement can be addressed adequately with current stent designs and materials, and an emphasis on precision in technique. Future changes in ureteral stents will need to maintain the current standard that has been set with existing devices in these regards. In contrast, new advances are sorely needed in encrustation and infection associated with ureteral stents. The main target for future development in ureteral stent materials lies in a biodegradable stent that degrades either on demand or degrades reliably within one-month with predictable degradation patterns that do not predispose to urinary obstruction, discomfort or need for secondary procedures. The main target for future development in ureteral stent design is improved patient comfort.

Keywords: endourology; ureteral stent
PACS: 01.30.Cc

INTRODUCTION

What is a stent? A stent is defined as a catheter, rod, or tube within a tubular structure that is used to maintain luminal patency or protect an anastomosis or graft. Our current "double-J" or "pigtail" ureteral stents have changed little since their introduction into the urologic armamentarium in 1978 [1,2]. Indeed, one might argue that they have served their purpose well for the last 30 years.

From that perspective might come the question, what clinical needs have driven research and development in ureteral stents, and what deficiencies deserve further innovative approaches? The ideal ureteral stent would be stiff at insertion and have a low coefficient of friction to facilitate placement. It would soften at body temperature while maintaining its resistance to extrinsic compression to prevent kinking and maintaining its coil strength to prevent stent migration. It would maintain intraluminal flow and avoid encrustation with prolonged exposure to urine. It would dissolve on demand and be a "silent partner"—causing no pain. As such, the two main areas of focus for ureteral stent research have been improvement in stent function and improvement in patient comfort.

CP1049, *Renal Stone Disease 2, 2nd International Urolithiasis Research Symposium,*
edited by A. P. Evan, J. E. Lingeman, J. A. McAteer, and J. C. Williams, Jr.

STENT FUNCTION

Stent function can be characterized by ease of placement, flow properties in intrinsic or extrinsic obstruction, risk of migration, risk of encrustation, promotion of stone passage, and ease of removal including biodegradable properties.

Ease of Placement

Ureteral stents are made of silicone, polyurethane, or proprietary co-polymers such as C-flex, Percuflex, or Silitek. Polyurethane is associated with urothelial ulceration and erosion, while silicon stents have higher biocompatibility [3]. Most ureteral stents have a hydrophilic coating that facilitates placement by decreasing the coefficient of friction. We have previously evaluated the coefficient of friction of commercially available ureteral stents, and demonstrated that the Microvasive Percuflex had the lowest coefficient of friction of stents tested, while the Cook Soflex had the highest (Figure 1).

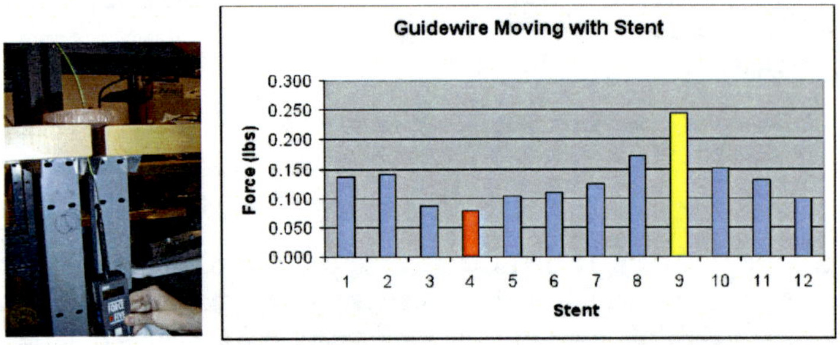

1= Surgitek Quadracoil
2= Microvasive Contour
3= Applied Vertex
4= Microvasive Percuflex
5= Circon Double Pigtail
6= Bard Lubricious
7= Bard Inlay
8= Cook Double Pigtail
9= Cook Soflex
10= Cook Endosof AQ
11= Cook Black Silicone
12= Cook C-Flex

FIGURE 1. Assessment of ease of stent placement by measuring coefficients of friction.

Another physical characteristic of stents that can impact the ease of placement is the stiffness or durometer—with softer stents tending to buckle especially if faced with resistance from an obstructing stone or stricture. In this regard, physical testing has demonstrated that the Cook C-flex has a stiffer Young's modulus (1472 kPa) while the Cook Silicone is a very soft stent (122 kPa) [4]. However, it has been hypothesized that the hardness of the stent may correlate with patient discomfort (see section below on patient comfort).

Flow properties

In vitro analyses have been conducted to compare flow characteristics through multiple stent designs, and to help delineate relative contributions of intraluminal and extraluminal flow [5,6,7]. While these studies did not demonstrate a superior stent design, they did identify certain stents that had inferior flow characteristics (Tower stent [5], Spiral stent [6], and Resonance stent [7] respectively).

A specific condition of concern with regards to maintenance of urinary stent flow is the clinical scenario of extrinsic compression (Figure 2). Early studies of ureteral stent compression suggested that the Cook C-Flex was the most resistant to compression, while the Silicone stents were least resistant [8]. In addition, when the outer diameter of the stent (8F, 10.2F) was increased without increasing the wall thickness, we noted a higher susceptibility to compression. Recent modifications to stents such as the Applied Silhouette with an impregnated coil and the lumenless Cook Resonance metallic stent have provided alternatives that appear to be resistant to extrinsic compression. Specifically, the force required to compress an Applied Silhouette (105 kPa) or the Cook Resonance (63 kPa) is significantly greater than the stiffest traditional stent (Cook C-Flex, 30 kPa) [9].

The Cook Resonance stent, though it may have lower flows under normal conditions, has been demonstrated to maintain superior flow in the face of extrinsic compression in an animal model [7]. Other alternatives to facilitate ureteral stent drainage in the face of extrinsic compression have included the development of a double-ureteral stent with two lumens [10] and the development of a Open-lumen ureteral stent [11]. The Open configuration of the I-beam geometry is thought to provide multiple potential channels for flow if faced with encrustation or compression, resulting in preservation of flow even though the cross-sectional areas for flow are similar to traditional stents.

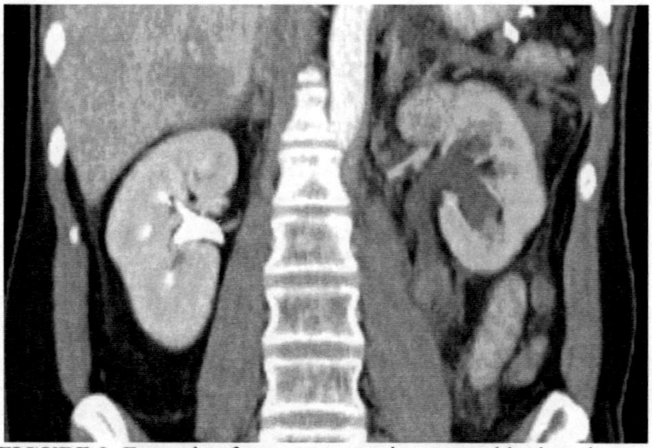

FIGURE 2. Example of stent compression, caused by lymphoma.

Stone expulsion and retrieval

Phan et al. in 1993 described a Spiral ureteral stent with a beveled helical ridge that was demonstrated to facilitate stone passage in a porcine model and facilitate extraluminal flow in an in vitro model [12,13]; however, later studies suggested that flow was diminished with this stent [6].

A radially expanding Stone Sweeper® 5 F or 6.5 F ureteral stent was introduced by Fossa Medical. This stent contains 15-17 four-strand, helical baskets along the length of the stent that open up to 21Fr. The baskets act to passively dilate the ureter over time, and can capture up to 5 mm stones. In a study of 50 patients with ureteral stones or stone fragments, 20/50 (40%) of patients had stones caught in the basket on removal, 27/50 (54%) passed stone fragments spontaneously, and all were cleared of ureteral stones after stent removal [14]. Of note, two patients required anesthesia for stent removal secondary to pain. Concerns were also encountered with regards to "entrapped" stents that caught larger fragments. To address this, the manufacturers have developed the Open-Pass modification, with a longitudinal load release slit that has been proposed to facilitate release of the stone fragments [15].

Risk of migration

The risk of migration of a ureteral stent is primarily related to the selection of the appropriate length stent with careful attention to the placement of the retention coils in the renal pelvis and bladder. We have compared the strength of the stent coils, and found that the Cook C-Flex and Cook Black silicone stents required significantly more force to release the coil (0.480 lb). After 4 weeks of exposure to urine the Applied Vertex had the weakest coil strength (0.088 lb), suggesting that it might be more prone to stent migration after a prolonged indwelling time [4].

Encrustation

The risk of stent encrustation correlates with the duration of indwelling in the patient (Figure 3). Indeed, it has been reported that 76% of ureteral stents will be encrusted if left for greater than 3 months [16]. The bulk of research on preventing stent encrustation has been centered on stent coatings, and as such will be discussed in a separate chapter.

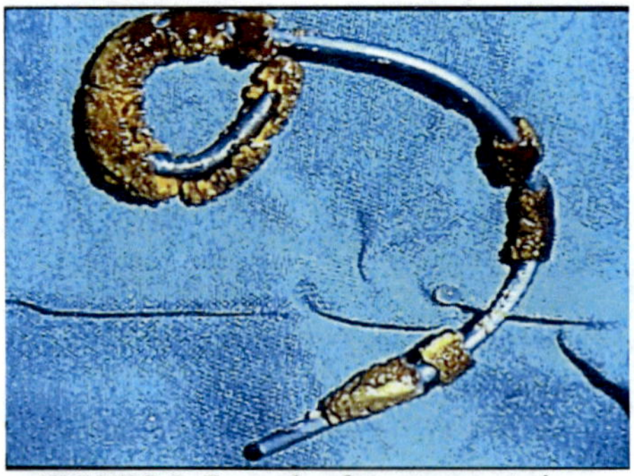

FIGURE 3. Example of stent encrustation.

Ease of removal & Biodegradable stents

All ureteral stents currently available come with a string tether that allows the patient to remove the ureteral stent without the need for cystoscopy. Studies suggest that the use of this tether has no impact on patient morbidity compared to cystoscopy and stent removal [17].

The Boston Scientific Looped Polaris stent was designed with the hope of improving patient comfort (see section below). Though it has not been demonstrated to accomplish this, a randomized clinical trial reported that the short loop significantly improved the ease of stent removal as compared to a traditional pig-tail configuration [18].

Clinical trials utilizing biodegradable ureteral stents were first reported by Boston Scientific [19]. The TUDS (Temporary urinary drainage system) was studied in 88 patients, however unpredictable dissolution, including some fragments that required ureteroscopic extraction, led to discontinuation of the concept. A new generation of biodegradable stent, the Uriprene, is currently under development by Indevus and Poly-Med. Hadaschik et al. reported in a porcine model that reliable 100% degradation was noted at 10 weeks with this stent [20]. The Uriprene incorporates a coil configuration to provide compression strength along with a woven mesh to provide axial strength.

Investigators have evaluated the use of Magnetic tipped retrievers to facilitate stent removal without the need for cystoscopy. Early renditions were successful in 76% of males [21]; however, the use of a rare-earth magnet on the retrieval catheter and a stainless steel bead on the ureteral stent proved more successful (97%) [22].

STENT COMFORT

Up to 80% of patients with indwelling ureteral stents will report stent discomfort, with a significant proportion also reporting urinary symptoms (78%), flank pain (25%), and hematuria (18%) [23,24]. These symptoms impact the ability to engage in work activities (58%) and activities of daily living. Unfortunately the etiology of stent discomfort is elusive. Factors thought to contribute to stent discomfort include the smooth muscle tone in the transmural ureter, increased pressures in the bladder during voiding resulting in reflux pain, and bladder irritation by the distal portion of the ureteral stent.

It has been hypothesized that the durometer of the stent correlates with stent discomfort. Indeed, some companies have developed dual durometer composite stents (Boston Scientific Polaris, Surgitek Sof-Curl), which have a stiff renal coil for ease of placement and a soft bladder coil for improved stent comfort; however, clinical trials are lacking to support this claim.

Early studies suggested that stents of softer durometer (Soflex) decreased dysuria, renal and suprapubic pain compared to a harder durometer stent (polyurethane) [25]. Other investigators, comparing Silitek, polyurethane, C-Flex and the Vantec Soft stent reported no difference in stent comfort based on durometer [17]. Similarly, a more recent randomized clinical trial using a validated stent questionnaire failed to demonstrate any difference in comfort between firm (Microvasive Percuflex) and soft (Microvasive Contour) ureteral stents [26].

In 2002, we asked manufacturers to provide the stent they made that they considered the best with regards to stent comfort. In a randomized clinical trial using a validated stent questionnaire, we were unable to identify any differences in pain; however, the Bard Inlay stent was associated with less urinary symptoms at Days 1 and 3 [27].

Investigators have attempted to modify the bladder retention mechanism to diminish patient discomfort. Dunn et al. reported that replacing the traditional bladder coil with a lumen-less 4F tail led to a 21% decrease in irritative voiding symptoms [28]. Though one would anticipate that the lumen-less 3F tail would lead to less ureteral reflux compared to traditional stents, there was no significant difference in flank pain noted with this design.

Preminger et al. reported on a large randomized clinical trial of 236 patients using a validated stent questionnaire. Evaluating a long-loop and short-loop configuration to modify the bladder retention mechanism, they reported no significant difference in body pain or urinary symptoms [18].

Ureteral stent comfort studies are challenging due to the subjectivity of the primary endpoint—pain and the risk of confounding variables. Commonly patients are excluded from enrollment if they have evidence of a urinary tract infection, neurological disorders that may impede their ability to sense or report pain, or voiding dysfunction that may predispose to prolonged need for urethral catheter drainage. In addition, many patients with urinary calculi are recurrent stone formers who now face issues of chronic pain and narcotic dependency—this can be difficult to screen for during enrollment, resulting in outliers with regards to pain scores and narcotic use. The pain associated with the primary pathology (e.g., obstructing stone) or primary intervention (e.g., ureteroscopy, SWL) often confounds the cause-effect analysis of the presence of a ureteral stent. The ideal stent comfort study would enroll healthy volunteer subjects who would be randomized between stent placement and sham cystoscopy.

New Innovations

Over 800 patents related to ureteral stents can be identified using the web-based database of the U.S. patent office. Indeed, many novel ideas have been proposed to address stent comfort and function. We are currently evaluating the use of diamond-shaped holes in along the ureteral stent shaft. Finite element modeling of non-linear deformation with axial strain suggest that with the appropriate number, distribution and configuration of such holes (Figure 4) we may be able to account for the 2-5 cm of movement of a stent that has been described with changes in the patient's body position [29]. This could lead to greater patient comfort.

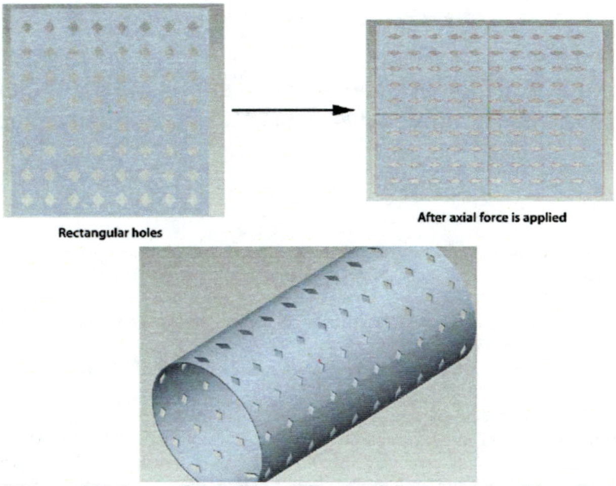

FIGURE 4. Diamond Hole configuration to allow axial expansion with patient movement.

CONCLUSION

Though great strides have been made in developing validated questionnaires to assess stent outcomes, a more robust tool is needed to evaluate the impact of changes in stent design, material, coating or adjuvant therapy on patient comfort. Issues of stent migration and challenges of stent placement can be addressed adequately with current stent designs and materials, along with an emphasis on precision in technique. Future changes in ureteral stents will need to maintain the current standard that has been set with existing devices in these regards.

In contrast, new advances are sorely needed in preventing the encrustation and infection associated with ureteral stents; however, these issues can be addressed to a certain degree by limiting the indwelling time of the stent. As such, the prevalence of these entities with the judicious use of oral antibiotics is relatively low such that industry must tailor their investments in these areas to the potential return. Clearly these two issues become of paramount importance as stents are developed with the target of longer dwell times (>4 months).

The main target for future development in ureteral stent materials lies in a biodegradable stent that degrades either on demand (perhaps in response to changes in urinary pH) or degrades reliably within one-month with predictable degradation patterns that do not predispose to urinary obstruction, discomfort or need for secondary procedures. The main target for future development in ureteral stent design is improved patient comfort; yet this search has eluded investigators for 30 years.

ACKNOWLEDGEMENTS

I gratefully acknowledge the rich collaborative efforts of Drs. William Durfee, Kari Hendlin and Krishna Vedula, my colleagues in Mechanical Engineering.

REFERENCES

1. Finney RP. Experience with new double-J ureteral catheter stent. J Urol 1978;120:678
2. Hepperlen TK, Mardis HK. Pigtail stent termed means of lessening ureteral surgery. Trends Clin Urol 1978;1:405.
3. Marx M, Bettmann MA, Bridge S, et al.: The effects of various indwelling ureteral catheter materials on the normal canine ureter. J Urol 139: 180, 1988
4. Hendlin K, Dockendorf K, Horn C, Lund B, Monga M: Ureteral stents – Coil strength and Durometer. Urology 68: 42-45, 2006
5. Brewer AV, Elbahnasy AM, Bercowsky E, Maxwell KL, Shalhav AL, Kahn SA, McDougall EM, Clayman RV. Mechanism of ureteral stent flow: a comparative in vivo study. J Endourol. 1999 May;13(4):269-71.
6. Olweny EO, Portis AJ, Afane JS, Brewer AV, Shalhav AL, Luszczynski K, McDougall EM, Clayman RV. Flow characteristics of 3 unique ureteral stents: investigation of a Poiseuille flow pattern. J Urol. 2000 Dec;164(6):2099-103.
7. Blaschko SD, Deane LA, Krebs A, Abdelshehid CS, Khan F, Borin J, Nguyen A, McDougall EM, Clayman RV. In-vivo evaluation of flow characteristics of novel metal ureteral stent. J Endourol. 2007 Jul;21(7):780-3
8. Hendlin K, Vedula K, Horn C, Monga M: In vitro evaluation of ureteral stent compression. Urology 67: 679-82, 2006
9. Pedro RN, Hendlin K, Kriedberg C, Monga M: Wire-based ureteral stents: impact on tensile strength and compression . Urology 70:1057-9, 2007
10. Hafron J, Ost MC, Tan BJ, Fogarty JD, Hoenig DM, Lee BR, Smith AD. Novel dual-lumen ureteral stents provide better ureteral flow than single ureteral stent in ex vivo porcine kidney model of extrinsic ureteral obstruction. Urology. 2006 Oct;68(4):911-5
11. Kolb GR, Mitchell ME: Open lumen ureteral stent demonstrates improved flow despite equal encrustation compared to single lumen stents in vitro. J Urol 173 (suppl.) Abstract 1161, 2005
12. Phan CN, Stoller ML. Helically ridged ureteric stent facilitates the passage of stone fragments in an experimental porcine model. Br J Urol. 1993 Jul;72(1):17-9.
13. Stoller ML, Schwartz BF, Frigstad JR, Norris L, Park JB, Magliochetti MJ. An in vitro assessment of the flow characteristics of spiral-ridged and smooth-walled JJ ureteric stents. BJU Int. 2000 Apr;85(6):628-31
14. Albala AD, Rickner T, Hoenig AD, et al. Human results of ureteral stone extraction with the stone sweeper (abstract). J Urol. 2004; 171:444.
15. L'Esperance JO, Rickner T, Hoenig D, Bamberger M, Albala DM. Ureteral expanding stent: a new device for urolithiasis. J Endourol. 2007 May;21(5):533-7
16. El-Faqih SR, Shamsuddin AB, Chakrabarti A, Atassi R, Kardar AH, Osman MK, Husain I. Polyurethane internal ureteral stents in treatment of stone patients: morbidity related to indwelling times. J Urol. 1991 Dec;146(6):1487-91.
17. Pryor JL, Langley MJ, Jenkins AD. Comparison of symptom characteristics of indwelling ureteral catheters. J Urol. 1991 Apr;145(4):719-22
18. Preminger GM, Lingeman JE, Goldfischer E, Monga M, et al: A prospective randomized clinical trial comparing levels of symptoms and discomfort associated with two investigational and two currently marketed ureteral stents. J Urol 173(Suppl) 2005, Abstract 1683
19. Lingeman JE, Preminger GM, Berger Y, Denstedt JD, Goldstone L, Segura JW, Auge BK, Watterson JD, Kuo RL. Use of a temporary ureteral drainage stent after uncomplicated ureteroscopy: results from a phase II clinical trial. J Urol. 2003 May;169(5):1682-8.
20. Hadaschik BA, Paterson RF, Chew BH: Investigation of a novel biodegradable ureteral stent in a porcine model. J Urol 179(Suppl) abstract 1722, 2008
21. Macaluso JN, Deutsch JS, Goodman JR et al: The use of the Magnetip double-J ureteral stent in urological practice. J Urol 142: 701, 1989
22. Taylor WN, McDougall IT: Minimally invasive ureteral stent retrieval. J Urol 168: 2020, 2002
23. Damiano R, Oliva A, Esposito C, De Sio M, Autorino R, D'Armiento M. Early and late complications of double pigtail ureteral stent. Urol Int. 2002;69(2):136-40.

24. Joshi HB, Newns N, Stainthorpe A, MacDonagh RP, Keeley FX Jr, Timoney AG. Ureteral stent symptom questionnaire: development and validation of a multidimensional quality of life measure. J Urol. 2003 Mar;169(3):1060-4
25. Lennon GM, Thornhill JA, Sweeney PA, Grainger R, McDermott TE, Butler MR. 'Firm' versus 'soft' double pigtail ureteric stents: a randomised blind comparative trial. Eur Urol. 1995;28(1):1-5
26. Joshi HB, Chitale SV, Nagarajan M, Irving SO, Browning AJ, Biyani CS, Burgess NA. A prospective randomized single-blind comparison of ureteral stents composed of firm and soft polymer. J Urol. 2005 Dec;174(6):2303-6.
27. Lee C, Best S, Premoli J, Monga M: A Randomized prospective evaluation of ureteral stents using a validated symptom questionnaire. Journal of Endourology 19: 990-3, 2005
28. Dunn MD, Portis AJ, Kahn SA, Yan Y, Shalhav AL, Elbahnasy AM, Bercowsky E, Hoenig DM, Wolf JS Jr, McDougall EM, Clayman RV. Clinical effectiveness of new stent design: randomized single-blind comparison of tail and double-pigtail stents. J Endourol. 2000 Mar;14(2):195-202
29. Chew BH, Knudsen BE, Nott L, Pautler SE, Razvi H, Amann J, Denstedt JD: Pilot Study of Ureteral Movement in Stented Patients: First Step in Understanding Dynamic Ureteral Anatomy to Improve Stent Comfort. Journal of Endourology. September 1, 2007: 1069-1076.

Ureteral Stent Coatings: What's Here and What's Coming

Hassan Razvi

The Schulich School of Medicine and Dentistry, University of Western Ontario, London, Ontario, Canada

Abstract. Ureteral stents have become an indispensable tool to the urologist in the management of various disorders afflicting the urinary tract. While the ideal stent remains elusive, novel technical advances in stent coating technology offer the potential of enhancing stent biocompatibility and clinical application. Currently available stent coatings as well as new and emerging devices will be reviewed.

Keywords: Biomimetics; stent coatings
PACS: 01.30.Cc

INTRODUCTION

Since the development of the modern double-pigtail stent in the late 1970's, these devices have assumed an ever-increasing role in the management of various urological problems [1]. The development and application of ureteral stents has, in many ways mirrored the evolution of the subspecialty of endourology, particularly with respect to the management of urinary stone disease. Without the ability to ensure a relatively simple and effective method of ensuring adequate urinary tract drainage, shock wave lithotripsy, ureteroscopy and percutaneous stone removal would not have had the clinical impact they have today.

Despite their widespread use and importance in modern urological practice, stents remain plagued by problems related to encrustation, biofilm formation, infection and patient discomfort. Needless to say, the development of the ideal ureteral stent remains an elusive goal. In an effort to eliminate some of these stent-related issues, research and manufacturing have focused on stent material, design and configuration modification and more recently stent coatings. As the technology to apply stent coatings evolves, one can envision not only the potential to improve upon the mechanical properties of currently available stents but a paradigm shift in thinking such that these devices may have expanded applications through drug elution capabilities. The potential to treat upper tract transitional cell cancer with a stent containing a chemotherapeutic coating, or to minimize the pain patients experience, are just a few of the potential applications we might envision. The use of drug eluting stents in cardiology serves as some inspiration along these lines [2]. This chapter will focus on some of these exciting possibilities.

CP1049, *Renal Stone Disease 2, 2nd International Urolithiasis Research Symposium,*
edited by A. P. Evan, J. E. Lingeman, J. A. McAteer, and J. C. Williams, Jr.

WHAT'S HERE

Various stent coatings have been investigated. At the present time most of the major manufacturers do, in fact, market a device with a proprietary coating. These stents were developed in an effort to ease insertion and to reduce the risk of encrustation, biofilm formation and infection. The elements common to the available coated stents include enhanced lubricity and a more hydrophilic surface, characteristics proven to lessen the risk of mucosal injury at least in urethral catheter research [3]. It is theorized that if mucosal injury can be minimized, the risk of infection may also be reduced. Similarly, stents with a hydrogel coating have been shown to resist encrustation, biofilm development and infection better than uncoated polyurethane stents [4].

Other coatings have also been developed to attempt to prevent similar complications on various medical devices including ureteral stents employing the use of silver, polyvinyl pyrollidone and heparin [5-7]. The use of a silver coating with *in vitro* models showed high antibacterial activity, but was not found to be as effective *in vivo* [5,8]. The clinical experience with heparin in particular was shown in a small series of patients to be quite effective in reducing stent encrustation even with indwell times of up to 12 months [7].

WHAT'S COMING

The field of biomimetics—the science of applying designs from nature to solve problems in engineering and medicine—offers the promise of novel and potentially more effective medical device coatings. Our research group has begun *in vitro* and animal testing on a novel antifouling coating inspired by the adhesive proteins produced by the common blue mussel, *Mytilus edulis.* These organisms have developed opportunistic attachment strategies in wet environments by secreting a unique set of mussel adhesive proteins (MAPs) containing 3,4-dihydroxyphenyl-alanine (DOPA). When covalently coupled to a proven, biocompatible antifouling polymer such as polyethylene glycol (PEG), it has been shown with *in vitro* testing that treated surfaces resist attachment to serum proteins, fibroblasts and *Staphylococcus epidermidis* [9,10,11].

Our group was the first to assess this peptide conjugate in the form of mPEG-$DOPA_3$ in relation to urologic devices [12]. In an *in vitro* study, titanium dioxide (TiO_2) coated silicon disks were either coated with mPEG-$DOPA_3$ or left uncoated and then challenged with six major uropathogens incubated in pooled human urine. After a 24 hour incubation period adherent bacteria were quantified using dilution plating. Representative disks were examined using scanning electron microscopy (SEM), energy dispersive x-ray analysis (EDX) and live/dead organism viability staining.

Our results revealed that the mPEG-$DOPA_3$ coated disks significantly resisted the attachment of all the test uropathogens, especially for *Escherichia coli* GR-12, *Enterococcus faecalis* 23241 and *Proteus mirabilis* 296. SEM and viability staining analyses also demonstrated the ability of the coating to resist encrustation with urinary constituents as well. These preliminary data have encouraged us to assess this coating on polyurethane stents employing an animal model. We envision the mPEG-DOPA$_3$ as a possible template for the addition of other molecules that might provide other pharmacologic properties as well.

Another novel stent coating under evaluation involves the application of the enzyme oxalate decarboxylase. This coating holds the promise of providing a more effective method of inhibiting calcium oxalate stone encrustation [13]. Through enzymatic degradation the precipitation of oxalate and the formation of encrustation on the stent surface could be avoided.

Carbon has been used in a variety of medical device applications. Its application in the form of diamond-like carbon (DLC) has a number of properties that are attractive to stent coating technology, including a low coefficient of friction, resistance to wear, and biocompatibility [14]. The application of DLC onto polyurethane in an *in vitro* study confirmed the coating's ability to resist encrustation and microbial adherence [15]. A small clinical trial reported similar findings with a reduction in biofilm formation and bacterial attachment to the stent surface. The authors also suggested that the patients found the stents easy to tolerate [16].

The concept of drug elution is an exciting evolution in the development of ureteral stents and offers the potential to expand the clinical applications of these devices. The application of the antimicrobial triclosan at least in an *in vitro* model demonstrated an inhibition of growth of several uropathogenic bacteria [17]. Clinical results however were less impressive and the triclosan coated stent that was manufactured for human clinical use is no longer marketed.

At the present time clinical trials are either ongoing or soon to be initiated to evaluate the efficacy and safety of stents with analgesic or anti-inflammatory drug coatings. The results of these trials are anxiously awaited. Future coatings employing chemotherapeutic, antispasmodic or smooth muscle relaxation properties can also be envisioned.

SUMMARY

This chapter has touched on some of the currently available and potential stent coatings. The concept of coating ureteral stents has obvious clinical appeal and will remain a topic of intense research in the years to come. In addition to minimizing the potential complications related to the stent, the possibility of additional therapeutic effect is tantalizing. Before coated stents become part of the standard urologic armamentarium however, a number of manufacturing challenges must first be overcome. Paramount is ensuring a reproducible manufacturing process that reliably permits adequate surface coverage, homogeneous distribution, resistance to mechanical effects and wear and the assurance of therapeutic concentration of the agent.

Without a doubt, the field of stent coatings using drug elution technology is the "holy grail" of future stent development and its success is anxiously awaited by patients and urologists alike.

REFERENCES

1. R.P. Finney, *J. Urol.* **120**, 678-681 (1978).
2. J.F. Granada, G.L. Kaluza, A. Raizner, *Curr. Atheroscler. Rep.* **5**, 308-316 (2003).
3. J.M. Vapnek, F.M. Maynard, J. Kim, *J. Urol.* **169**, 994-998 (2003).
4. S.P. Gorman, M.M. Tunney, P.F. Keane et al, *J. Biomed. Mater. Res.* **39**, 642-649 (1998).
5. D.K. Riley, D.C. Classen, L.E. Stevens, J.P. Burke, *Am. J. Med.* **98**, 349-358 (1995).
6. M.M. Tunney, S.P. Gorman, *Biomaterials* **23**, 4601-4608 (2002).
7. F. Cauda, V. Cauda, C. Fiori et al, *J. Endourol.* **23**, 465-472 (2008).
8. D.G. Maki, L. Cobb, J.K. Garman, J.M. Shapiro et al, *J.A.M.A.* **127**, 267-274 (1988).
9. J.L Dalsin, B.H. Hu , B.P. Lee et al, *J. Am. Chem. Soc.* **125**, 4253-4258 (2003).
10. J. L. Dalsin, S. Tosatti, J. Voros et al, *Langmuir* **21**, 640-646 (2005).
11. A.R. Statz, R.J. Meagher, A.E. Barron, *J. Am. Chem. Soc.* **127**, 7972-7973 (2005).
12. R. Ko, P.A. Cadieux, J.L. Dalsin et al, *J. Endourol.* **in press** (2008).
13. J.D. Watterson, P.A. Cadieux, D.T. Bieko et al, *J. Endourol.* **17**, 269-274 (2003).
14. D.P. Monaghan, K.C. Laing, P.A. Logan, *Mater. World* **1**, 347-349 (1993).
15. D.S. Jones, C.P. Garvin, D. Dowling et al, *J. Biomed. Mater. Res. B. Appl. Biomater.* **78**, 230-236 (2006).
16. Laube et al, *J. Urol.* **177**, 1923-1927 (2007).
17. M. Mittelman, W. Bucay-Cuto, J. Li et al, *J. Urol.* **171**(4 suppl), 443 (2004).

IV. CLINICAL BIOLOGY OF STONE FORMERS

Bariatric Surgery and Stone Disease

John C. Lieske[a] and Rajiv Kumar[b]

[a]*Division of Nephrology and Hypertension, Department of Internal Medicine, Department of Laboratory Medicine and Pathology, Mayo Clinic, Rochester, MN*
[b]*Division of Nephrology and Hypertension, Division of Endocrinology, Diabetes, Metabolism and Nutrition, Department of Internal Medicine, Department of Biochemistry and Molecular Biology, Mayo Clinic, Rochester, MN*

Abstract. Bariatric surgery is an effective treatment strategy for patients with morbid obesity that can result in effective weight loss, resolution of diabetes mellitus and other weight related complications, and even improved mortality. However, it also appears that hyperoxaluria is common after modern bariatric surgery, perhaps occurring in up to 50% of patients after Roux-en-Y gastric bypass. Although increasing numbers of patients are being seen with calcium oxalate kidney stones after bariatric surgery, and even a few with oxalosis and renal failure, the true risk of these outcomes remains unknown. The mechanisms that contribute to this enteric hyperoxaluria are also incompletely defined, although fat malabsorption may be an important component. Since increasing numbers of these procedures are likely to be performed in the coming years, further study regarding the prevalence and mechanisms of hyperoxaluria and kidney stones after bariatric surgery is needed to devise effective methods of treatment in order to prevent such complications.

Keywords: Bariatric Surgery, Calcium Oxalate, Hyperoxaluria, Nephrolithiasis, Roux-en-Y Gastric Bypass
PACS: 01.30.Cc

COMPLICATIONS OF OBESITY: THE CASE FOR BARIATRIC SURGERY

Morbid obesity, defined as a BMI >38 kg/m^2 in men and 41 kg/m^2 in women, is an increasing problem in the United States (US). Potential complications include diabetes (38-fold increased risk), heart disease (37-fold increased risk) and peripheral vascular disease (105-fold increased risk) (*1*). Because of these ominous statistics, bariatric surgical procedures to promote weight loss have increased in popularity over the last decades. These procedures can be categorized as purely restrictive (e.g., vertical banded gastroplasty or adjustable gastric band), restrictive/malabsorptive (e.g., Roux-en-Y gastric bypass [RYGB]), or resective/malabsorptive (e.g., biliopancreatic diversion-duodenal switch [BPD-DS]). Evidence suggests that each of these procedures can be effective to facilitate loss of between 50 to 70% of excess weight, with resulting improvements in diabetes, dyslipidemia, hypertension and obstructive sleep apnea in a majority of treated patients (*2*). Weight loss results are less durable after restrictive procedures which also result in less net reduction of excess body weight (*3*). Therefore, RYGB accounts for close to 90% of all bariatric procedures

CP1049, *Renal Stone Disease 2, 2nd International Urolithiasis Research Symposium,*
edited by A. P. Evan, J. E. Lingeman, J. A. McAteer, and J. C. Williams, Jr.

performed for morbid obesity in the US (*4*). Importantly, long-term results of the Swedish Obesity Subjects Study confirm that patients undergoing bariatric surgery have reduced long-term mortality compared to un-operated obese controls (*3*).

MORBID OBESITY AND THE KIDNEY

Obesity is associated with an increased relative risk of end-stage renal failure that approaches seven-fold when BMI exceeds 40 kg/m^2 (*5*). Recent kidney biopsy studies have shown that morbidly obese patients have an increased prevalence of glomerulomegaly, focally sclerotic glomeruli, globally sclerotic glomeruli, and interstitial fibrosis prior to bariatric surgery when compared to nonobese controls (*6*). Such morbidly obese subjects manifest renal functional changes that include hyperfiltration and elevated albuminuria, and these kidney parameters improve within two years post bariatric surgery when successful weight loss occurs (*7*). Studies have also confirmed that the morbidly obese population manifests an increased prevalence of hypercalciuria, hyperoxaluria, hyperuricosuria, hypocitraturia, and low urinary pH (*8*), parameters that might contribute to the known association of obesity and kidney stone risk (*9*). However, until recently it was unknown what affect, if any, bariatric surgery might have on these urinary lithogenic parameters.

JEJUNOILEAL BYPASS

Between 1963 and 1981 approximately 25,000 jejunoileal bypass procedures were performed in the US for obesity. Although this malabsorptive procedure clearly promoted weight loss, complications were recognized that included calcium oxalate kidney stones, and even kidney failure in a subset of patients. This and other complications led centers to abandon the procedure in the early 1980s when it was actually banned by the US government. Among patients post jejunoileal bypass surgery, urinary oxalate excretion directly correlated with fecal fat content (*10*), and this enteric hyperoxaluria appeared to be the result of colonic calcium complexation by unabsorbed fatty acids that resulted in increased bioavailability of dietary oxalate. Indeed administration of calcium supplements with meals (2800 mg/day) effectively reduced absorption of a radiolabeled oxalate, as well as renal oxalate excretion in a group of such patients (*11*).

LITHOGENIC CHANGES AND NEPHROLITHIASIS AFTER BARIATRIC SURGERY

Although it was known that jejunoileal bypass surgery caused extensive fat malabsorption and enteric hyperoxaluria, this was generally not considered a complication of modern bariatric surgery until relatively recently. Indeed, limited published data documents that while as little as 15% of a fat load might be absorbed in patients after jejunoileal bypass, as much as 97% might be absorbed after a restrictive procedure (**Table 1**) (*4*). BPD-DS patients have fat absorption capacity that is comparable to jejunoileal bypass subjects, while RYGB patients are intermediate. However, it is important to note that the data in **Table 1** was derived in a very small number of patients (e.g., only nine subjects after gastric bypass (*12*)).

TABLE 1. Degree of fat malabsorption after categories of bariatric surgery.

Procedure	Type	Fat absorption
Jejunoileal bypass	Malabsorptive	15%
Gastric bypass (RYGB)	Restrictive/malabsorptive	62%
Biliopancreatic Diversion with Duodenal Switch	Restrictive/malabsorptive	19%
Vertical Banded Gastroplasty	Restrictive	97%
Adjustable gastric band	Restrictive	97%

Adapted from (*4*)

In 2005, clinicians at Mayo Clinic Rochester reported on a series of 60 patients that presented with new onset nephrolithiasis after RYGB (*13*). Although only approximately 20% of patients at this medical center undergo a more extensive "distal" RYGB (one that is designed to promote greater weight loss), approximately half of the stone patients identified had undergone this procedure. A mail out survey suggested that the prevalence of new stones post-procedure approached 20% in this sub population. Most disturbingly, two patients were recognized that had developed end-stage renal failure and oxalosis after RYGB.

TABLE 2. Urinary lithogenic factors in obese patients before and after RYGB. Values expressed as mean (SD).

	Reference range	Obese base	Obese base	6 mo after RYGB	12 mo after RYGB	SF after RYGB	Male SF after RYGB	Female SF after RYGB
Reference		(*14*)	(*8*)	(*14*)	(*14*)	(*14*)	(*15*)	(*15*)
Number of subjects		20	45	8	13	31	28	104
Volume		1.94 (0.76)	1.53 (0.72)	1.41 (0.89)	1.63 (0.83)	1.61 (0.69)	1.75 (0.14)	1.52 (0.08)
pH		5.95 (0.38)	5.80 (0.50)	5.81 (0.92)	5.76 (0.59)	5.6 (0.6)	5.71 (0.07)	5.75 (0.04)
Oxalate	<45 mg	34 (18)	29 (10)	31 (15)	72 (43)	65 (40)	92 (11)	73 (4)
Citrate	>400 mg	660 (227)	679 (379)	563 (449)	444 (376)	394 (361)	524 (85)	396 (27)
Calcium	< 275 mg	206 (111)	187 (118)	111 (86)	112 (92)	132 (96)	140 (14)	143 (8)
Uric Acid	< 750 mg	708 (255)	559 (288)	426 (108)	461 (166)	456 (207)		
CaOx SS (DG)	<1.77	1.51 (0.78)	1.50 (0.78)	1.49 (1.31)	2.38 (0.49)	2.23 (0.52)		
CaOx SS (RSS)	<8.1(Male) <6.6(Fem.)						10.6 (1.3)	13.6 (0.9)

Subsequently, the metabolic profile of 31 post RYGB patients seen in the Mayo Kidney Stone Clinic were evaluated and reported (*14*). Patients presented a mean of 2.2 years after the surgery, at a time when they had lost a mean of 17.5 kg/m^2. The majority had calcium oxalate stones (27/29 analyzed), while the remainder had uric acid (2/29). Hyperoxaluria, hypocitraturia, and hypocalciuria were all commonly present, as was an increased calcium oxalate supersaturation (**Table 2**). The five patients that presented with their first stone less than six months postoperatively all lacked hyperoxaluria, but still manifested an increased urinary calcium oxalate supersaturation secondary to very low urine volumes. Asplin and Coe have reported very similar urinary findings amongst a group of bariatric surgery patients being worked up for kidney stone events through a referral lab (**Table 2**) (*15*). Of note, in the latter report even though urinary oxalate was not quite as high in the RYGB patients with stones as in the older JI-bypass group, urinary calcium oxalate supersaturation was slightly higher among the modern RYGB patients (*15*).

Although this evidence suggested that hyperoxaluria might be a cause of kidney stones after RYGB, it did not provide any information regarding the prevalence of these urinary changes. Therefore we completed a small prospective study amongst patients before, six months and 12 months after RYGB. Alarmingly, eight of 13 patients were hyperoxaluric 12 months postoperative (mean 0.74 mmol/day), and mean calcium oxalate supersaturation was high in this group (**Table 2**). Paralleling our observation amongst RYGB patients that presented with clinical kidney stones, hyperoxaluria was not prevalent in the six-month group. This observation suggests that it may take a period of time for this complication of RYGB to develop, perhaps due to dietary adaptations and/or other physiological changes post operative.

CONCLUSIONS

Observations to date suggest that hyperoxaluria is indeed common after modern bariatric surgery. Fat malabsorption may be an important contributing factor. However, not all patients seem to develop hyperoxaluria and/or stones after RYGB, suggesting that other modifying factors might influence risk. The risk of kidney stones, and/or renal oxalosis after modern RYGB is entirely unknown, but might be significant. Previous experiences of the medical community after jejunoileal bypass suggest that the risk of renal complications could be long-standing and progressive, even over a period of decades (*16*). Given the epidemic of obesity in the US, and the evidence cited above that modern bariatric surgery is one effective treatment strategy, it seems likely that increasing numbers of these procedures will be performed in the coming years. Therefore, it behooves us to study this potential complication thoroughly, in order to determine mechanisms and the optimal treatment strategies.

ACKNOWLEDGMENTS

The authors acknowledge the contributions of our collaborators Maria Colazzo-Clavell, Mukesh Sinha, Michael Sarr, and Wayne Nelson to these studies.

REFERENCES

1. Sjostrom, L., Larsson, B., Backman, L., Bengtsson, C., Bouchard, C., Dahlgren, S., Hallgren, P., Jonsson, E., Karlsson, J., Lapidus, L., and et al. (1992) Int J Obes Relat Metab Disord 16, 465-79.
2. Buchwald, H., Avidor, Y., Braunwald, E., Jensen, M. D., Pories, W., Fahrbach, K., and Schoelles, K. (2004) Jama 292, 1724-37.
3. Sjostrom, L., Narbro, K., Sjostrom, C. D., Karason, K., Larsson, B., Wedel, H., Lystig, T., Sullivan, M., Bouchard, C., Carlsson, B., Bengtsson, C., Dahlgren, S., Gummesson, A., Jacobson, P., Karlsson, J., Lindroos, A. K., Lonroth, H., Naslund, I., Olbers, T., Stenlof, K., Torgerson, J., Agren, G., and Carlsson, L. M. (2007) N Engl J Med 357, 741-52.
4. Puzziferri, N., Blankenship, J., and Wolfe, B. M. (2006) Endocrine 29, 11-9.
5. Hsu, C. Y., McCulloch, C. E., Iribarren, C., Darbinian, J., and Go, A. S. (2006) Ann Intern Med 144, 21-8.
6. Serra, A., Romero, R., Lopez, D., Navarro, M., Esteve, A., Perez, N., Alastrue, A., and Ariza, A. (2008) Kidney Int 73, 947-55.
7. Navarro-Diaz, M., Serra, A., Romero, R., Bonet, J., Bayes, B., Homs, M., Perez, N., and Bonal, J. (2006) J Am Soc Nephrol 17, S213-7.
8. Duffey, B. G., Pedro, R. N., Kriedberg, C., Weiland, D., Melquist, J., Ikramuddin, S., Kellogg, T., Makhlouf, A. A., and Monga, M. (2008) J Urol 179, 1401-6.
9. Curhan, G. C., Willett, W. C., Rimm, E. B., Speizer, F. E., and Stampfer, M. J. (1998) J Am Soc Nephrol 9, 1645-1652.
10. Modigliani, R., Labayle, D., Aymes, C., and Denvil, R. (1978) Scand J Gastroent 13, 187-192.
11. Hylander, E., Jarnum, S., and Nielsen, K. (1980) Scand J Gastroent 15, 349-352.
12. Gagner, M., and Matteotti, R. (2005) Surg Clin North Am 85, 141-9, x-xi.
13. Nelson, W. K., Houghton, S. G., Milliner, D. S., Lieske, J. C., and Sarr, M. G. (2005) Surgery for Obesity and Related Diseases 1, 481-485.
14. Sinha, M. K., Collazo-Clavell, M. L., Rule, A., Milliner, D. S., Nelson, W., Sarr, M. G., Kumar, R., and Lieske, J. C. (2007) Kidney Int 72, 100-7.
15. Asplin, J. R., and Coe, F. L. (2007) J Urol 177, 565-9.
16. Requarth, J. A., Burchard, K. W., Colacchio, T. A., Stukel, T. A., Mott, L. A., Greenberg, E. R., and Weismann, R. E. (1995) Arch Surg 130, 318-25.

Type 2 Diabetes and Uric Acid Nephrolithiasis

Naim M. Maalouf

Center for Mineral Metabolism and Clinical Research,
University of Texas Southwestern Medical Center, Dallas, Texas

Abstract. Type 2 diabetes is associated with an increased propensity for uric acid nephrolithiasis. In individuals with diabetes, this increased risk is due to a lower urine pH that results from obesity, dietary factors, and impaired renal ammoniagenesis. The epidemiology and pathogenesis of uric acid stone disease in patients with diabetes are hereby reviewed, and potential molecular mechanisms are proposed.

Keywords: Type 2 diabetes; uric acid; nephrolithiasis; urine pH
PACS: 87.19.xk

EPIDEMIOLOGY OF NEPHROLITHIASIS IN TYPE 2 DIABETES

Several studies have suggested an association between kidney stone disease and type 2 diabetes (T2DM). In a cross-sectional study of 3 large cohorts including over 200,000 participants, the prevalence of nephrolithiasis was significantly greater among individuals with T2DM compared to individuals without T2DM [1]. In the same study, the incidence of nephrolithiasis over a combined 44 years of follow-up was also significantly greater among individuals with T2DM [1]. Conversely, patients with nephrolithiasis are more likely to suffer from T2DM compared to non-stone formers [2] (Figure 1). At least two studies have suggested a specific predisposition to uric acid stones among with patients with T2DM [3,4] (Figure 2). In a retrospective examination of registries of stone formers, nephrolithiasis patients with T2DM were significantly more likely to have passed uric acid stones compared with non-diabetic stone formers [3]. Examining stone composition in over 4,500 patients, Daudon *et al.* noted a significantly greater prevalence of uric acid stones among diabetic than non-diabetic patients [4].

LOW URINE PH IN TYPE 2 DIABETES

A low urine pH is the principal factor predisposing to uric acid formation in the general stone population [5]. An overly acidic urine (pH<5.5) increases the concentration of relatively insoluble undissociated uric acid which tends to precipitate, leading to the formation of uric acid stones [6]. Recent studies have shown a lower urine pH in patients with T2DM, both among non-stone forming [7] and stone-forming T2DM patients [8] (Figure 3). One factor that could lead to the more acidic urine with T2DM is a higher body weight [7,9]. However, T2DM stone formers are

CP1049, *Renal Stone Disease 2, 2nd International Urolithiasis Research Symposium,*
edited by A. P. Evan, J. E. Lingeman, J. A. McAteer, and J. C. Williams, Jr.

more likely to form uric acid stones at any given BMI [8], suggesting that obesity alone does not account for the increased risk for uric acid nephrolithiasis in T2DM. Consumption of a diet with greater acid ash content by T2DM could potentially account for the more acidic urine, although patients with T2DM have persistently more acidic urine even after controlling for urine sulfate, a marker of dietary acid ash content [7].

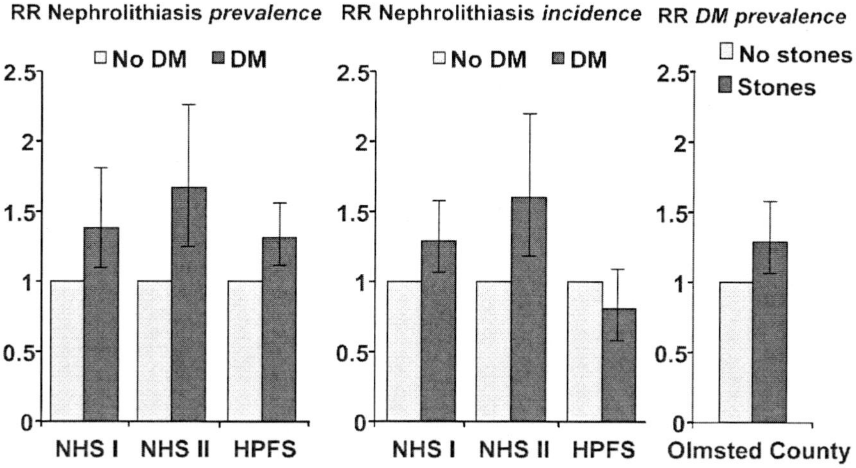

FIGURE 1. Prevalence and incidence of nephrolithiasis among individuals with diabetes mellitus (DM) compared to individuals without DM (left and middle panels). Right panel, prevalence of DM in stone formers and non-stone formers. Data adapted from Taylor *et al.* [1] and Lieske *et al.* [2]. NHS, Nurses' Health Study; HPFS, Health Professionals Follow-up Study.

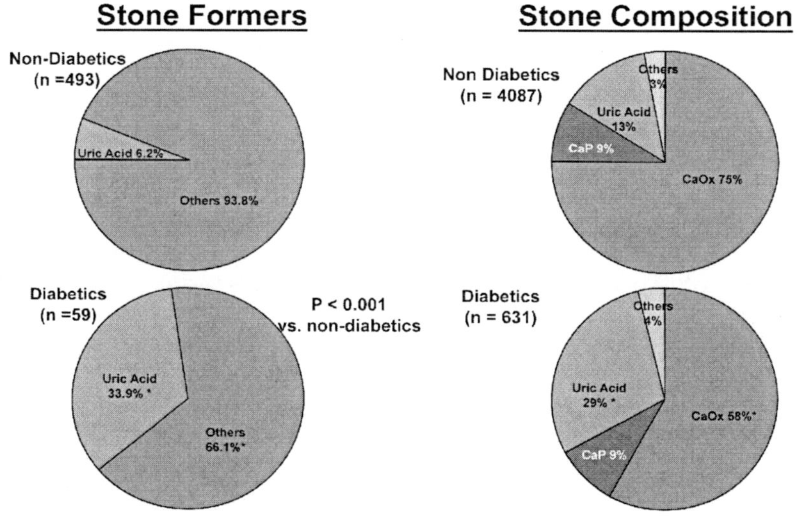

FIGURE 2. Stone formers are more likely to have uric acid stones if they are diabetic. Data from Pak *et al.* [3] and Daudon *et al.* [4].

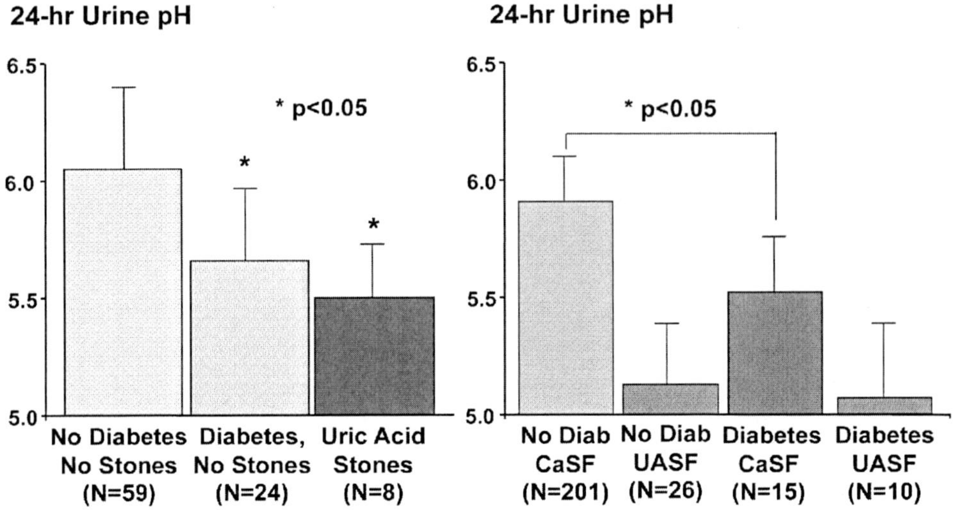

FIGURE 3. Urine pH in non-stone formers, calcium stone formers (CaSF), and uric acid stone formers (UASF), with and without diabetes (Diab). Data from Cameron *et al.* [7], and from Daudon *et al.* [8].

PATHOGENESIS OF URIC ACID NEPHROLITHIASIS IN TYPE 2 DIABETES

The persistently lower urine pH in T2DM independent of dietary acid intake suggests a potential defect in buffering of urine. Urine ammonia is one of the major urinary buffers, and a defect in urinary ammoniagenesis has previously been reported in patients with uric acid nephrolithiasis [10]. It is likely that the more acidic urine in T2DM is also a result of defective renal ammoniagenesis, as we have recently reported a lower urine pH and urine ammonium excretion per net acid excretion (NH_4^+/NAE) with increasing number of features of the metabolic syndrome [11]. These features, which are associated with obesity and insulin resistance, are very common in patients with T2DM.

Excess fat accumulation outside adipose tissue (steatosis) can alter metabolism and lead to toxicity in different organs (lipotoxicity, e.g. hepatic steatosis leading to steatohepatitis and cirrhosis) [12]. Lipotoxicity was recently shown to occur in the animal kidney *in vivo*, and renal cells *in vitro* [13]. Compared with pair-fed lean control rats, Zucker diabetic fatty rats were found to have higher renal triglyceride content (steatosis) and decreased urinary ammonium and pH, features of humans with uric acid nephrolithiasis. The direct effect of fat accumulation was assessed in opossum kidney (OKP) cells *in vitro*. Incubation of these cells with a mixture of long-chain fatty acids led to accumulation of intracellular lipids with concomitant dose-dependent decrease in the activity of Na(+)/H(+) exchanger-3 (NHE3), a major mediator of ammonium excretion. These findings suggest that renal steatosis decreases ammonium secretion in the proximal tubule, in part by reducing NHE3 activity. Our preliminary studies suggest the occurrence of renal steatosis in humans, although its role in the pathogenesis of uric acid nephrolithiasis remains to be proven.

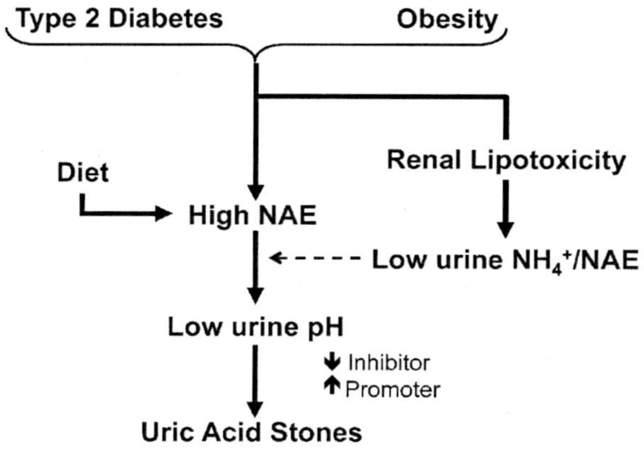

FIGURE 4. Hypothesis showing the various factors that may play a part in the formation of uric acid stones in type 2 diabetes.

CONCLUSIONS

In conclusion, type 2 diabetes is strongly associated with nephrolithiasis in general and uric acid stones in particular. A lower urine pH that cannot be entirely explained by obesity or dietary factors is responsible for the higher predisposition to uric acid stone formation in patients with type 2 diabetes. The overly acidic urine is in part explained by impaired ammoniagenesis, likely due to accumulation of lipids in the renal cortex (renal lipotoxicity). A low urine pH appears to be necessary, but not sufficient, for uric acid stone formation, suggesting that additional factors, possibly inhibitors or promoters of uric acid stone precipitation, also play a pathogenetic role (Figure 4).

ACKNOWLEDGMENTS

This work is in part supported by the National Institutes of Health (K23-RR21710, P01-DK20543, and R01-DK48482).

REFERENCES

1. Taylor EN, Stampfer MJ, Curhan GC. Diabetes mellitus and the risk of nephrolithiasis. Kidney Int. 2005 Sep;68(3):1230-5.
2. Lieske JC, de la Vega LS, Gettman MT, Slezak JM, Bergstralh EJ, Melton LJ 3rd, Leibson CL.Diabetes mellitus and the risk of urinary tract stones: a population-based case-control study. Am J Kidney Dis. 2006 Dec;48(6):897-904.
3. Pak CY, Sakhaee K, Moe O, Preminger GM, Poindexter JR, Peterson RD, Pietrow P, Ekeruo W. Biochemical profile of stone-forming patients with diabetes mellitus. Urology. 2003 Mar;61(3):523-7.

4. Daudon M, Lacour B, Jungers P. High prevalence of uric acid calculi in diabetic stone formers. Nephrol Dial Transplant. 2005 Feb;20(2):468-9.
5. Pak CY, Sakhaee K, Peterson RD, Poindexter JR, Frawley WH. Biochemical profile of idiopathic uric acid nephrolithiasis. Kidney Int. 2001 Aug;60(2):757-61.
6. Maalouf NM, Cameron MA, Moe OW, Sakhaee K. Novel insights into the pathogenesis of uric acid nephrolithiasis. Curr Opin Nephrol Hypertens. 2004 Mar;13(2):181-9.
7. Cameron MA, Maalouf NM, Adams-Huet B, Moe OW, Sakhaee K. Urine composition in type 2 diabetes: predisposition to uric acid nephrolithiasis. J Am Soc Nephrol. 2006 May;17(5):1422-8.
8. Daudon M, Traxer O, Conort P, Lacour B, Jungers P. Type 2 diabetes increases the risk for uric acid stones. J Am Soc Nephrol. 2006 Jul;17(7):2026-33.
9. Maalouf NM, Sakhaee K, Parks JH, Coe FL, Adams-Huet B, Pak CY. Association of urinary pH with body weight in nephrolithiasis. Kidney Int. 2004 Apr;65(4):1422-5.
10. Sakhaee K, Adams-Huet B, Moe OW, Pak CY. Pathophysiologic basis for normouricosuric uric acid nephrolithiasis. Kidney Int. 2002 Sep;62(3):971-9.
11. Maalouf NM, Cameron MA, Moe OW, Adams-Huet B, Sakhaee K. Low urine pH: a novel feature of the metabolic syndrome. Clin J Am Soc Nephrol. 2007 Sep;2(5):883-8.
12. Unger RH. Reinventing type 2 diabetes: pathogenesis, treatment, and prevention. JAMA. 2008 Mar 12;299(10):1185-7
13. Bobulescu IA, Dubree M, Zhang J, McLeroy P, Moe OW. Effect of renal lipid accumulation on proximal tubule Na+/H+ exchange and ammonium secretion. Am J Physiol Renal Physiol. 2008 Jun;294(6):F1315-22

Stone Morphology: Implication for Pathogenesis

Michel Daudon[1], Paul Jungers[2] and Dominique Bazin[3]

[1]*Service de Biochimie A, Hôpital Necker, 149 Rue de Sèvres, 75015 Paris, France*
[2]*Service de Néphrologie, Hôpital Necker, 149, Rue de Sèvres, 75015 Paris, France*
[3]*Laboratoire de Physique des Solides, Bat. 510, Université Paris-Sud, 91405 Orsay, France*

Abstract. Urinary stones of similar crystalline composition as identified by X-ray diffraction or Fourier transform infrared spectroscopy (FT-IR) may exhibit distinct structures, which are reflected in distinctive stone morphology. Among factors involved in stone morphology—some reflecting lithogenic activity, others depending on the crystal shape, or on the propensity of crystalline phases to form large aggregates, finally the environment where the stone is growing—all of these factors influence the inner structure of the stone and its superficial characteristics. We present here examples of the clinical interest of refined morphologic examination of stones, in addition to X-ray diffraction or FT-IR identification of its components. Such combination of methods allows the identification of specific etiologies among calcium oxalate stones, especially a morphological type pathognomonic of primary hyperoxaluria and other types related to distinct conditions of stone formation. Among phosphatic stones—in addition to stone composition, which must be considered not only on the basis of the main component, but also taking into account the minor crystalline phases, which often are clinically relevant—morphological types also contribute to diagnosis of the underlying etiology, especially for stones related to distal tubular acidosis. Finally, common purine stones also exhibit different morphologies related to stone composition and etiology: two main structures for uric acid and two for ammonium urate help to distinguish risk factors and lithogenic conditions involved in the formation of these calculi. Morphologic examination is a simple, rapid and cheap method that points to specific diseases or lithogenic factors. Better awareness of its clinical relevance should lead to wider utilization.

Keywords: Stone morphology, etiology, pathophysiology, calcium oxalates, calcium phosphates, purines
PACS: 01.30.Cc; 61.66.–f

INTRODUCTION

Nephrolithiasis is a very common condition in industrialized countries and its prevalence is relentlessly increasing [1-3]. In most cases, stones are made of calcium salts, mainly calcium oxalates which account for nearly 80% of kidney stones. Calcium oxalate in stones presents in two different crystalline forms: calcium oxalate monohydrate (COM) or whewellite, and calcium oxalate dihydrate (COD) or weddellite. Calcium oxalate stones often contain some proportion of calcium phosphate. On the other hand, in about 10% of cases, calcium phosphate—as carbapatite or other crystalline forms—is the main component of stones which often contain also some proportion of calcium oxalate [4]. Thus, stone analysis solely based on chemical composition is of limited clinical relevance, because it cannot

CP1049, *Renal Stone Disease 2, 2nd International Urolithiasis Research Symposium,*
edited by A. P. Evan, J. E. Lingeman, J. A. McAteer, and J. C. Williams, Jr.

discriminate among these different crystalline forms, which involve different pathogenic factors [5]. Physical methods such as X-ray diffraction and Fourier transform infrared spectroscopy (FT-IR), now commonly applied to stone analysis, provide a more accurate identification of the stone composition, including qualitative distinction between crystalline phases and quantitative assessment of the proportions of the various phases. However, useful additional information that is not given by the stone composition alone is provided by examination of stone morphology, which may differ between stones of similar chemical and crystalline composition [6, 7].

The aim of this review is to highlight the interest of considering stone morphology in addition to mineral composition, because morphology reveals specific lithogenic processes, orients the physician to peculiar etiological factors, and reflects the lithogenic activity of the disease.

Based on morphological analysis, we have proposed a classification of stones according to their main crystalline phase into 6 types and 21 subtypes, as previously reported [8]. Briefly, COM stones correspond to type I, COD to type II, purine stones to type III, phosphate stones to type IV, cystine to type V and protein stones to type VI. More recently, a new subtype (Ie) was added to type I stones to describe the peculiar morphology of COM stones observed in cases of heavy enteric hyperoxaluria.

FACTORS INFLUENCING STONE MORPHOLOGY

The morphology of urinary stones is determined by a number of factors, namely nature of the crystalline phase, kinetics of crystallization, existence of anatomical anomalies, presence of other stones in the same anatomical site, permanent or transient expression of urinary metabolic disorders, etc. As a consequence, a given crystalline species may induce stones with different morphological characteristics reflecting the factors involved in its formation. Results reported here are based on coupled FT-IR analysis and stone morphological examination of more than 56,000 stones from 1977 to 2007.

Morphology and Size of the Crystals

The first relevant factor able to significantly influence the stone morphology is the habit and size of the urinary crystals. For example, uric acid crystals present under very different forms that influence the organization of the stone. The same is true of other crystalline species such as calcium oxalate. As seen in figure 1, COD may present either as octahedral crystals, the most common form of this species, or dodecahedral crystals mainly observed in cases of heavy hypercalciuria [9]. Octahedral crystals of COD present as very small or, conversely, large crystals with size ranging from 1 to 50 µm. Moreover, this type of crystal is prone to form large aggregates which can be especially damaging to the kidney. In contrast, the dodecahedral form of COD has generally a crystal size less than 25 µm and it is often poorly aggregated.

The type of COD crystals influences the morphology of stones. Figure 2a shows a typical COD stone made of dodecahedral crystals (arrows), in a patient with heavy hypercalciuria. Figure 2b shows another COD stone made of small octahedral crystals, in a patient with moderate hypercalciuria, whereas figure 2c is a stone of same size made of large octahedral crystals, passed by a patient with hypercalciuria associated with hyperoxaluria and hypocitraturia.

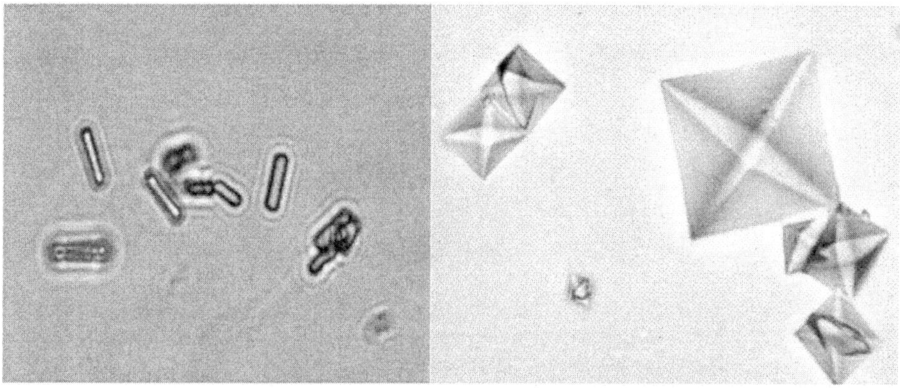

FIGURE 1: Different morphologies of crystals made of calcium oxalate dihydrate (COD), examined at same magnification (x 400). **Left panel**: dodecahedral COD crystals. **Right panel**: octahedral COD crystals. Note that dodecahedral crystals are of rather homogeneous size (about 10 μm), whereas octahedral crystals exhibit a wide range of size (5-50 μm).

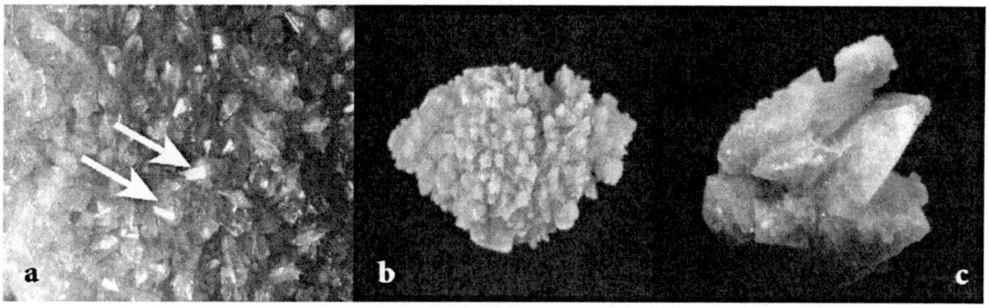

FIGURE 2: various morphologies of COD stones. **a**) typical COD stone made of dodecahedral crystals; **b**) COD stone made of small octahedral crystals; **c**) COD stone made of large octahedral crystals.

As shown in Figure 3, the percentage of urine specimens that contain dodecahedral crystals of COD sharply increases with increasing levels of urinary calcium concentration.

Kinetics of Crystal Growth and Agglomeration

The second important factor is the kinetics of crystal growth and, especially, the ability of crystals to rapidly form large aggregates. Some crystalline species are

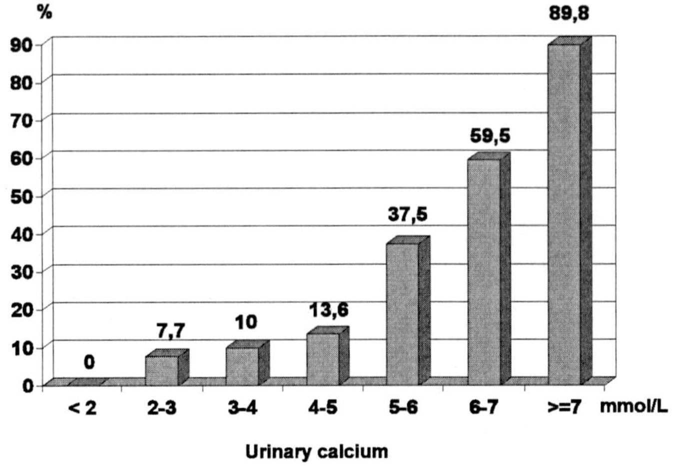

FIGURE 3. Percentage of urine specimens containing dodecahedral COD crystals in urines of differing calcium concentrations. The percentage of urine specimens containing dodecahedral crystals markedly increases with increasing calcium concentration.

susceptible to quickly develop aggregates in urine, such as uric acid dihydrate in acidic urine or brushite in the pH range 6-7 (Figures 4a and 4b). In such cases, the core of stones is poorly organized, because stone nucleation results from random agglomeration of large and/or numerous aggregates of crystals. With respect to calcium oxalate crystals, the propensity to form aggregates depends on the respective concentration of calcium and oxalate in urine and on the degree of hyperoxaluria. While few aggregates form in cases of heavy hypercalciuria facing a normal or moderately increased oxalate concentration (Figure 4f), hyperoxaluria is an important, but not the only, factor favoring the formation of large aggregates, commonly composed of mixed calcium oxalate phases, especially when the molar ratio of calcium to oxalate is low (Figures 4c and 4d). In most cases, calcium oxalate crystalluria is made of octahedral COD crystals when urine calcium concentration is moderately increased (4-7 mmol/L) and oxalate concentration in the normal range or only slightly increased ($\leq$0.45 mmol/L). In such cases, few COD aggregates are formed (Figure 4e), and rarely exceeds 50-60 μm.

It is well known that urinary calculi are composed of crystals admixed with an organic material containing macromolecules such as proteins and glycosaminoglycans, which may act as a cement and also contribute to the structure of the stone. Crystals result from urine supersaturation. They can grow and aggregate. However, the presence of crystals in urine is not always indicative of a stone process because crystals are commonly found in urine of healthy subjects and stone formers as well. In fact, stone nucleation results in most cases from retention of large crystals or aggregates or from large amounts of tiny crystals agglomerated within the lumen of a tubule. They may be retained because of their size, or shape, or due to adhesion to the epithelium, urine stasis or trapping in a narrow calyceal infundibulum. Therefore, stones may grow either by collecting new ions from the supersaturated urine or by capture of crystals newly formed in urine. When few crystals are formed, most are voided with urine and only some of them may fix on the initial nucleus, contributing to its growth. This slow process of stone formation essentially results in intermittent and slow stone growth, typically reflected by a well-organized structure made of a number of concentric layers. According to their morphological characteristics and relation to macromolecules, the crystals within each layer may be ordered, defining a radiating structure (Figure 5a).

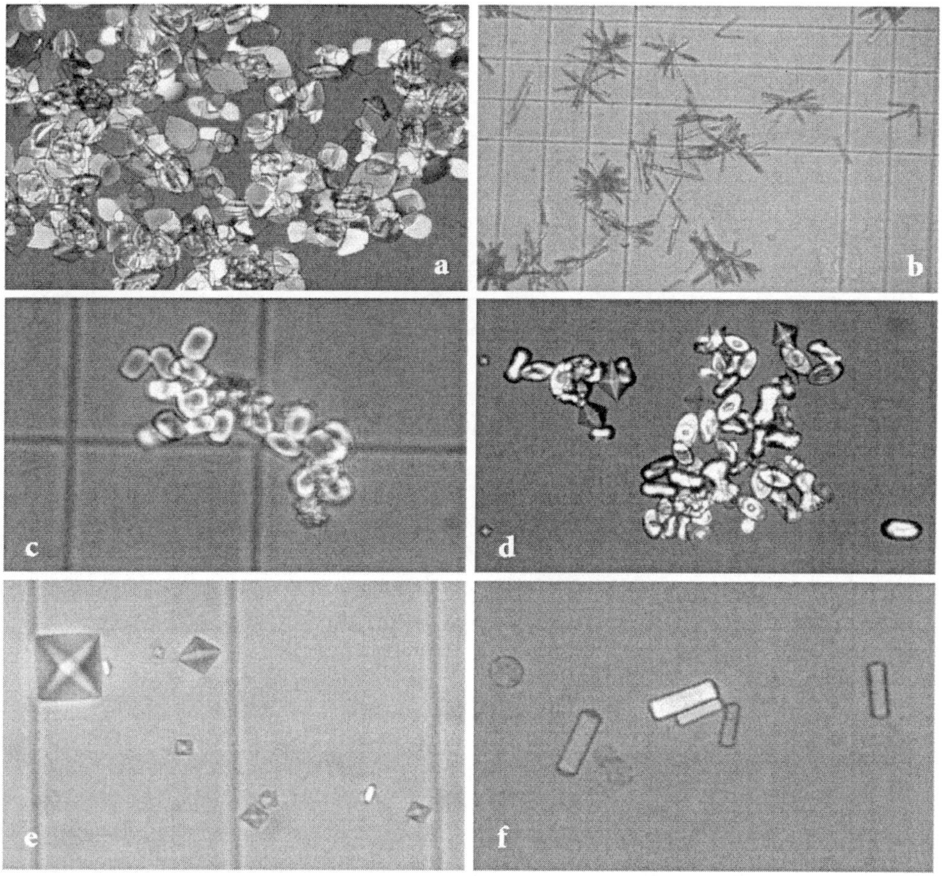

FIGURE 4: a) large aggregates of uric acid dihydrate crystals; b) radiating aggregates of brushite crystals; c) aggregate of COM crystals in a patient with primary hyperoxaluria type 1; d) large aggregates of COM and COD crystals; e) small and large octahedral crystals of COD in the same urine; f) long dodecahedral crystals of COD in a case of heavy hypercalciuria (calcium=15 mmol/L). Note that COD crystals have low propensity to form aggregates, whereas uric acid dihydrate, brushite and COM readily form aggregates.

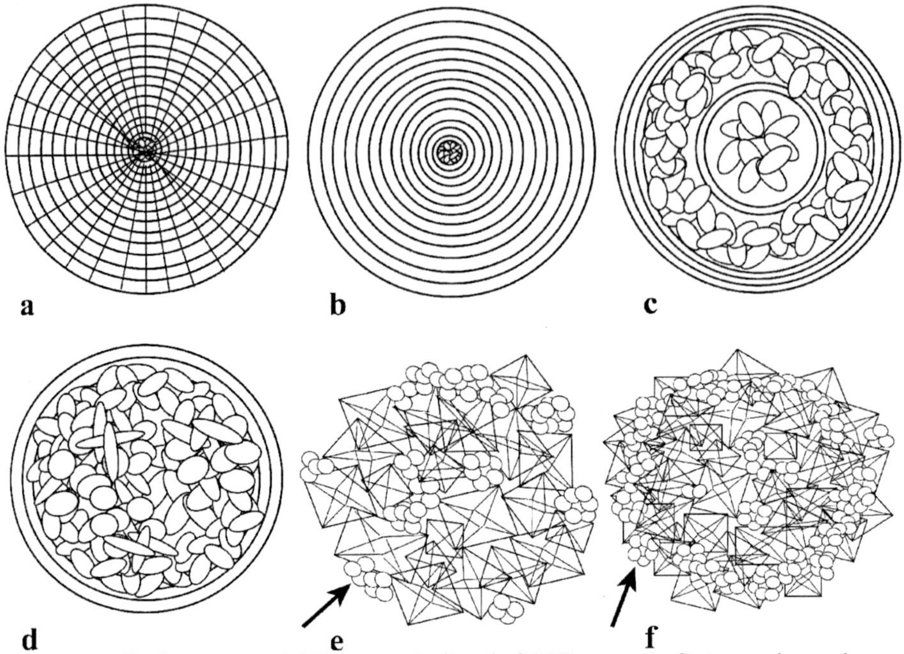

FIGURE 5. Stylized structures of COM stones (a-d) and of COD stones (e, f). Arrows in panels e and f show small deposits of apatite (in the form of small spherules) which are often observed between COD crystals.

When crystals are numerous or form large aggregates, the rapid agglomeration of these elements results in the formation of stones without any apparent organization (Figure 5d). Metabolically active lithogenic processes are often responsible for such poorly organized structures (Figure 5c and 5d). In contrast, intermittent weak metabolic disorders linked to imbalance in dietary habits are mainly associated with well organized structures (Figure 5a and 5b). COD crystals, due to their bipyramidal shape and often large size, cannot easily form concentric layers. They are aggregated and generally accompanied by deposits of small grains of carbapatite which locally accumulate in spaces not filled by the COD crystals (Figure 5e). When calcium phosphate deposits are abundant, they may coat COD crystals, thus forming an irregular layer which serves as support for new deposits of COD crystals, thus resulting in a structure typically made of grossly alternating layers of carbapatite and COD (Figure 5f). Such a structure is commonly found in cases of resorptive hypercalciuria such as in primary hyperparathyroidism [10].

Figure 6 presents common calcium oxalate stones made of COM developed on a Randall's plaque. The dark brown color of the surface (Figure 6a) and the well-organized section showing concentric layers with a radiating organization (Figure 6c) both suggest a slow and intermittent lithogenic process, mainly dependent on environmental factors. The dark color of the stone reflects the secondary incorporation of urine macromolecules and pigments into the stone during the slow lithogenic process. (Indeed, COM crystals themselves are white in color.)

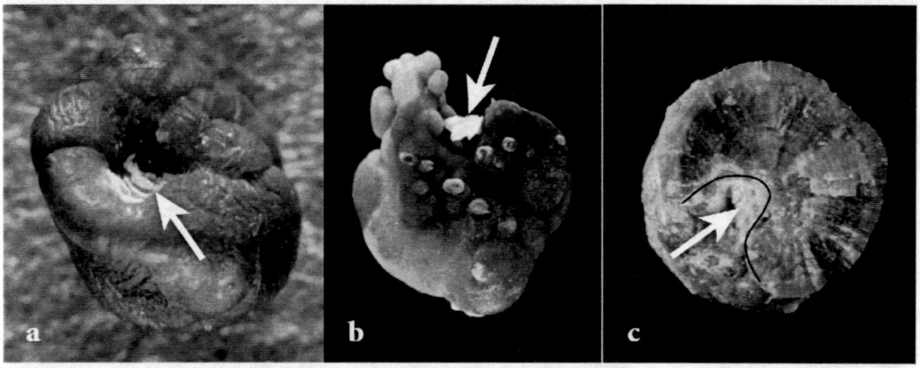

FIGURE 6: COM stones with a Randall's plaque (white arrows). The section (right panel) is made of concentric layers with a radiating structure converging on the plaque.

In contrast, COM stones formed in cases of a very active crystallization process, such as primary hyperoxaluria or enteric hyperoxaluria, are usually of light color and even white in some children (Figure 7a). Thus, the color of COM calculi is an important criterion reflecting the activity of the lithogenic process. Moreover, in cases of rapid crystallization, crystals are agglomerated without order, inducing a poorly organized core structure (Figure 7d) and a budding surface of the stone (Figure 7c). These morphologic criteria are highly suggestive of heavy hyperoxaluria from a genetic or other origin being responsible for the stone formation, especially in primary hyperoxaluria, characterized by permanent, massive hyperoxaluria present from birth. Figure 7 shows several examples of stones developed in patients suffering from primary hyperoxaluria type 1. They have common morphological characteristics including light color, budding surface and unorganized section. This typical morphology corresponds to type Ic of the classification and was found in all stone formers with primary hyperoxaluria [11].

When hyperoxaluria is less marked and intermittent, such as in enteric hyperoxaluria, stone morphology (type Ie) reveals the coexistence of poorly organized areas and locally concentric layers with radiating organization. As expected, unorganized layers, which correspond to active phases of crystallization, are less pigmented than those formed during slow lithogenic phases.

PECULIAR LITHOGENIC PROCESSES

Stone morphology and superficial characteristics may be influenced by specific lithogenic processes which induce stone formation or come before it and favor lithogenesis in conjunction with other factors.

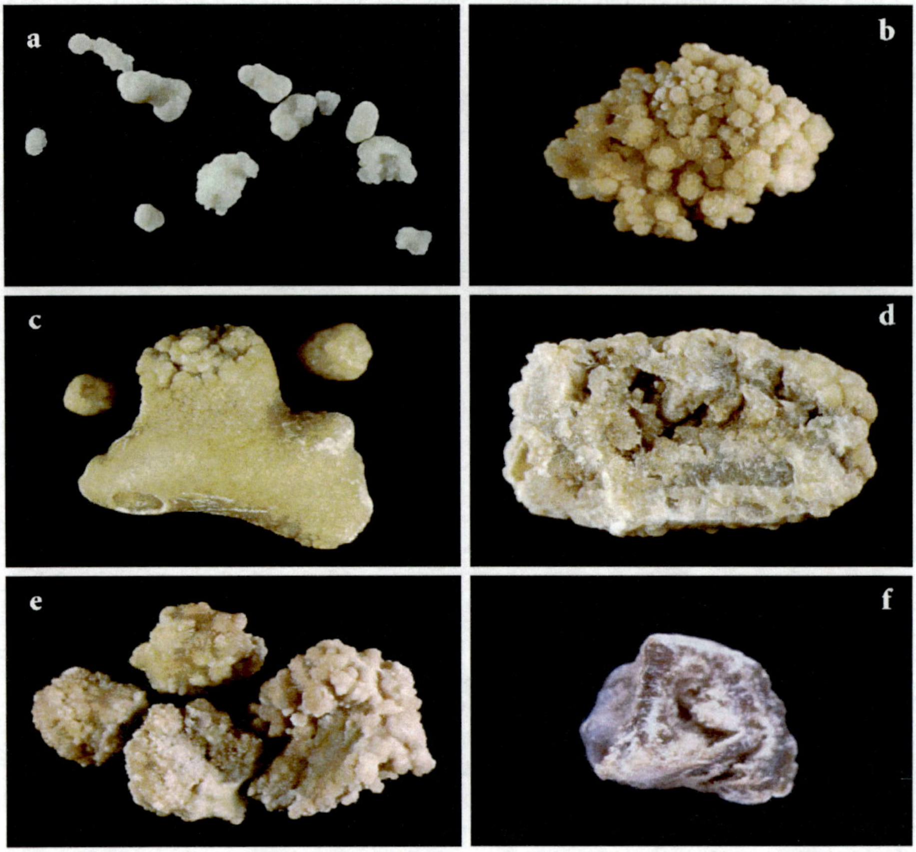

FIGURE 7. Morphology of COM stones from patients with primary hyperoxaluria type 1 (PH1) (a-d) or with enteric hyperoxaluria (e, f): a) whitish stones from an infant with PH1; b) typical clear COM stone from a young PH1 adult patient with severely recurrent stone formation; c) large pelvic COM stone in a child with PH1; d) section of a PH1 stone with a typical loose, unorganized inner structure; e) COM stone from a patient with ileal resection and heavy oxaluria; f) section of a COM stone from the same patient. Note the coexistence of clear, loose, unorganized areas and of more structured and dark areas.

Randall's plaque

The most common of these factors that lead to stone formation is the Randall's plaque, a calcification process resulting in deposition of carbapatite crystals in the inner medulla. The spread of these deposits up to the papillary epithelium induces its disruption and therefore exposure of the carbapatite deposits to the supersaturated urine, which may produce crystals able to form stones by fixing on the surface of the plaque. As shown in Figure 6, these stones are first made of COM and grow slowly in the absence of patent metabolic disorder. They typically exhibit a superficial morphology characterized by an irregular dip (umbilication) which contains a whitish mineral deposit (Randall's plaque) made of carbapatite (white arrow) [12-14] onto which COM crystals may be anchored. In hypercalciuric patients, the first layers of calcium oxalate crystals beneath the plaque are usually made of COM, whereas the rest of the stone is mainly composed of poorly organized crystals of COD (Figure 8).

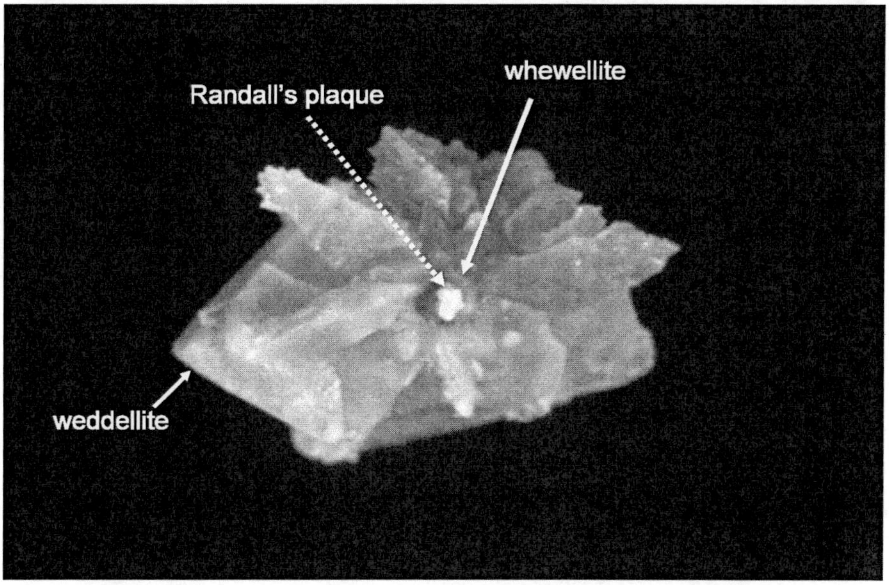

FIGURE 8. COD stone developed on a Randall's plaque in a hypercalciuric patient. Note that the Randall's plaque (made of carbapatite) is surrounded by some layers of COM, which themselves are covered by COD.

Medullary Sponge Kidney

Medullary sponge kidney has a variable influence on stone formation, according to the degree of anatomical anomalies and the presence of metabolic disorders. In some patients, tubule dilatations are limited to a small part of one kidney, for example one lower calyx, without associated metabolic abnormalities. In such cases, localized stasis is the main factor for stone formation. Crystallization occurs in the dilated parts of the nephrons where the urine flow is slowed down, and crystals may agglomerate to form stones within the tubule or may fix on a Randall's plaque close to the tubule end, thus leading to a stone on the tip of the papilla. In more severe cases, several caliceal units are affected and various metabolic disorders may accompany anatomical deformations of the tubules, including hypercalciuria and local tubular acidification defects. Often, this diffuse form of sponge kidney is the cause of an active lithogenic process resulting in the passage of multiple stones. The numerous stones retained within tubular ectasias produce a radiological aspect of medullary nephrocalcinosis. As shown in Figure 9, stones formed within the tubules have a typical "cylindrical" shape. In other cases, intratubular lithogenesis induces the formation of multiple nuclei made of carbapatite subsequently covered by new carbapatite layers and finally by calcium oxalate crystals.

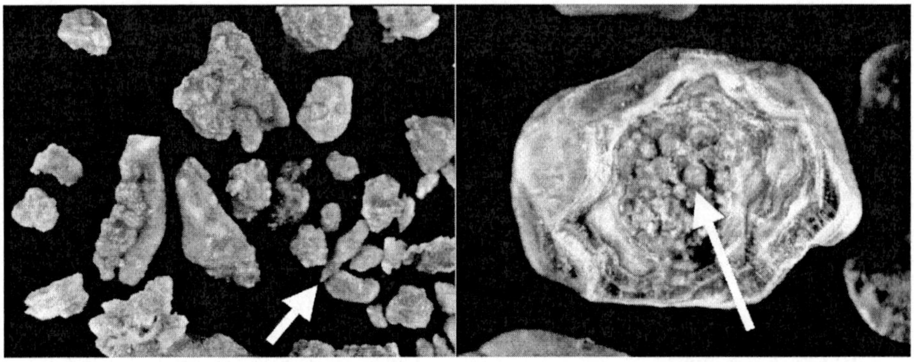

FIGURE 9. Stones passed by a patient with medullary sponge kidney. In the **left panel**, the arrow points to a cylindrical stone developed within a spindle-shaped tubular ectasia. **Right panel**: section of a stone showing multiple carbapatite nuclei formed in an ectasia and secondarily covered by new layers of carbapatite.

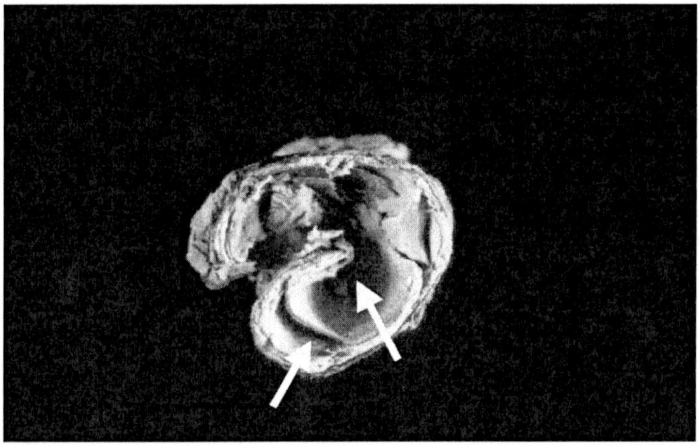

FIGURE 10. Section of an infection stone initiated by a protein matrix and secondarily mineralized Note the presence of typical cavities (arrows) due to protein retraction.

Matrix Lithogenic Process

In cases of urinary tract infection, a number of microorganisms are able to produce a proteoglycan matrix, which favors adhesion to the epithelium, creates a favorable environment for their development and protects against antibodies produced by the patient and antibacterial agents. This matrix constitutes a physical support for crystal fixation. In addition, local changes in urine biochemistry due to the enzymatic material of the microorganisms create conditions favorable to the crystallization of phosphates, including magnesium ammonium phosphate, carbapatite, amorphous carbonated calcium phosphate and whitlockite. These crystals may cover the matrix and thus form a solid mineral layer which is the first step of a mineralized stone. The layer of crystals may be covered in turn by protein matrix which is further covered by new crystals, and so on. Progressively, the inner layers are isolated from the urine and may lose some proportions of water, the consequence of which being a retraction of protein layers and formation of cavities within the stone. After surgical removal, *in vitro* dehydration of proteins present within the stones creates large voids between mineral layers. Figure 10 illustrates an example of such a very loose concentric organization typical of an infectious stone process.

Anatomical Anomalies of the Urinary Tract

Anatomical anomalies such as caliceal diverticula or megaureter favor stone formation, the former because of local stasis, the latter because of urinary tract infection [15-17]. In both cases, stone morphology is strongly influenced by the anatomical context. As shown in Figure 11, stasis within a diverticulum may induce formation of multiples stones which are often small, spherical with a smooth surface. Sometimes, there are thousand stones in a diverticulum. Depending on urine biochemistry, the stones may be composed of COM, carbapatite or other calcium salts. When the stone forms in a megaureter, irrespective to its composition, it presents as a cylindrical cast of the ureter. In most cases, it results from an infectious lithogenic process and is mainly composed of calcium and magnesium phosphates.

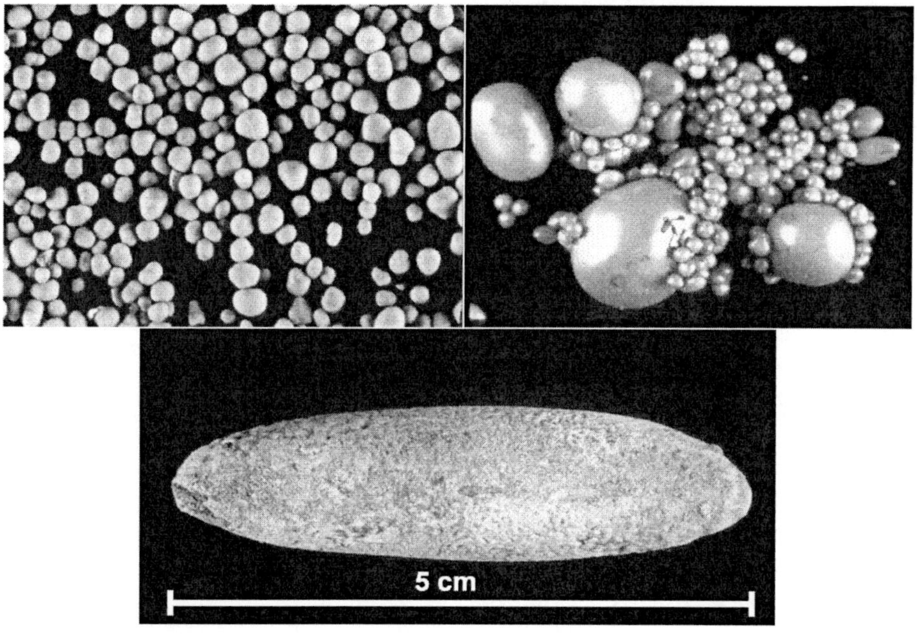

FIGURE 11. Multiple stones developed in caliceal diverticuli (upper left: COM calculi; upper right: carbapatite calculi) or in a megaureter (lower panel).

Crystalline Conversion

Several chemical compounds present as crystalline species with various levels of hydration. As a rule, the most thermodynamically stable form has the lowest content in water molecules. So, among crystalline phases of a given substance, the most hydrated ones spontaneously tend toward a less hydrated state. Among calcium oxalate species, COD frequently converts to COM by crystalline conversion [18-20]. Morphological changes that result from conversion are visible in the structure of the stone as shown in Figure 12.

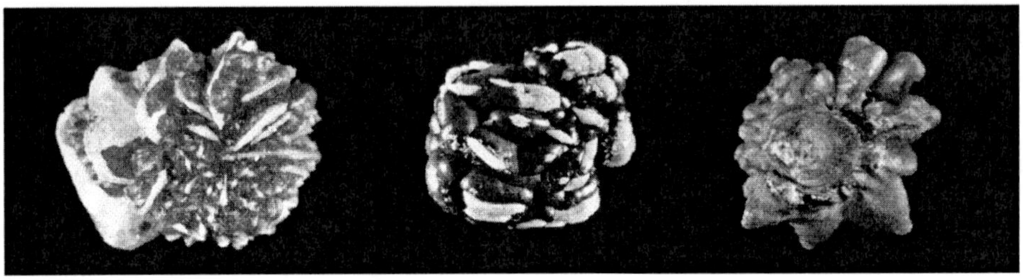

FIGURE 12. Crystalline conversion from COD to COM. (left to right)

SIGNIFICANCE OF MORPHOLOGICAL CHANGES FROM THE CORE TO THE SURFACE OF THE STONES

Examples of stones characterized by morphological changes from the core to the surface highlight the interest of examining the structures both at the surface and the section of calculi. The first example (Figure 13) is a 20 mm pelvic stone surgically removed from a boy aged 9 years. Urine biochemistry examination revealed hypercalciuria as the unique metabolic disorder. This agreed with the surface of the stone made of aggregated crystals of COD mixed with whitish carbapatite deposits. However, section of the stone revealed successive concentric zones with various color and organization. The core was composed of pure ammonium acid urate (morphological type IIId); the median part of the stone, which presented as a dark-brown ring was made of pure COM of Ib type, and the peripheral part of the stone was made of COD mixed with carbapatite corresponding to a mixed type IIa+IVa1. These findings were in keeping with the history of this young patient who initially lived in North Africa. First, because of chronic infectious diarrhea associated with low diuresis, low phosphate and protein intake (lack of dairy products), all conditions which favor high ammonia excretion and hyperuricosuria, the crystallization process was initiated by ammonium acid urate. Subsequently, during several years, the diet was mainly based on cereals and vegetables rich in oxalate, in a context of insufficient water intake and low diuresis in a hot country, thus favoring COM crystallization. Finally, the child migrated with his parents to France where abundant intake of dairy products resulted in dietary hypercalciuria and addition of COD and carbapatite to the stone.

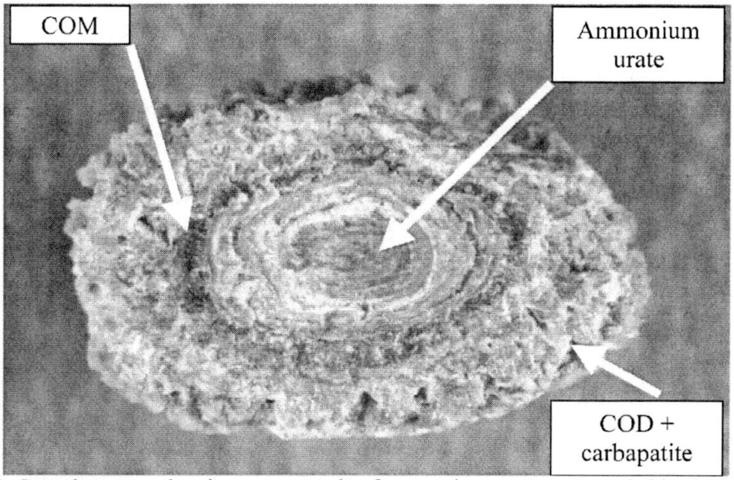

FIGURE 13. Complex stone showing a core made of ammonium urate, surrounded by COM layers and finally covered with a mixture of COD and carbapatite

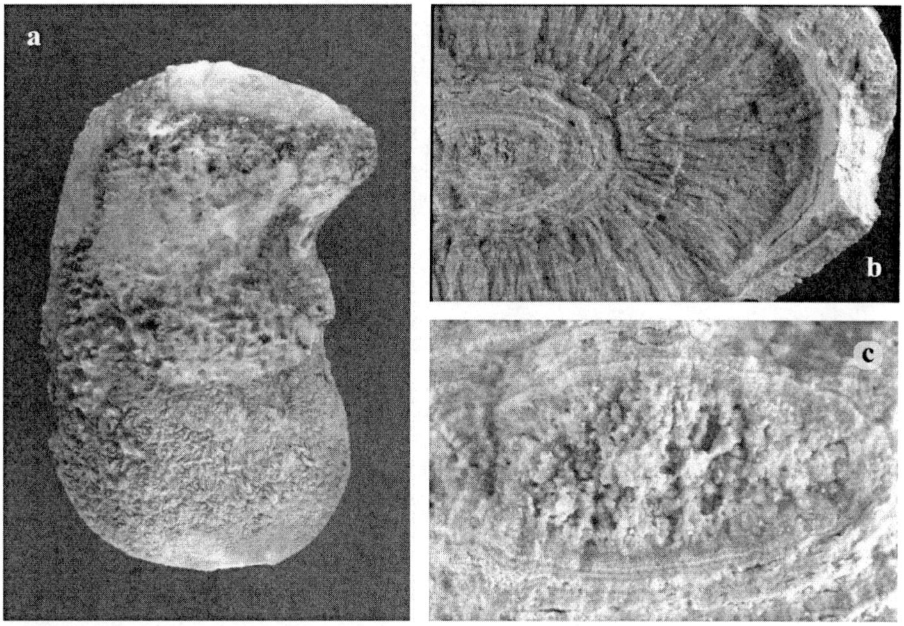

FIGURE 14. Complex stone from a patient with primary hyperoxaluria. The surface (a) is made of struvite. The section (b) is made of COM with radiating structure. The core (c) shows a clear, loose unorganized structure (type Ic) highly suggestive of primary hyperoxaluria 1.

The second example is that of a young man aged 26 years who had a chronic urinary tract infection by *Proteus mirabilis* who presented with a unique, very large bladder stone (Figure 14). The stone was surgically removed; its dimensions were 12 x

8 cm and its weight was 420 grams. Its surface (Figure 14a) was of IVc morphology and mainly composed of magnesium ammonium phosphate hexahydrate (struvite) mixed with some proportions of carbapatite, COM and proteins. The section revealed, under the peripheral layers of phosphate salts, a wide, compact structure looking like type Ia, mainly radiating and fairly concentric, which was pale brown in color (Figure 14b) and made of pure COM. However, the core of the stone was typically unorganized and loose, with a pale color and also composed of pure COM, suggesting a type Ic structure (Figure 14c). This finding oriented the diagnosis toward a genetic disease, namely primary hyperoxaluria type 1. Specific metabolic investigations including measurements of oxalate, glycolate and L-glycerate excretion in 24h-urine confirmed the diagnosis.

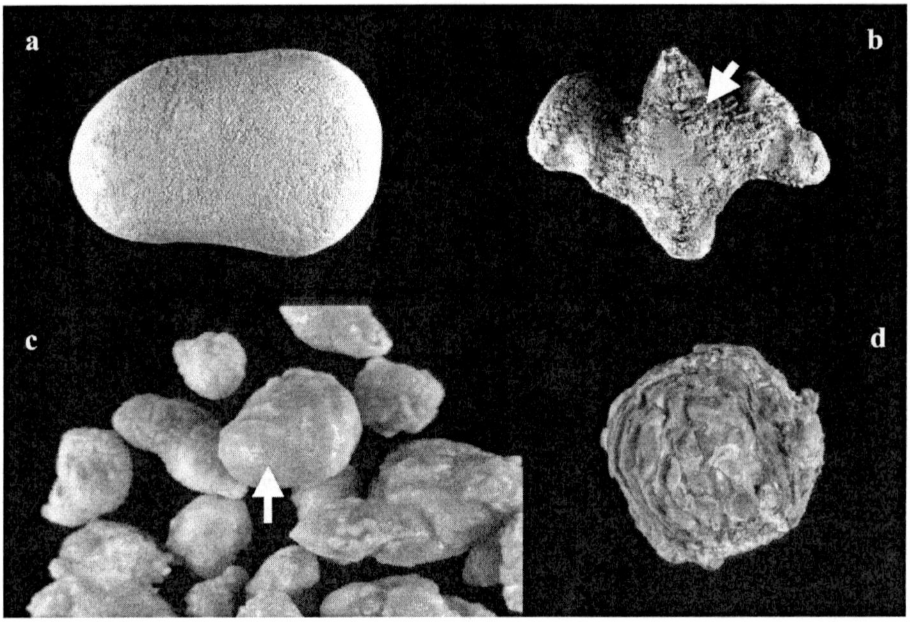

FIGURE 15. Various morphologies of phosphate stones with carbapatite as main component. a) carbapatite mixed with some struvite. b) Large branched pelvic stone in a patient with primary hyperparathyroidism, made of carbapatite admixed with COD (arrow); c) type IVa2 carbapatite stones from a patient with distal tubular acidosis (Sjögren syndrome). Note the typical cracks at the surface of stones (arrow); d) section of a IVa2 stone

VARIOUS MORPHOLOGIES OF CARBAPATITE STONES

Among calcium phosphate stones, various morphologies may help to suspect specific causes of the calculus. Figure 15 illustrates some typical cases. First, Figure 15a shows a type IVa1 stone with a slightly rough, whitish surface. The stone section (not shown) is poorly organized, with whitish, roughly concentric layers. Commonly, this type of stone is observed in cases of urinary tract infection associated or not with hypercalciuria [21].

Figure 15b shows a large pelvic stone of IVa1 type, associated with crystals of COD (arrow) corresponding to type IIb morphology. Such an association is highly suggestive of combined hypercalciuria and hyperphosphaturia, as observed in primary hyperparathyroidism. Figure 15c illustrates a peculiar aspect of carbapatite stones with a glazed and locally embossed surface with cracks. The stone section (Figure 15d) resembles the surface with a more or less glazed aspect. Inner structure is made of irregular concentric layers of various brown-yellow colors. Often, the organization of such stones reveals multiple independent concentric structures in the core, highly suggestive of multiple nuclei. This morphology corresponds to type IVa2 of our classification and it is mainly observed in patients with inherited or acquired distal tubular acidosis. In our experience, 89.5% of stone formers with Sjögren syndrome had stones exhibiting this IVa2 morphology.

VARIOUS MORPHOLOGIES OF URIC ACID AND URATE STONES

Similarly, distinct morphology of purine stones orients toward different risk factors and causes. For example, Figures 16a and 16b illustrate the case of multiple stones of type IIIa found in the bladder of an older man with a benign prostate hypertrophy. The surface of stones is smooth, homogeneous, with a pale orange color. The section is well organized, showing concentric layers and a radiating organization of the crystals. This type of stone mainly results from urine stasis.

In contrast, type IIIb stones (Figures 16c and 16d) have a heterogeneous surface with a poorly organized section, suggesting a more active lithogenic process. Indeed, type IIIb stones often are associated with the metabolic syndrome or with type 2 diabetes. Figure 16e shows a typical IIIc stone, made of ammonium acid urate. This morphology is a marker of three possible biochemical conditions: hyperuricosuria, high ammoniagenesis and high urine pH. Often, high ammonia excretion and high urine pH result from urinary tract infection by urea-splitting bacteria. In contrast, type IIId stones as presented in Figure 16f illustrate a complex lithogenic process involving metabolic disorders due to low dietary phosphate intake, loss of electrolytes due to chronic or intermittent episodes of diarrhea or, in Western countries, laxative abuse. In the latter, stones often exhibit a violet color.

MAIN RELATIONSHIPS BETWEEN STONE MORPHOLOGY AND ETIOPATHOGENY

In total, stone morphology appears to be of clinical relevance to orient etiologic diagnosis. In most cases, the morphological type of the stone is indicative of the main biochemical disorder(s) involved in stone formation. Table 1 presents the main etiological factors in relation to the morphological stone types. For example, type II is found in about 94% of calcium oxalate stones associated with hypercalciuria.

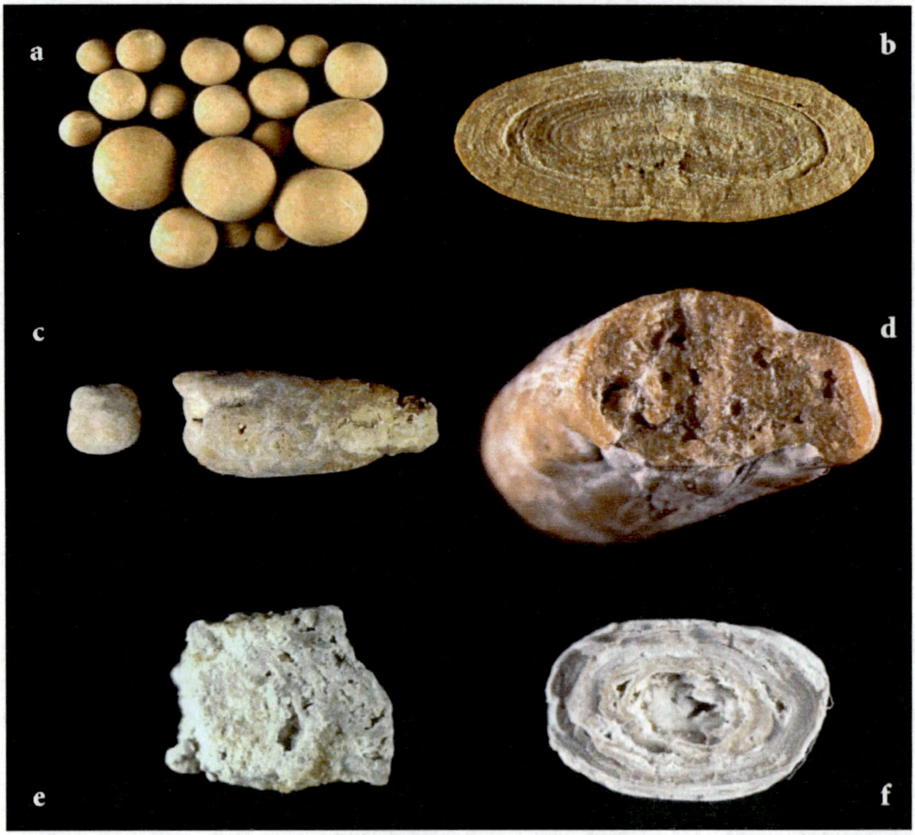

FIGURE 16. Various aspects of purine stones. a) typical orange, spherical anhydrous uric acid stones (type IIIa) from a patient with bladder urolithiasis; b) section of a IIIa uric acid stone showing a concentric structure; c) Uric acid stones (type IIIb) made of mixed anhydrous and dihydrate uric acid, from a patient with type 2 diabetes; d) section of a IIIb stone with an unorganized structure; e) section of an ammonium urate stone (type IIIc) from a patient with uric acid nephrolithiasis treated by excessive alkalinization; f) section of a IIId stone made of ammonium urate in a child originating from a developing country.

In case of primary hyperparathyroidism, the most frequent morphology is the mixed type II + IVa1, found in more than 50% of stones, whereas type IVd, which corresponds to stones mainly composed of brushite, was found in 14.2% of cases, an unusually high rate for this rare stone component.

In conclusion, characterization of stone morphology provides useful etio-pathogenic information, in addition to stone composition, to identify metabolic factors involved in stone formation. Stone morphology is of special interest for early diagnosis of severe inherited or acquired stone diseases that in the absence of proper management, may lead to progressive loss of renal function and ultimately end-stage renal failure. Morphological analysis is rapid, cheap and easily performed by skilled staff involved in stone analysis and should merit to be more largely used in addition to the determination of stone composition.

TABLE 1. Relationships between stone morphology and etiopathogenic conditions

Pathogenic conditions	No. of cases	Stone morphology	Frequency (%)
Idiopathic hypercalciuria	850	Type IIa	83.2
		Mixed type IIa + Ia	10.8
Primary hyperparathyroidism	226	Mixed type II + IVa1	51.8
(Main component of stones:		Type IVd	14.2
COD = 84; Carbapatite = 74;		Type IVa1	12.4
COM = 36; Brushite = 32)		Type IIa	11.7
Idiopathic hyperoxaluria	342	Type Ia	88.1
Primary hyperoxaluria type 1	87	Type Ic	100
Enteric hyperoxaluria	59	Type Ie	81.4
Sjögren syndrome	57	Type IVa2	89.5
Type 2 diabetes in stone formers: male	669	Type IIIb	30.9*
female	193	Type IIIb	37.0*
Diarrhea and low phosphate intake	46	Type IIId	91.3

* type IIIb stones were found in 23.7% of male stone formers and in only 13% of female stone formers without diabetes matched for age

REFERENCES

1. A. Trinchieri, F. Coppi, E. Montanari, A. Del Nero, G. Zanetti and E. Pisani, *Eur Urol* **37**, 23-25 (2000).
2. A. Hesse, E. Brandle, D. Wilbert, K.U. Kohrmann and P. Alken, *Eur Urol* **44**, 709-713 (2003).
3. K.K. Stamatelou, M.E. Francis, C.A. Jones, L.M. Nyberg and G.C. Curhan, *Kidney Int* **63**, 1817-1823 (2003).
4. M. Daudon, R. Donsimoni, C. Hennequin, S. Fellahi, G. Le Moel, M. Paris, S. Troupel and B. Lacour, *Urol Res* **23**, 319-326 (1995).
5. C.Y.C. Pak, J.R. Poindexter, B. Adams-Huet and M.S. Pearle, *Am J Med*; **115**, 26-32 (2003).
6. M. Daudon, L. Estepa, B. Lacour and P. Jungers, *J Nephrol* **11 Suppl 1**, 51-55 (1998).
7. M. Daudon and P. Jungers, *Nephron Physiol* **98**, 31-36 (2004).
8. M. Daudon, C.A. Bader and P. Jungers, *Scanning Microsc* **7**, 1081-1106 (1993).
9. M. Daudon, F. Barbey and P. Jungers, *Rev Med Suisse Romande* **124**, 455-459 (2004).
10. L. Cifuentes Delatte, A. Rapado, M. Santos, M.L. Traba and L.M. Castrillo, *Rev Clin Esp* **138**, 305-311 (1975).
11. M. Daudon, P. Jungers P and D. Bazin, *NEJM* **359**, 100-102 (2008).
12. L. Cifuentes Delatte, J. Minon-Cifuentes and J.A. Medina, *J Urol* **137**, 1024-1029 (1987).
13. M. Daudon, O. Traxer, P. Jungers and D. Bazin, In: A.P. Evan, J.E. Lingeman and J.C. Williams Jr (eds), Renal Stone Disease. *American Institute of Physics Conference Proceedings, Melville, New York,* **900**, pp. 26-34 (2007).
14. A.P. Evan, F.L. Coe, J.E. Lingeman, Y. Shao, A.J. Sommer, S.B. Bledsoe, J.C. Anderson and E.M. Worcester. *Anat Rec* **290**, 1315-1323 (2007).
15. R.L. Vereecken and W. Proesmans, *Eur Urol* **36**, 342-37 (1999).
16. M. Daudon, F. Cohen-Solal, B. Lacour and P. Jungers, *Prog Urol* **13**, 1320-1329 (2003).
17. B.K. Auge, M.E. Maloney, B.J. Mathias, P.K. Pietrow and G.M. Preminger, *BJU Int* **97**, 1053-1056 (2006).
18. L. Cifuentes Delatte, A. Hidalgo, J. Bellanato and M. Santos, In: Cifuentes Delatte L, Rapado A, Hodgkinson A (eds), *Urinary calculi. Recent advances in aetiology, stone structure and treatment. Karger, Basel,* pp.220-230 (1973).
19. W. Berg, P. Lange, C. Bothor and D. Rössler, *Eur Urol* **5**, 136-143 (1979).
20. G. Schubert and G Brien, *Int Urol Nephrol* **13**, 249-260 (1981).
21. L. Maurice-Estepa, P. Levillain, B. Lacour and M. Daudon, *Scand J Urol Nephrol* **33**, 299-305 (1999).

V. PROGRESS IN SHOCK WAVE LITHOTRIPSY

The Advantage of a Broad Focal Zone in SWL

Robin O. Cleveland

Department of Mechanical Engineering, Boston University, Boston, MA 02215

Abstract. The evolution of lithotripters over the past 20 years has lead to the production of lithotripters with smaller focal zones (diameters 4-8 mm) than the first generation lithotripters (~12 mm diameters) and with higher peak pressures (~100 MPa compared to ~40 MPa). At first glance it may seem beneficial to focus the acoustic energy more tightly onto the stone however clinical reports suggest that the narrower focal zones have poorer outcomes and more side effects. Here the impact of focal spot size on energy delivered to stones and the intensity delivered to tissue is considered by numerical modeling. It is shown that lithotripters with focal spots much larger than a stone are able to deliver similar energy to a stone as a narrow high pressure focal spot lithotripter. The reduction of energy delivered to the stone is exacerbated in the presence of motion. The larger focal spot lithotripters result in reduced incident intensity to the tissue. These results suggest that wide focal spot lithotripters have the potential to adequately fragment stones with a lower risk of side effects.

Keywords: Shock waves, lithotripsy, kidney stone fragmentation, ultrasound bioeffects.
PACS: 43.80.Gx, 87.54.Hk, 43.20.Gp.

INTRODUCTION

The first lithotripter introduced in the US was the Dornier HM3. This was an electrohydraulic lithotripter which produced a waveform with a peak pressure of around 40 MPa—as shown in Figure 1. The "focal zone" as determined by the location where the positive pressure drops to 50% of the peak value (also referred to as the 6 dB width, as a 50% drop in pressure corresponds to -6dB on the decibel scale [1]) was 12 mm wide and 85 mm long [2]. Many newer lithotripters employ an electromagnetic source which can produce higher peak pressures and smaller focal spots. Figure 1 also shows a waveform measured in a Storz Modulith SLX. The waveform is morphologically similar to that of the HM3 but the amplitude is much higher with a peak positive pressure of 115 MPa. The focal zone is also much smaller: 4 mm wide by 35 mm long—although it should be noted that the -6 dB pressure is 57 MPa which is higher than the peak pressure in the HM3 [2,3].

It is the pressure that describes the acoustic field; however the pressure is not perhaps the best metric for determining how shock waves break stones or how shock waves damage tissue. Indeed there is little agreement in the literature as to the mechanisms by which shock waves fragment stones or damage tissue and so it is not clear what metrics should be employed [2,4,5]. The approach used in this study was to calculate the energy delivered to the stone which is likely related to the fragmentation process. The peak pressure was used as a proxy for tissue damage.

CP1049, *Renal Stone Disease 2, 2nd International Urolithiasis Research Symposium,*
edited by A. P. Evan, J. E. Lingeman, J. A. McAteer, and J. C. Williams, Jr.

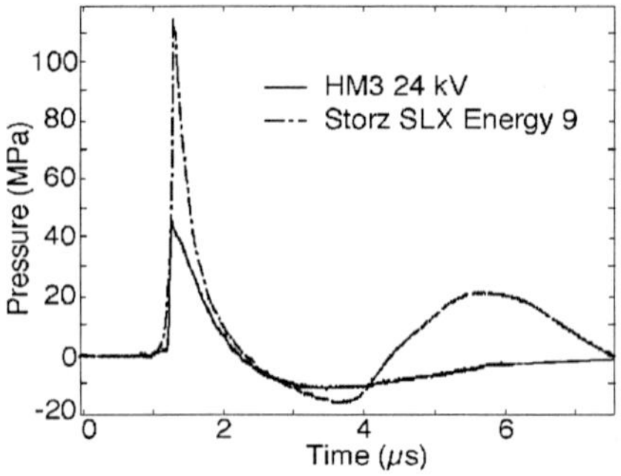

FIGURE 1. Comparison of waveforms measured in a Dornier HM3 and a Storz Modulith SLX.

METHOD

Analysis of the difference between wide and narrow focal zones was carried out numerically. The peak pressure was assumed to decay following a Gaussian distribution in the lateral direction, that is,

$$p_+(r) = p_+(0)e^{-(r/r_0)^2} \tag{1}$$

where $p_+(0)$ is the peak positive pressure on the axis and r_0 governs the width. The radius and which the pressure drops by 50% (6dB) from the peak is given by r_{6dB}=0.83 r_0 and therefore the focal width (which is reported in what follows) is 1.66 r_0.

The energy delivered to a stone can be calculated as follows [1,2]. First at each point on the surface of the stone the pulse intensity integral (PII) or energy flux density (EFD) needs to be calculated. This is obtained by integrating the square of the pressure over the duration of the pulse in time, *viz*:

$$PII = \int \frac{p^2(t)}{\rho_0 c_0} dt \tag{2}$$

where ρ_0=1000 kg/m^3 is the density and c_0=1540 m/s is the sound speed of the medium. For the HM3 waveform shown in Figure 1, PII=0.4 mJ/mm^2. The energy is then obtained by integrating the PII over the area of the stone:

$$E = \iint PII(x,y)dxdy \tag{3}$$

The units of energy are joules (J). For the HM3 waveform shown in Figure 1 the energy delivered to a 10 mm diameter stone is 30 mJ.

In what follows the only parameters of the shock wave that will be changed are the focal width and the peak pressure. That is, it is assumed that the shape of the SW is the same for all different lithotripters and at all radial locations. This means that the PII is proportional to peak pressure squared and therefore once $p_+(r)$ is specified, as in Eq. 1, the impact of the focal characteristics can be accounted for in the surface integral needed for the energy calculation.

RESULTS

Figure 2 shows the energy incident on a stone as a function of the width of the focal zone of the lithotripter. In this case the peak pressure is held constant at 40 MPa for all focal widths. Curves are shown for stones of diameter 4, 6, 8 and 10 mm. It can be seen that for each stone the incident energy gets larger as the focal zone becomes wider because more of the surface of the stone sees a high pressure. For the cases where the focal width is greater than twice the size of the stone (e.g., the 4 mm and 6 mm stones) the energy approaches a constant value because the amplitude of the pressure over the stone is almost uniform. For a given focal width the energy increases with stone diameter because there is more area of the stone to absorb the energy.

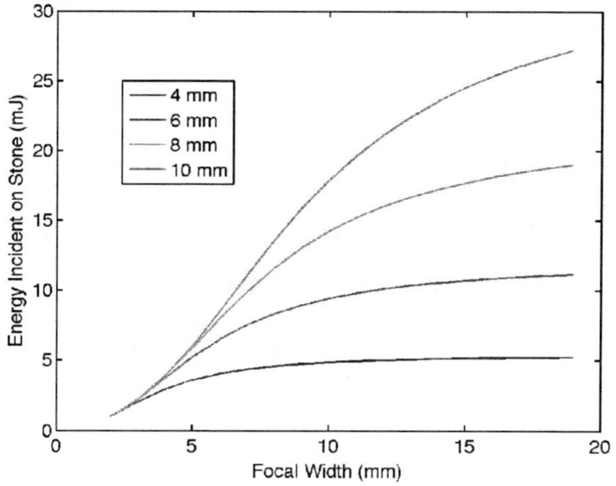

FIGURE 2. Energy delivered to a stone of different sizes as a function of the focal width.

For the data shown in Figure 2 the peak pressure amplitude remained at 40 MPa independent of focal width. In reality narrow-focus lithotripters have higher peak pressures. If one assumes that the energy delivered to the stone should remain constant, then it is possible to calculate the peak pressure required as the focal width is decreased. Figure 3 shows plots of the required peak pressure to maintain constant energy as a function of focal width for the four stones sizes considered previously. The constant energy value was calculated for the case of an infinitely wide focal zone with a peak pressure of 40 MPa. It can be seen that as the focal width gets smaller the required peak pressure increases dramatically. For a 6 mm stone the data suggest that a lithotripter with a focal width of 5 mm would need a peak pressure in excess of 200 MPa. For larger stones the effect is more pronounced. These results are consistent with the fact that narrow focal zone lithotripters have peak pressures in excess of 100 MPa.

However, narrow focal zone lithotripters do not generate the high peak pressures suggested in Figure 3, which indicates that energy delivered to a stone may not be the perfect metric for determining stone comminution. Although the predictions are not quantitatively in agreement it is clear that small focal zone lithotripters do have an increase in peak pressure, with no real gain in energy delivered to the stone. These high pressures may not be a good strategy with respect to side effects. Data suggest that tissue damage is strongly dependent on peak pressure [6] and therefore a 100 MPa SW may induce more side effects than a 40 MPa SW.

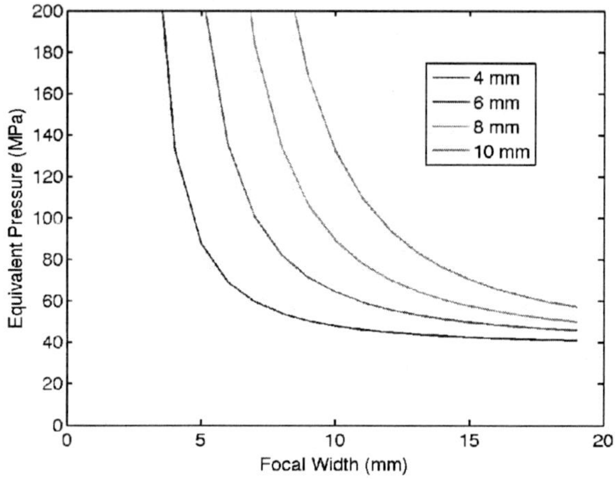

FIGURE 3. Peak focal pressure required to deliver the same energy to the stone as a function of focal width. As the focal width becomes narrower the peak pressure needs to be higher.

The results shown here assume that the stone is perfectly localized at the focus. In reality the stone will not be perfectly targeted and motion of the stone, primarily due to respiration, will lead to displacements that can be larger than the size of the focal region. *In vitro* fragmentation studies indicate that the narrow focus Modulith is much less effective at breaking stones that are moving; for example, motion of ±5 mm results in a 50% decrease in fragmentation efficiency [7].

The impact of motion was considered by simulating the motion of a stone lateral to the SW path and determining the energy delivered to the stone as it moved. Figure 4 shows an example from the simulations for the cases of a 4.5 mm diameter stone and a 12 mm diameter focal width. For reference a kidney and renal pelvis have been included in the image. The left image shows a snap-shot when the stone is aligned with the focus and the right image shows a time when the kidney and stone have moved 10 mm to the left. In the latter case it can be clearly seen that the stone is no longer within the focal zone. Below each image the time history of the relative energy (normalized to the value when the stone is at the focus) delivered to the stone is shown. It can be seen that when the stone is at the focus the energy is 100% but when it is off-axis the energy is less than 10%. The relative energy delivered to the stone

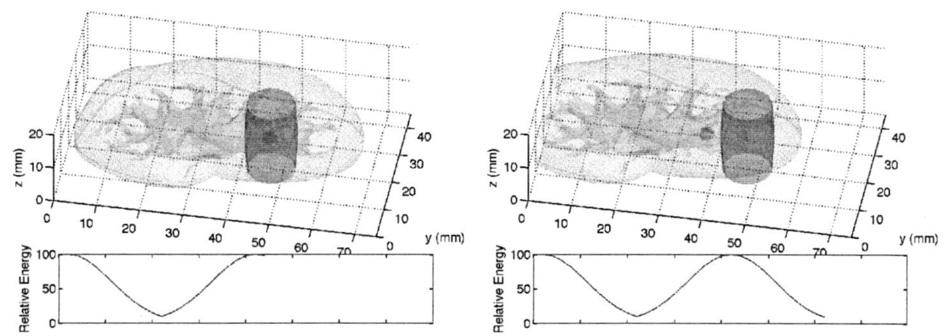

FIGURE 4. Snap-shots of a simulations showing the energy delivered to a stone within the renal pelvis as the kidney moves. Image showing the kidney (cyan), renal pelvis (magenta), stone (blue) and focal volume (red). The focal region is taken to be 12 mm wide. Left: Snapshot when the stone is in the focal region. Right: Snapshot when the kidney and stone have moved 10 mm laterally. Below each image is the time trace of the relative energy (in percent) as a function of time.

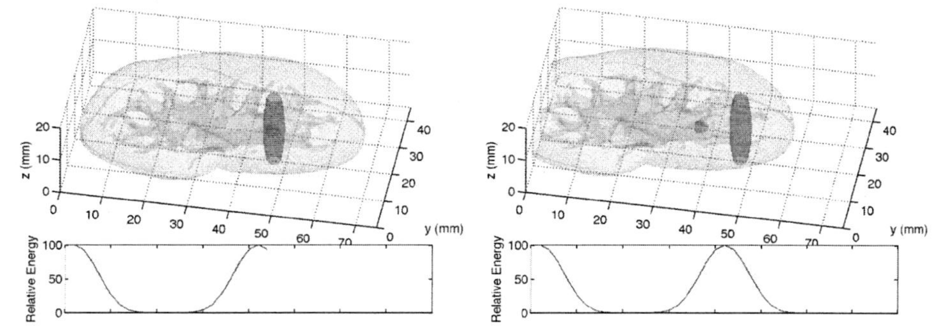

FIGURE 5. Snap-shots of a simulations showing the energy delivered to a stone within the renal pelvis for a narrow (6 mm diameter) focal width.

varies smoothly between these values through the motion. Figure 5 shows equivalent data but for the case of a 6 mm focal width. It can been seen from the relative energy traces that as the stone moves away from the focus the energy quickly drops away and is close to zero for almost half of the time.

Table 1 shows the mean relative energy delivered to the stone for three different motions, two different focal widths and two different stone diameters. For the case of ±2.5 mm of motion the 12 mm wide focal width delivers a relative energy in excess of 90%. For the narrower focus (width 5 mm) a little less energy is delivered to the stones; in particular for the smaller stone the relative energy is at 85%. As the motion increases to ±5 mm the wide focal zone is still able to deliver about 80% of the energy to both stones but the narrow focal zone lithotripter delivers only 56% to the small stone. This is consistent with the reduction in fragmentation efficiency reported for the Modulith [7]. For motion of ±10 mm the wide focal zone delivers about 50% of the energy but the narrow focal zone delivers less than 30% of the energy to the small stone. This data indicates that the broad focus is capable of delivering significant energy to the stone for motion up to ±10 mm. The corollary to the fact that less energy reaches the stone is that the remaining energy will impact the tissue. This implies for the case when the stone moves that a narrower focus will lead to greater impact on the tissue and could potentially induce greater tissue damage.

TABLE 1. The relative energy delivered to a stone that is undergoing motion. Energy has been averaged over one complete cycle of motion.

Focal Width	**12 mm width**		**5 mm width**	
Stone Diameter	**6 mm**	**10 mm**	**6 mm**	**10 mm**
Motion ±2.5 mm	93%	98%	85%	95%
Motion ±5 mm	78%	84%	56%	83%
Motion ±10 mm	48%	55%	29%	47%

DISCUSSION AND CONCLUSIONS

The analysis presented here describes how the energy delivered to a kidney stone and the surrounding tissue is affected by the width of the focal zone of the lithotripter. The analysis was carried out assuming that the pressure distribution in the focal zone could be treated as Gaussian in shape and that there were not significant changes in the waveform shape with lateral position.

The results show that to achieve sufficient energy deposition into a stone one should use a lithotripter with a focal zone larger than the diameter of the stone. For stones in the range up to 10 mm this implies use of a "wide-focus" lithotripter, for example, the HM3 with a focal width of 12 mm. For a lithotripters with a smaller focal width, equivalent energy deposition could be obtained by increasing the peak pressure but for typical values of a narrow focal zone lithotripter (~4 mm) the required increase was dramatic—in excess of 100%. Data suggests that high peak pressures may result in greater tissue damage [6] and therefore the increase in pressure may not be an ideal strategy.

In the case where a stone is moving distances of up to ±10 mm (as one might expect due to respiration) the wider focal zone was able to interact with the stone enough to ensure that at least 50% of the energy was delivered to the stone. In the case of the narrow focal zone the energy was typically less than 50% for motion of ±5 mm and more. This indicates that either more SWs or even greater peak pressures would be needed to compensate for the number of SWs that miss the stone. Also as more SWs miss the stone there will be greater insult to the surrounding tissue, an effect that will be exacerbated by the higher peak pressures and greater number of shock waves.

In conclusion, a theoretical analysis is presented to support the hypothesis that a broad focal zone lithotripter may be advantageous in shock wave lithotripsy by providing sufficient energy for stone fragmentation but with reduced insult to the surrounding tissue. The predictions are qualitatively consistent with reports of better fragmentation achieved clinically with a broad focus, specifically retreatment rates are in the range 4%-7% for the HM3 and 22%-49% for the SLX [8]. The prediction of higher side effects for a narrow focal zone lithotripter due to the higher peak pressures and number of SWs is consistent with the hematoma rates of 0.8% for the HM3 and 3% for the Modulith reported in the manufacturers' operating manuals.

ACKNOWLEDGMENTS

I would like to acknowledge important discussions on this work with numerous members of the Consortium for Shock Waves in Medicine in particular: Michael Bailey, Andrew Evan, James Lingeman, James McAteer, Oleg Sapozhnikov, and James Williams. This work was funded in part by the National Institutes of Health through grant DK-43881.

REFERENCES

1. IEC61846, IEC 61846 Ultrasonics - Pressure pulse lithotripters - Characteristics of fields. 1998, International Electrotechnical Commission: Geneva, Swizterland.
2. Cleveland, R.O. and J.A. McAteer, The Physics of Shock Wave Lithotripsy, in Smith's Textbook on Endourology, G.H.B. A. D. Smith, D. H. Bagley, R. V. Clayman, S. G. Docimo, G. H. Jordan, L. R. Kavoussi, B. R. Lee, J. E. Lingeman, G. M. Preminger, J. W. Segura, Editor. 2007, BC Decker: Hamilton, ON, Canada. p. 317-332.
3. Wess, O., Shock Wave Lithotripsy (SWL) and Focal Size, in Therapeutic Energy Applications in Urology, C. Chaussy, et al., Editors. 2005, Verlag: Thieme. p. 26-35.
4. Zhu, S., F.H. Cocks, G.M. Preminger, and P. Zhong, The role of stress waves and cavitation in stone comminution in shock wave lithotripsy. Ultrasound in Medicine & Biology, 2002. 28(5): p. 661-671.
5. Cleveland, R.O. and O.A. Sapozhnikov, Modeling elastic wave propagation in kidney stones with application to shock wave lithotripsy. J. Acoust. Soc. Am., 2005. 118: p. 2667-2676.
6. Connors, B.A., A.P. Evan, L.R. Willis, P.M. Blomgren, J.E. Lingeman, and N.S. Fineberg, The effect of discharge voltage on renal injury and impairment caused by lithotripsy in the pig. Journal of the American Society of Nephrology, 2000. 11(2): p. 310-318.
7. Cleveland, R.O., A. R, and R.K. Babayan, Effect of stone motion on in vitro comminution efficiency of a Storx Modulith SLX. J. Endourology, 2004. 18: p. 629-633.
8. Kerbl, K., J. Rehman, J. Landman, D. Lee, C. Sundaram, and R.V. Clayman, Current management of urolithisasis: Progress or regress? Journal of Endourology, 2002. 16(5): p. 281-288.

Standards for Lithotripter Performance

Reiner Schultheiss[a] and Michael Doerffel[b]

[a]*TRT Tissue Regeneration Technologies LLC, 110 Arnold Mill Park, Suite 400 Woodstock, Georgia 30188, USA*
[b]*MTS Europe GmbH, Robert-Bosch-Str. 18, D-78467 Konstanz, Germany*

Abstract. Standards for lithotripsy have been developed by the International Electrotechnical Commission (IEC) and the FDA. In addition to the existing regulations and norms for the manufacturers, special standards were developed to address a treatment method developed in the early 1980's using extracorporeal shock waves. Initially, the FDA regulated the premarket approval process for lithotripters as a Class III device but reclassified lithotripters in 2000 to a Class II device. The corresponding guidance document for showing the substantial equivalence of new devices with predicate devices will be described in detail. The FDA guidance document is very useful in helping device manufacturers: (i) develop technical performance testing for a shock wave lithotripter within the parameters of an FDA submission, and (ii) conduct clinical performance testing via at least one clinical confirmation study with a small number of subjects. Unfortunately although the submitted data are available at the FDA they are not available in the marketplace and this causes difficulties for physicians in deciding which device to use. The results of the technical performance testing of the LithoGold™ are provided.

Keywords: IEC, Regulations, LithoGold, performance testing, pressure measurements, lithotripter, FDA.
PACS: 43.80.Vj

WHY DEFINE STANDARDS FOR EXTRACOPOREAL LITHOTRIPTER PERFORMANCE?

In the early 1980's a new treatment modality of disintegrating urinary concrements by highly focused and high-pressure acoustic impulses made its way from the laboratory (i.e., testing implanted concrements in pig and dog kidneys) into clinical use for humans.

With respect to medical products, regulations and norms have always played an important role in establishing certain safety levels for patients, users (physicians), and third-party individuals such as nurses or technical service personnel. Because using focused high energy shock waves to disintegrate concrements in the kidney was a brand new treatment modality and new energy form (being different from ultrasound) it raised a lot of questions concerning the: (1) technical safety, specifically the safety of shock wave generation and application, and (2) medical safety, specifically the biological effects of the transmitted waves on the different tissue in front of or behind the target (the brittle non-vital concrement material).

CP1049, *Renal Stone Disease 2, 2nd International Urolithiasis Research Symposium,*
edited by A. P. Evan, J. E. Lingeman, J. A. McAteer, and J. C. Williams, Jr.

The concept of disintegration was clear: 1) use the compressional and shear forces and energies generated by the extracorporeally generated acoustic shock; 2) focus the energy on a small focal volume related to the size of the stone (preferably smaller than the stone); 3) locate the concrement precisely in 3-dimensional space; 4) position the patient and the concrement to match exactly with the position of the shock wave focal point; 5) generate a good acoustical coupling (avoid air bubbles) for transmission of the extracorporeal shock wave into the patient's body; and 6) release up to a few thousand shock waves to disintegrate the stone by mechanical forces and cavitation processes.

Standards Set by the International Electrotechnical Commission (IEC)

Technical standardization was relatively straightforward because the technical committees of the IEC organization had working groups already experienced in the field of ultrasound. The technical working group SC 62D [1], which is still active today, generated some of the necessary standards for extracorporeal shock wave lithotripsy. The standard generated in the early 1980's was the *IEC 60601-2-36: Medical electrical equipment - Part 2-36: Particular requirements for the safety of equipment for extracorporeally induced lithotripsy*, which was issued 1997 [2].

In the process of harmonization, this standard was accepted within the European Community and was released as the European Version EN 60601-2-36. The important regulated technical features in this norm must be fulfilled by lithotripter manufacturers. Further, the international Standard *IEC 61846 Ultrasonics – Pressure pulse lithotripters – Characteristics of fields* was released in 1998 [3] for the specification of the measured and defined data for a lithotripter shock wave field, as well as for hydrophones and the measurement process itself. IEC 61846 defines the test equipment such as the test chamber, the characteristics and frequency range of the hydrophone, and the spatial intervals for the field measurements. The measurement procedure for gaining the spatial, temporal and energy information are also defined.

Measured properties of the shock wave include peak-positive pressure amplitude, peak-negative pressure amplitude, shock rise time and duration of the compressive phase of the shock pulse (Figure 1). Additional features of the acoustic field (maximum focal width, orthogonal focal width, focal extent, focal volume, distance between focus and target location, focal energy of the acoustic pulse) must be determined, and are defined and illustrated later (see Figure 4).

Further IEC standards have to be taken into consideration for medical products and must be followed in the design and manufacturing phases. The most important regulations are listed below and those especially assigned for lithotripters are indicated.

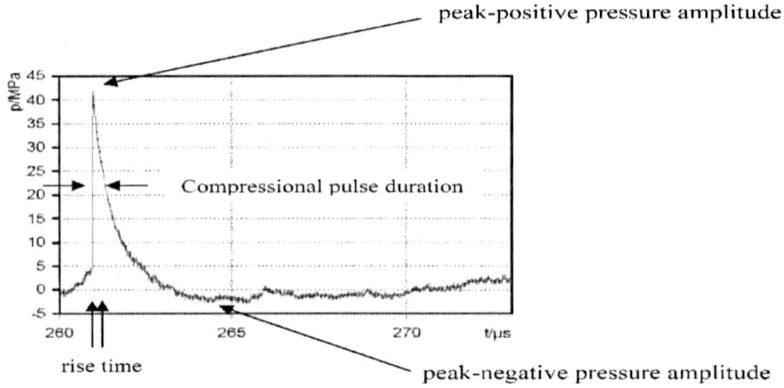

FIGURE 1. A typical lithotripter pressure-time signal. The rise time of the shock wave is the time for positive pressure to increase from 10% to 90% of peak amplitude, while the pulse duration is the time during which positive pressure is at least half the peak amplitude. This waveform is from a LithoGold LG380 lithotripter operated at its highest power setting (E11). In this example, P^+ (~42 MPa) is ~5 MPa higher than the mean value for shock waves recorded for this setting at the acoustic focus (point along the acoustic axis where the maximum value for positive pressure is measured) (see also Table 3).

FDA Process for Premarket Approval (PMA)

Premarket approval (PMA) is the FDA process of scientific and regulatory review to evaluate the safety and effectiveness of Class III medical devices [5]. Class III devices are those that support or sustain human life, are of substantial importance in preventing impairment of human health, or which present a potential, unreasonable risk of illness or injury. Due to the level of risk associated with Class III devices, the FDA has determined that general and special controls alone are insufficient to assure their safety and effectiveness of Class III devices. Therefore, these devices require a premarket approval (PMA) application under section 515 of the FD&C Act in order to obtain marketing clearance.

In 2000 the FDA reclassified extracorporeal shock wave lithotripters as Class II devices [Federal Register/Vol. 65, No. 154/ Wednesday, August 9, 2000/ Rules and Regulations, page 48609]. The summary states:

> "*The Food and Drug Administration (FDA) is issuing a final rule to reclassify from class III to class II the extracorporeal shock wave lithotripter, when intended for use to fragment kidney and ureteral calculi. [6]*
>
> *FDA is taking this action on its own initiative in order to assure that these devices are regulated according to the appropriate degree of regulatory control needed to provide reasonable assurance of their safety and effectiveness. Elsewhere in this issue of the Federal Register, FDA is publishing a notice of availability of a guidance document, which will serve as the special control for the reclassified device. This rule is effective September 8, 2000.*"

TABLE 1. List of basic IEC standards [4] which are requested for a medical device. (*) Market regulations especially assigned to lithotripters

Title of the standard	IEC identification	Year
Medical Electrical Equipment- Part 1 General requirements for Safety	IEC 60601 – 1	2005
Medical Electrical Equipment- Part 1 Electromagnetic Compatibility;	IEC 60601 - 1 - 2	2007
Medical Electrical Equipment- Part 1 Programmable Electrical MD;	IEC 60601- 1 - 4	2000
*Medical electrical equipment -- (Part 2: Particular requirements for the safety of equipment for extracorporeal induced lithotripsy	IEC 60601 - 2 – 36	1997
Medical electrical equipment - Part 6: General requirements for Safety; Collateral standard: Usability	IEC 60601 - 1 – 6	2006
Biological evaluation of medical devices	ISO 10993 - 1	2003
*Pressure Pulse Lithotripters	IEC 61846	1998
Risk Management	ISO 14971	2007

FDA reclassification from a class III to a class II device means that extended clinical studies and trials are no longer necessary for gaining market access. In a class II submission to the FDA the sponsor must provide sufficient information to the FDA following a 510(k) premarket notification process and using the related guidance documents of the FDA. The FDA investigates and evaluates the technical and medical comparison provided by the sponsor showing the substantial equivalence to an already registered predicate device.

With the 510(k) premarket notification process the FDA has, since the first "Draft Guidance on information of clinical safety and effectiveness data for extracorporeal shock wave lithotripsy of upper urinary tract calculi 1992," taken a path that requires the manufacturers and distributers of lithotripters to provide detailed information on the clinical application, safety and efficacy of the device.

The FDA 510(k) premarket notification process is intended to set standards for the technology and the medical efficacy of the device and to clarify risks involved in the form of contraindications and side effects.

TABLE 2. List of special guidance documents issued and requested by the FDA for extracorporeal shock wave lithotripters (actual version August 9, 2000).

Title	Year
Draft Guidance for Information on Clinical Safety and Effectiveness Data for Extracorporeal Shock Wave Lithotripsy of Upper Urinary Tract Calculi	February 5, 1992
Guidance for the Content of Premarket Notifications (510(k)s) for Extracorporeal Shock Wave Lithotripters Indicated for the Fragmentation of Kidney and Ureteral Calculi	February 8, 1999
Guidance for the Content of the Premarket Notifications (510(k)s) for Extracorporeal Shock Wave Lithotripters Indicated for the Fragmentation of Kidney and Ureteral Calculi [7]	August 9, 2000

TABLE 3. Information on acoustical output and derived values for the LithoGold™ (LG380) at minimum (E1), typical (E5) and maximum (E11) power settings at the acoustic focus according to IEC 61846. The peak positive pressure and peak negative pressure amplitudes are very low values indicating a low-pressure lithotripter. The focal width at F2 (geometrical focal point) is very broad (~20 mm). Because of the focal shift of the acoustical focus disintegration testing was used to verify the best stone disintegration capacity at several points along the z-axis (acoustic axis) of the lithotripter. Disintegration was highest at the geometrical focus F2 of the ellipsoid and this point was therefore defined as the target position. Additional acoustic data are provided at this target position. For additional clarification see also Fig 4. The maximum peak pressure (28.8 MPa) at the target position is about 8.1 MPa lower than at the acoustic focus (36.9 MPa). Larger focal width is one of the most important factors for the generation of stress within the stone and is one of the key important parameters for good stone disintegration. Low pulse amplitudes (both positive and negative pressure) help minimize tissue side effects. This concept (broad focus, low pressure) differs from many early lithotripters in which a narrow focal width was intended to maximize fragmentation efficiency and avoid delivering energy to the surrounding tissue.

Acoustic Output Characteristics:	Min.(E1)	Typical.(E5)	Max.(E11)
Peak-positive acoustic pressure (MPa)	24.6	30.7	36.9
Peak-negative acoustic pressure (MPa)	-3.1	-3.9	-4.6
Rise time (ns) +/- 5 ns	200	17	26
Compressional pulse duration (ns)	220	306	396
Maximum focal width (mm)	7.0	5.6	10.4
Orthogonal focal width (mm)	7.0	5.6	10.4
Focal extent (mm)	67.3	97.4	101.1
Focal volume (mm^3)	1726.7	1599.3	5725.5
Distance between the focus and target location (mm)	25	30	35
Derived focal acoustic pulse energy (mJ)	2.86	3.31	22.7
Additional information at target position F2 (geometrical focus)			
Peak-positive acoustic pressure (MPa)	14.2	21.7	28.8
Peak-negative acoustic pressure (MPa)	-3.5	-4.6	-5.9
Rise Time (ns) +/- 5 ns	431	105	280
Compressional pulse duration (ns)	326	507	538
Maximum focal width (mm)	16.6	17.1	19.9 (E9)
Derived focal acoustic pulse energy (mJ)	9.25	24.32	59.64 (E9)

Special Controls: Extracorporeal shock wave lithotripters are subject to the special control of the above listed guidance document. This guidance document describes a means by which shock wave lithotripsy ("SWL") devices may comply with the requirement of special controls for class II devices. Designation of this guidance document as a special control means that manufacturers attempting to establish that their device is substantially equivalent to a predicate SWL device should demonstrate that the proposed device complies with either the specific recommendations of this guidance or some alternate control that provides equivalent assurances of safety and effectiveness.

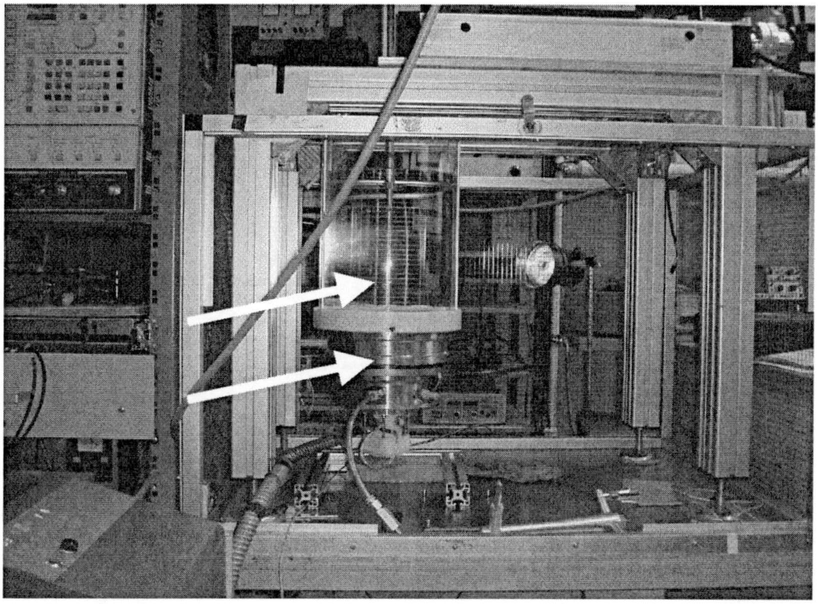

FIGURE 2. Laboratory setup for the measurement of the pressure pulse characteristics according to the requests defined within the IEC 61846. For the 3-dimensional distribution, field measurements must be taken to form a complete set of 3-dimensional data points around the acoustical focus, which is defined by the point of maximum pressure in the distribution. The general measurement procedure followed for the values presented later for the LithoGold in Table 3 was as follows. The shock wave is generated by a spark plug at the F1 focal point of a hemiellipsoidal reflector and the measurements are done in a water tank using an optical hydrophone. It is known from this principle that pulse to pulse variations in the pressure pulse shape as well as in the peak amplitude may occur. Against this background at least eight pressure pulses at each spatial position for a given intensity setting were recorded to assess these variations. The focal position (acoustical focus) was determined by scanning the x-y plane at different positions on the z-axis and calculations of the arithmetic mean value of the peak pressure amplitudes for each spatial point. The location of the acoustic focus was defined at that point where the maximum average peak pressure amplitude value was measured. This procedure was repeated for every intensity setting. At the beginning of the measurements the geometrical focus F2 of the reflector was determined by the use of a focal gauge, provided by the manufacturer. The geometrical focus of the F2 of the hemiellipsoidal reflector is used as a reference point during the measurements (see Fig 6). Spatial sampling increments: lateral (dx, dy): 1 mm, extended up to 5 mm axial (dz): 5 mm extended to 10 mm. The lateral and axial sampling increments were chosen in accordance to IEC 61846 as approximately 1/5 of the corresponding –6 dB beam widths and were extended during lateral measurements since the amplitude decrease was less than 10% at larger distances from the focus.

Classification/Product Code in the 510(k): The Code of Federal Regulations (CFR) number, regulatory class, and product code applicable to the extracorporeal shock wave lithotripter (listed below) should be provided:

CFR Number: 21 CFR 876.5990

Regulatory Class: Class II (special controls)

Product Code: 78 LNS

Devices Not Included: This guidance document only addresses other shock wave delivering devices that are indicated for the fragmentation of urinary calculi in the kidney or ureter. Devices with other indications, such as biliary/gallstone lithotripsy or orthopedic lithotripsy, are currently class III and are not included within the scope of this guidance.

Predicate Device: Predicate devices are the legally marketed device(s) to which the proposed device is being compared. To be as specific as possible, the 510(k) should include the following information to identify each predicate device and support the claim of substantial equivalence:

- Trade/proprietary name
- Model number
- Manufacturer
- 510(k)/PMA reference number (if known)
- Intended use
- Technological characteristics/performance specifications
- Labelling

TECHNOLOGICAL CHARACTERISTICS/PERFORMANCE SPECIFICATIONS

Following the above approach and using the FDA 510(k) guidance document [7] the technical parameters analyzed in relation to the shock generating component of the lithotripter include performance testing, localization accuracy and road testing:

Performance Testing

The purpose of performance testing is to quantify those shock wave characteristics that are believed to contribute to stone fragmentation and adverse tissue effects, and, thus, are indicators of clinical performance. These acoustic quantities (listed below) should be measured/calculated using the methodology described in the consensus standard *IEC 61846 "Ultrasonics - Pressure pulse lithotripters - Characteristics of fields"* (1998). Furthermore, these acoustic quantities should be reported for minimum, typical, and maximum shock wave generator output settings, and (to the extent possible) compared to those reported for the predicate device(s).

The results of these measurements are used to draw the pressure isobaric curves and to define the shape and volume of the characteristic shock wave field. Besides the measured values for the pressure pulse signal which include the peak-positive pressure amplitude, the peak-negative pressure amplitude, the rise time and the compressional pulse duration, the following values give the 2-dimensional field dimensions when using the -6dB isobaric line - marking the region where the pressure is at least half the maximum positive pressure (pressure half maximum)-in the x,y plane and repeating the same in the x,z plane. By combining these two axial extensions the focal volume is defined by the focal length $f_{z(-6dB)}$, and orthogonal focal widths $f_{x(-6dB)}$ and $f_{y(-6dB)}$.

Providing the FDA with all required data leads to an extensive set of acoustical and derived values. These values are disclosed for the LithoGold™ (TRT Tissue Regeneration Technologies LLC, Woodstock, Georgia, USA) in Table 3.

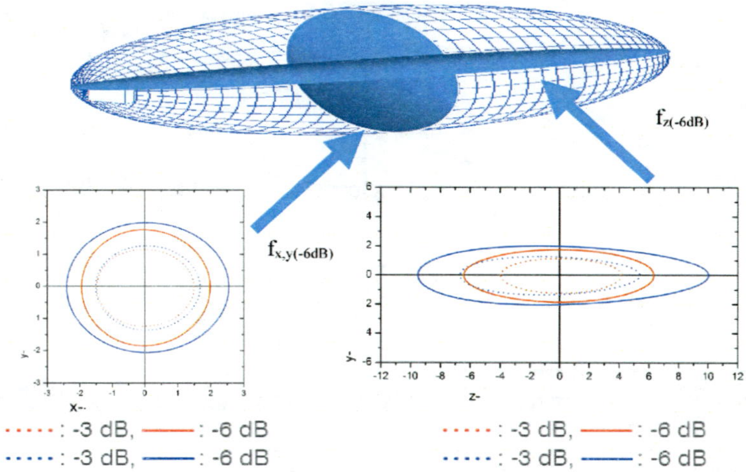

FIGURE 3. Plots of shape characteristics of a hypothetical lithotripter acoustic field. (Top) Focal volume (-6dB) with the two planes (filled areas), one indicating focal width in x,y (fx,y(-6dB)) and one showing focal length (fz(-6db)). (Lower left) Pressure distribution (2-d) in the x,y plane at the point of maximum positive pressure along the acoustic axis (z). The dotted line in red (innermost dotted line) indicates the -3dB distribution for positive pressure while the blue dotted line marks -3dB negative pressure. Solid lines mark the -6dB distribution (red positive, blue negative). (Lower right) Pressure distribution (2-d) in the y,z plane showing -3dB (dotted red positive, dotted blue negative) and -6dB (solid red positive, solid blue negative) fields. The -3dB distribution indicates a reduction of the peak pressure by about a factor of 1.41 and is included for comparison with the -6dB zone to aid in estimating the fall in acoustic pressure. [Note: For all diagrams the x, y and z values displayed are artificial.]

Localization Accuracy

To ensure the positioning of the stone within the focal area and as close as possible to the target point, the dimensions of the stone, the overall accuracy of the target point and the accuracy of the adjustment of the locating system (x-ray C-arm with crosshair for the target position in most cases) must be considered.

The manufacturer has to provide testing to verify that the localization/stone targeting system is capable of locating the shock wave focus with sufficient accuracy to target stones as small as 4 mm in largest dimension within the focal volume. For this test, the manufacturer should quantitatively assess the maximum deviation of the "target location" (*i.e., the location in space where the manufacturer intends the operator to locate the stone*) from the "shock wave focus" (*i.e., the point of peak-positive acoustic pressure*) after aligning the localization/stone targeting system with the shock wave focus in accordance with the pre-treatment procedures described in the device's instructions for use. This evaluation includes measurement of the distance between the focus and target location, along with an assessment of the errors/uncertainties inherent in the localization/stone targeting system and acoustic measurements.

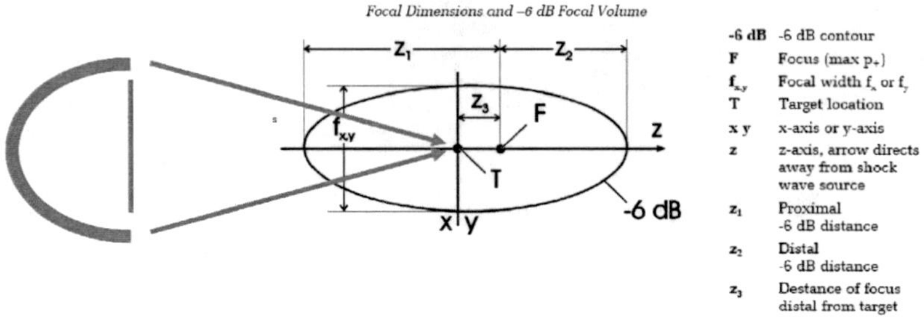

Energy level		Z1 (mm)	Z2 (mm)	Z3 (mm)
Minimum	1	38.3	29.0	25
Typical	5	46.3	51.1	30
Maximum	11	53.9	47.2	35

FIGURE 4. Definitions for dimensions used in the lithotripter positioning procedure. The focal volume extends along the beam axis from Z_1 mm proximal to Z_2 mm distal to the target location (T). The maximum and orthogonal focal widths are fz, fx and fy, respectively. The focus is z_3 mm distal to the target location. The central black ellipse indicates the -6 dB contour of the focal volume with acoustic focus in F. This information must be provided to users by the manufacturer in the operation manual. The acoustical focus F does not necessarily correspond with the target position T. The stone positioning remains at target position T. In most cases using higher energy settings, the focal shift occurs away from the acoustical source indicated by the ellipsoid on the left. This holds true at least for electro-hydraulic lithotripters. The focal extensions Z_1 and Z_2 are not exactly symmetrical; typically Z_3 is distal to the aperture of the ellipsoid. Also see Fig 6 for the shape of the focal volume.

To reiterate, "The manufacturer has to provide testing to verify that the localization/ stone targeting system is capable of locating the shock wave focus with sufficient accuracy to target stones as small as 4 mm in largest dimension within the focal volume." Figure 5 might help to illustrate this requirement. One of the difficulties in performing the treatment is the movement of the patient and the concrement during respiration, which means positioning is not a static situation.

Despite all these theoretical facts, the direction and dimensions of the focal volume on the screen of the x-ray imaging system is inexact. Often the dimension of the stone is unknown due to lack of a measuring scale.

For calibration and verification of the alignment between the target point and the locating system a metal ball is used in conjunction with a focus phantom. The magnification of the locating system can be calculated by measuring the diameter of the metal ball and its shadow on the x-ray monitor after the alignment procedure.

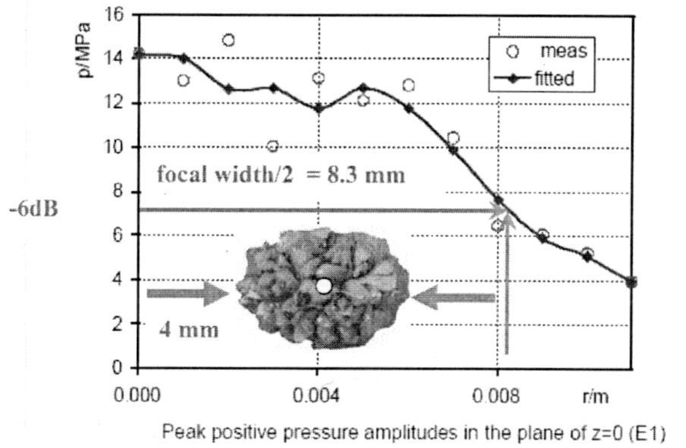

FIGURE 5. The 4 mm stone is positioned in the target position at the geometrical focus F2 of the LithoGold. The maximum focal width at lowest energy setting El reads 16.6/2 mm (see Table 3). The illustration shows that a 4 mm stone could completely be positioned within the focal volume (-6dB). The variance and accuracy of the LithoGold stone positioning is 2 mm while the -6dB orthogonal focal width is at the minimum energy setting a radius of 8.3 mm (total focal width 16.6mm) thus the stone is located within the focal volume at the target position.

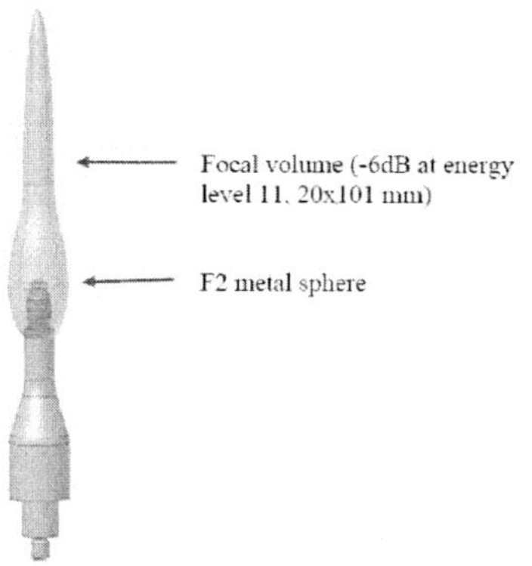

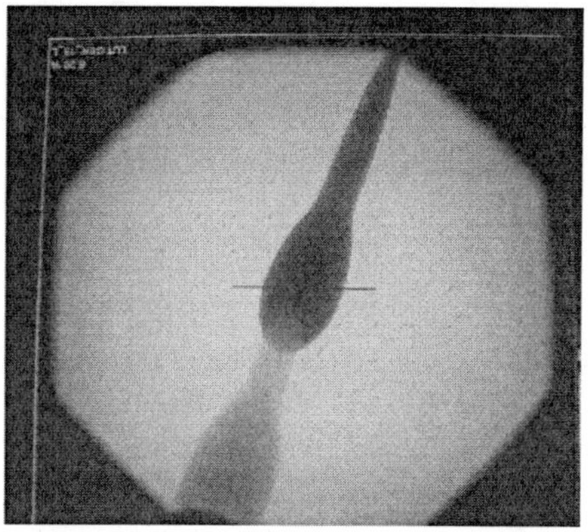

FIGURE 6. Focal volume phantom. Drawing at left shows a phantom which could be used for the alignment procedure of the target position with the locating system—indicated by the cross hair of the x-ray monitor. The metal ball is exchanged with a plastic phantom of the focal volume (-6dB contour). The center of the crosshair is adjusted to the target position. The direction of the focal volume represents the acoustical axis, were the shock waves are traveling from the lower left to upper right. The dilation in the base of the focal volume has also been calculated for electrohydraulic shock wave sources [8].

To illustrate how the focal volume is imaged a plastic phantom with the size and shape of the focal volume could be used instead of the simple metal ball. Figure 6 shows the x-ray image of such a focal volume for the LithoGold^{TM}.

Road Testing

The purpose of this test is to verify that the mobile/transportable SWL system can withstand the stresses and vibrations experienced during unloading, set-up, transportation, loading, and stowing without significant degradation in performance specifications.

Specific testing required is mainly to:

- Using a final lithotripter system, determine baseline measures of the: (1) mean peak-positive acoustic pressure at the shock wave focus at the typical shock wave generator output, (2) localization/stone targeting system accuracy, and (3) overall system functionality (only relative measures).
- Prepare the device for transport, consistent with the directions specified in the labelling.
- Perform a road test of the device by transporting the device for at least 1 hour. The course used for this test should represent a worst-case scenario, e.g., speed bumps, train tracks, sudden application of the breaks, highways, secondary and gravel roads, stop-and-go traffic, etc.
- Prepare the device for use, consistent with the directions specified in the labelling.
- Repeat the baseline tests of: (1) mean peak-positive acoustic pressure at the shock wave focus at the typical shock wave generator output, (2) localization/ stone targeting system accuracy, and (3) overall system functionality.

These test results should be compared to those obtained prior to the road test, and should demonstrate that there is no difference in system performance specifications before and after transportation.

Assessment of Technically Substantial Equivalence: After having addressed all the regulations and verified conformity to the medical IEC standards and after having performed special testing for lithotripters, including all acoustical characterization, localization/stone targeting system accuracy and road testing, the lithotripter is regarded to be safe and effective because its technical features are substantially equivalent to a referenced predicate device.

CLINICAL PERFORMANCE TESTING

If the proposed lithotripter employs a similar mechanism of action for the generation of shock waves as compared to predicate SWL systems and has shock wave characteristics that are within the range of predicate SWL systems, a confirmatory clinical study should be performed to demonstrate substantial equivalence. The following information should be considered when designing a confirmatory clinical study:

- The objectives of this clinical study are to confirm the functionality of the device and adequacy of the proposed labeling.

- The study should enroll a total of 20 patients with urinary stone disease at 2 investigational sites, with follow-up early post-procedure (e.g., 48 hours to 2 weeks). All subjects should be candidates for SWL and should satisfy the device's proposed indications and contraindications for use.
- Investigators should record appropriate data during the SWL treatment session and at the early post-procedure follow-up exam to document the operational status of the device, such as:
  - the incidence, cause, and resolution of device malfunctions;
  - treatment parameters used;
  - stone fragmentation results;
  - the incidence of complications;
  - anesthesia/analgesia usage;
  - radiation exposure; and
  - evaluation of system ergonomics.

Of central importance are the lithotripter's stone fragmentation results and side effects. The device will be tested according to the intended use defined within the operating manual of the lithotripter. FDA gives detailed labeling instructions which must be incorporated into the labeling of the device by the manufacturer.

RESUMÉ

The FDA Guidance document is a great tool and guideline for manufacturers to provide technical and medical information to the FDA. Unfortunately FDA does not require manufacturers to provide this information to the users or buyers of their devices. Most manufacturers are willing to provide their clinical results but many are unwilling to provide customers with all the technical specifications they provide to the FDA. Comparisons between devices would be much easier (or at least possible) when rigorous acoustic characterization data becomes available for all lithotripters.

REFERENCES

1. http://www.iec.ch/cgi-bin/procgi.pl/www/iecwww.p?wwwlang=e&wwwprog=dirwg.p&progdb=db1&ctnum=1217
2. http://www.iec.ch/cgi-bin/procgi.pl/www/iecwww.p?wwwlang=E&wwwprog=sea22.p&search=iecnumber&header=IEC&pubno=60601&part=&se=&submit=Submit
3. http://www.iec.ch/cgi-bin/procgi.pl/www/iecwww.p??wwwlang=e&wwwprog=TCpubs.p&progdb=db1&css_color=purple&committee=TCTC&number=87
4. http://www.iec.ch/
5. http://www.fda.gov/CDRH/DEVADVICE/pma/
6. http://www.fda.gov/OHRMS/DOCKETS/98fr/080900a.pdf
7. http://www.accessdata.fda.gov/scripts/cdrh/cfdocs/cfGGP/Results.CFM
8. R.O Cleveland and J.A. McAteer. The physics of shock wave lithotripsy. In: *Smith's Textbook on Endourology*. Smith AD, Badlani GH, Bagley DH, Clayman RV, Docimo SG, Jordan GH, Kavoussi LR, Lee BR, Lingeman JE, Preminger GM, Segura JW (eds), Hamilton, Ontario, Canada, BC Decker, Inc, pp: 317-332 (2007).
9. W. Eisenmenger. The mechanisms of stone fragmentation in ESWL, *Ultrasound Med Biol*, 27, 683–693 (2001).

The Characteristics of Broad and Narrow Focal Zone Lithotripters

Yuri A. Pishchalnikov, James A. McAteer, R. Jason VonDerHaar, Irina V. Pishchalnikova, and James C. Williams, Jr.

Department of Anatomy and Cell Biology, Indiana University School of Medicine, 635 Barnhill Drive, Indianapolis, IN 46202, USA

Abstract. The focal width of a lithotripter is a measure of the diameter of its focal zone, the region where acoustic pressures are at least half the maximum positive pressure generated at a given power level. Different lithotripters have different focal widths. The Dornier HM3, for example, has a focal width of ~10-12mm and for many years this was the widest focal zone among clinical machines. Electromagnetic lithotripters tend to have narrower focal zones, in the range of ~4-6mm. Recent studies suggesting that focal width plays an important role in stone breakage prompted this assessment of two electromagnetic lithotripters. Acoustical mapping using a fiber optic probe hydrophone (FOPH-500) and breakage of U-30 gypsum model stones were used to compare a conventional lithotripter (Dornier DoLi-50) and a broad focal zone device (XiXin XX-ES). FOPH mapping characterized the focal width of the DoLi to be about 5mm and that of the XX-ES to be much wider (~18mm). For stone breakage experiments the DoLi was fired at power level 3 (mid-range) and the XX-ES was operated at the recommended clinical setting of 9.3 kV. Both lithotripters were fired at 60 SW/min. U-30 model stones held in a 2mm mesh basket were positioned at the clinical target point on the acoustic axis and at 5mm steps laterally, and the number of SW's to complete fragmentation was counted. Breakage on-axis was similar for the two machines (DoLi 676±105 SW's versus XX-ES 644±123 SW's, $p>0.6$), but at 15mm the DoLi required nearly twice the number of SW's as the XX-ES (DoLi 3006±780 SW's versus 1726±972 SW's, $p<0.006$). This demonstrates that a broad focal zone lithotripter is more effective in breaking stones off axis and supports the idea that focal width is an important feature, likely to be relevant in the clinical setting where respiratory motion may limit the effectiveness of narrow focal zone machines.

Keywords: shock wave lithotripsy, focal width, peak pressure, stone breakage efficiency.
PACS: 43.80.Vj, 43.80. Gx, 43.35.Yb.

INTRODUCTION

Lithotripters differ in the characteristics of the focal zones they generate, and the width of the focal zone can vary from quite narrow to broad (i.e. ~3-4mm for the Storz Modulith, to ~18mm for the XiXin XX-ES). Others have demonstrated in vitro that the focal width of a lithotripter can affect its stone breakage efficiency, and the effect is most evident when the stone is moving. That is, when stones were placed in a motorized device that simulated stone movement during respiratory excursion, a lithotripter with a focal width of ~12mm showed significantly better breakage efficiency than a lithotripter with a focal width of ~3-4mm [1]. In the current study we, likewise assessed the role of focal width in the effectiveness of stone breakage,

CP1049, *Renal Stone Disease 2, 2nd International Urolithiasis Research Symposium,*
edited by A. P. Evan, J. E. Lingeman, J. A. McAteer, and J. C. Williams, Jr.

but in this case we used a static in vitro system in which the stones were purposely placed off-axis.

MATERIALS AND METHODS

This study was conducted using two clinical electromagnetic lithotripters, a DoLi-50 (Dornier MedTech America, Inc., Kennesaw, GA, USA) [2] and a XX-ES (Xi Xin Medical Instruments Co. Ltd., Suzhou, PRC) [3, 4]. The DoLi has 6 power levels and was operated at mid-range, power level 3. The XX-ES was operated at the recommended clinical setting 9.3kV. Both lithotripters were fired at 60 shock waves per minute.

The water cushion of the DoLi (Fig. 1) was coupled to the acoustic window of the test tank using LithoClear gel (Sonotech Inc., Bellingham, WA), as previously described [5]. The water cushion of the XX-ES lithotripter was submerged directly into the test tank (Fig. 2). The test tank was filled with tap water at room temperature. The water was continuously degassed using a pinhole degasser [2]. Dissolved oxygen remained at dynamic equilibrium at about 30% of saturation (or 2.7ppm).

Functional performance of the lithotripters was assessed using Ultracal-30 gypsum stones (6.5mm diameter by 7.5mm length) held in 2 mm mesh baskets (Figs. 1-2) [6]. The baskets were positioned at the clinical target point on the acoustic axis, and at 5 mm steps laterally, and the number of shock waves to complete breakage was counted. At least seven stones were broken at each position.

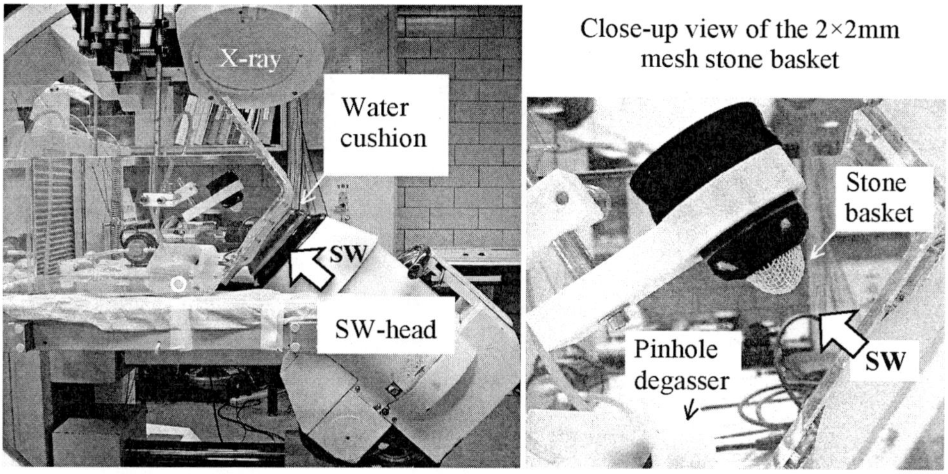

FIGURE 1. Experimental setup for stone breakage with the DoLi. DoLi shock waves (SW) propagate at 45° (arrow). Model stones were broken in the 2×2mm nylon mesh basket positioned on the acoustic axis, and at 5 mm steps laterally.

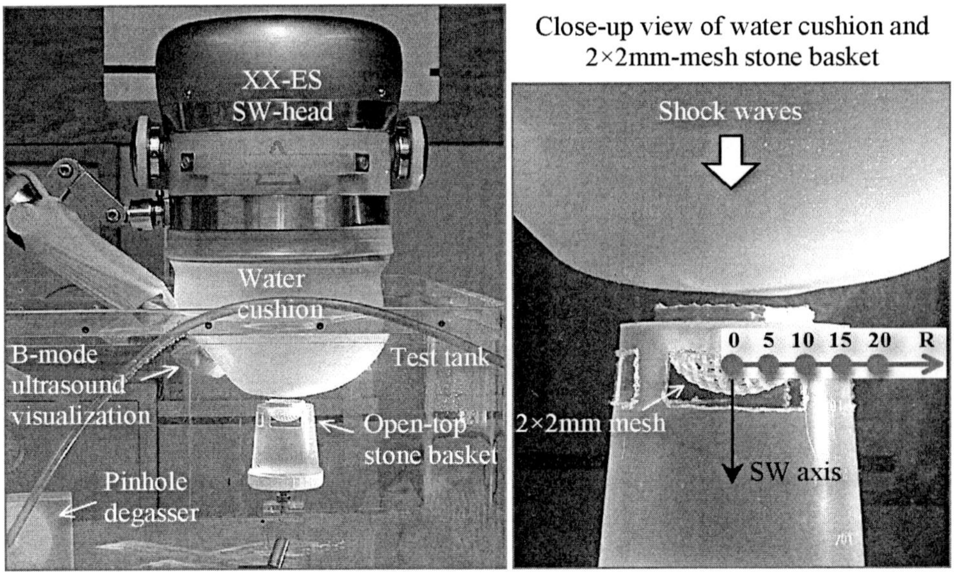

FIGURE 2. Experimental setup for stone breakage with the XX-ES lithotripter. The XX-ES shock wave head sits above the treatment table, so SWs propagate downward (vertical arrow). Model stones were broken in the open-top 2×2mm nylon mesh basket positioned at lateral distances (R) of 0, 5, 10, 15, and 20mm off-axis (right panel).

Except for differences in the physical configuration of the two lithotripters, test conditions (i.e. water quality, stone model) were very similar. Whereas the DoLi is a conventional device in which the shock head is below the treatment table (acoustic axis ~45°), the shock head of the XX-ES is above the table and SW's propagate downward (Fig. 2). As such, in stone breakage experiments with the DoLi—as is the case for typical lithotripters—SW's passed through the mesh basket to reach the stone. With the XX-ES, however, SW's impacted the stone directly from above. The potential effect of this difference in the experimental set-ups is described elsewhere in these proceedings [Pishchalnikov et al]. In that study it is shown that passage through a mesh reduces the negative tail of SW's but has virtually no effect on the positive pressure of the pulse. Therefore, we have assumed that the leading positive-pressure phase of SW's delivered to stones in mesh baskets can be characterized for both of these lithotripters using acoustic measurements performed in the free-field.

Free-field characterization of the acoustic field of these lithotripters was performed using a fiber-optic probe hydrophone (FOPH-500, RP Acoustics, Leutenbach, Germany). Waveforms were recorded in sets of 30-100 SW's collected at 1mm steps lateral to the acoustic axis in the targeting plane of the lithotripters [4]. Average temporal profiles were calculated by realigning individual SW's at the half amplitude of their shock fronts [2]. The spatial distribution of P+ was used to determine the widths of the focal zone, defined as the lateral distance at which the peak positive pressure drops by half of its maximum value measured on the acoustic axis of the lithotripter [7]. As the 50% decrease in amplitude corresponds to about -6dB on the decibel scale, the focal width is also referred as the -6dB zone of the lithotripter.

RESULTS

Lateral distributions of peak positive pressure with the DoLi and the XX-ES lithotripters are shown in Fig. 3. We assume cylindrical symmetry of the acoustic fields so the lateral distribution of P+ is shown as a function of the radial distance R from the axis. These measurements show that the focal width (or -6dB zone) was ~5mm diameter for the DoLi (Fig. 3a), and ~18mm diameter for the XX-ES lithotripter (Fig. 3b). Thus, the focal width of the XX-ES was 3.6 times wider than the -6dB zone of the DoLi.

Breakage of model stones showed that the lateral distribution of breakage efficiency fell faster for the narrow focal zone lithotripter (DoLi) than for the broad focal zone lithotripter (XX-ES), although breakage was not significantly different until 15mm lateral. At R=15mm, the DoLi required almost twice the number of SWs as the XX-ES (3006±780 SW's vs. 1726±972 SW's, P<0.006). The DoLi was entirely ineffective at R=20mm (no breakage with 10,000 SW's), while the broad focal zone XX-ES achieved breakage (3691±1618 SW's) even at this large distance off-axis. Thus, the broad focal zone lithotripter (XX-ES) had a broader region of stone comminution than the narrow focal zone machine (DoLi).

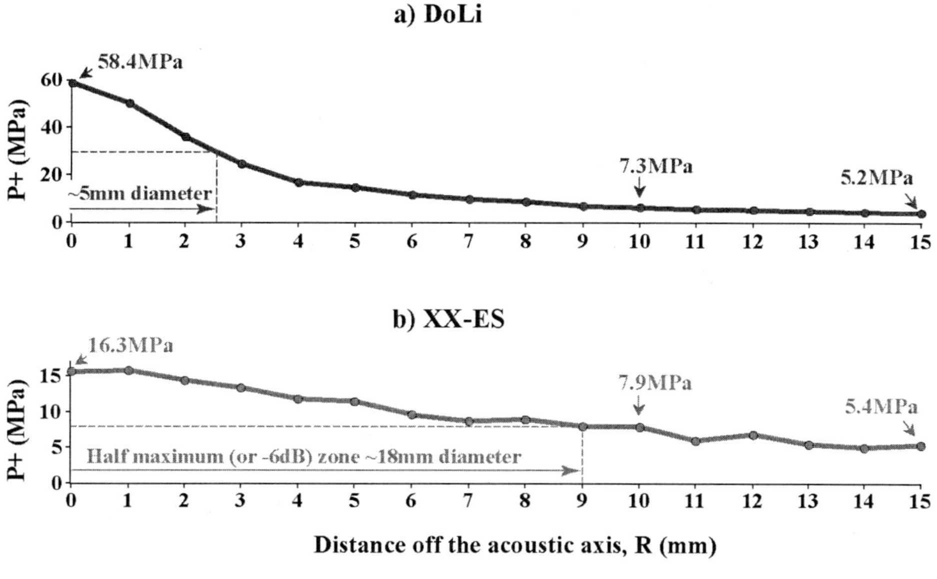

FIGURE 3. Lateral distribution of peak positive pressure (P+) with the Doli (a) and the XX-ES (b). The focal width (half maximum P+ or -6dB zone) was ~5mm diameter for the DoLi, and ~18mm diameter for the XX-ES. At the power levels used in this study (DoLi PL3; XX-ES 9.3kV) peak positive pressure on the DoLi axis (58.4MPa) was 3.6 times greater than P+ on the XX-ES axis (16.3MPa).

DISCUSSION

Several recent studies suggest that the width of the focal zone plays an important role in stone breakage. Laboratory experiments with model stones show that it takes fewer SW's to fracture a stone when the incident pulse is wider than the stone [8]. Likewise, numerical modeling has been used to demonstrate that shear stress within a stone is enhanced, and more energy is delivered to the stone interior, when the focal width is wider than the stone [9]. This, plus the finding that a wider focal zone is more effective than a narrow focal width at delivering effective energy to a moving stone, has focused attention to the potential benefit of a broad focal zone in SWL [1]. The present findings support the idea that a broad focal zone may, indeed, be an advantage. These data provide a functional correlate (stone breakage) to acoustic measurements of focal width, and show that a lithotripter with a broad focal zone is more effective at breaking stones further off axis than a lithotripter with a narrow focal width.

An obvious footnote to this study is that the waveforms of these two lithotripters exhibit somewhat different structure. That is, at its geometric focus the DoLi-50 shows a typical shock front—an instantaneous rise to maximum positive pressure with an overall duration of the compressive phase of only ~2 μs [2]. The XX-ES on the other hand has a pulse of low amplitude and long duration and only forms a true shock at the acoustic focus (distal to targeting point) [4]. Thus, the acoustic output of these two machines differs in more than just the dimensions of the focal zone. Clearly, further work is needed to determine the role of features of the waveform of these and other lithotripters in breaking stones on and off axis. Still, this is a solid indication that a broad focal zone lithotripter can deliver an effective acoustic field to a wider region than a narrow focal width machine.

ACKNOWLEDGMENTS

Supported by a grant from the National Institutes of Health (DK-43881).

REFERENCES

1. R. O. Cleveland, R. Anglade and R. K. Babayan, *J Endourol* **18 (7)**, 629-633 (2004).
2. Y. A. Pishchalnikov, J. A. McAteer, R. J. Vonderhaar, I. V. Pishchalnikova, J. C. Williams, Jr. and A. P. Evan, *J Urol* **176 (5)**, 2294-2298 (2006).
3. W. Eisenmenger, X. X. Du, C. Tang, S. Zhao, Y. Wang, F. Rong, D. Dai, M. Guan and A. Qi, *Ultrasound Med Biol* **28 (6)**, 769-774 (2002).
4. A. P. Evan, J. A. McAteer, B. A. Connors, Y. A. Pishchalnikov, R. K. Handa, P. Blomgren, L. R. Willis, J. C. Williams, Jr., J. E. Lingeman and S. Gao, *BJU Int* **101 (3)**, 382-388 (2008).
5. Y. A. Pishchalnikov, J. S. Neucks, R. J. VonDerHaar, I. V. Pishchalnikova, J. C. Williams, Jr. and J. A. McAteer, *J Urol* **176 (6 Pt 1)**, 2706-2710 (2006).
6. J. A. McAteer, J. C. Williams, Jr., R. O. Cleveland, J. Van Cauwelaert, M. R. Bailey, D. A. Lifshitz and A. P. Evan, *Urol Res* **33 (6)**, 429-434 (2005).
7. IEC61846, IEC 61846 Ultrasonics - Pressure pulse lithotripters - Characteristics of fields. 1998, International Electrotechnical Commission: Geneva, Switzerland.
8. O. A. Sapozhnikov, A. D. Maxwell, B. MacConaghy and M. R. Bailey, *J Acoust Soc Am* **121 (2)**, 1190-1202 (2007).
9. R. O. Cleveland and O. A. Sapozhnikov, *J Acoust Soc Am* **118 (4)**, 2667-2676 (2005).

Treatment Protocols to Reduce Injury and Improve Stone Breakage in SWL

James A. McAteer,[a] Andrew P. Evan,[a] Bret A. Connors,[a] Yuri A. Pishchalnikov,[a] James C. Williams, Jr.,[a] and James E. Lingeman[b]

[a]*Department of Anatomy and Cell Biology, Indiana University School of Medicine, Indianapolis, IN 46202-5120, USA; and*
[b]*Methodist Hospital Institute for Kidney Stone Disease, Indianapolis, IN 46202, USA*

Abstract: Here we provide a capsule summary of key observations showing that adverse effects can be reduced and stone breakage outcomes can be improved by the choice of the treatment protocol used in SWL. The take home message is—technique in lithotripsy can be used to significant advantage. SW-rate is key, and so is the sequence of SW delivery. Patient studies have shown that stone breakage is significantly improved at 60SW/min compared to a rate of 120SW/min, and laboratory experiments with pigs show that acute SWL injury to the kidney can be reduced dramatically by further slowing the SW firing rate to 30SW/min. The sequence of SW administration has a profound effect on the kidney, and renal injury is significantly reduced when the treatment protocol incorporates a priming dose of SW's followed by a brief pause before treatment is resumed. Continued developments in lithotripsy technology are welcome and will hopefully lead to improved SWL systems. Current experience suggests, however, that technology is not a substitute for expert technique, and attention to the fundamentals of SW delivery is essential to achieve the best possible outcomes regardless of the lithotripter at hand.

Keywords: shock wave lithotripsy, kidney, trauma, kidney stones, animal models
PACS: 43.25.Cb, 43.40.Jc, 87.19.rp

INTRODUCTION

Recent studies suggest that outcomes in shock wave lithotripsy (SWL) can be improved by attention to the treatment protocol, particularly the settings for power and SW-rate—and the sequence of SW delivery. Here we review this work with particular emphasis on those findings showing that the technique of how shock waves (SW's) are delivered can be used to improve stone breakage and reduce adverse effects. First, it seems useful to revisit the rationale for this effort—the challenge posed by adverse effects in SWL.

ADVERSE EFFECTS AND THE IMPORTANCE OF REDUCING ACUTE INJURY IN SWL

There is no longer any question that SW's have the potential to cause tissue damage. The spectrum of adverse effects in SWL has been thoroughly reviewed

CP1049, *Renal Stone Disease 2, 2nd International Urolithiasis Research Symposium,* edited by A. P. Evan, J. E. Lingeman, J. A. McAteer, and J. C. Williams, Jr.

elsewhere but, in brief, SW's can rupture blood vessels and this focal hemorrhage within the renal parenchyma leads to inflammation and scarring [1-6]. What is known about SWL injury to the kidney comes, for the most part, from studies with experimental animals where it is possible to use invasive methods to assess damage at the tissue level. Such studies with the pig model show that a clinical dose of SW's causes hemorrhage in the vicinity of the targeted region occupying roughly 5% of the functional renal volume (FRV) [7,8]. This is injury that is detectable by histologic analysis, might well be visible by sophisticated MRI or PET imaging, but which cannot be seen by routine x-ray or typical CT scanning. This is also a form of injury that is not directly related to the occurrence of subcapsular hematomas. That is, parenchymal hemorrhage in SWL-treated experimental animals is not always accompanied by subcapsular bleeds. Thus the absence of a hematoma does not rule out injury to the kidney, and lack of a hematoma by x-ray or CT—as would most often be used to assess patients following SWL—does not mean that the kidney did not sustain damage. As such, to say that an SWL treatment was perfectly safe because it did not cause a hematoma is basing an outcome on an insensitive marker. In this regard the hematoma rate is an incomplete indicator of treatment safety in SWL.

Whereas a great deal is now known about the characteristics of acute SWL injury to the kidney, long-term effects are not nearly as well defined. That is, few laboratory studies have followed the progression of the lesion, but those that have show a dose-dependent loss of functional renal volume [reviewed in 4, 5, 9]. It is a common perception that acute injury in SWL typically resolves rapidly (within weeks) and without lasting consequence [6]. This may, indeed, be the case for the vast majority of patients—particularly those individuals who receive a single SWL session. Patients who undergo multiple lithotripsies may, however, be at increased risk of long-term effects. The recent suggestion of a link between SWL and the onset of diabetes mellitus may be such an example as the occurrence of diabetes was related to SW dose (power and total number of SW's) [10]. There is also an apparent link between multiple lithotripsy sessions and the transition from calcium oxalate stones to calcium phosphate and brushite stones, where it has been theorized that repetitive SWL injury to the renal papilla affects tubular physiology driving the progression to a more complicated pathology [11].

In sum, acute SW damage to the kidney can progress to scar formation and perhaps lead to other long-term effects. This reality, that SWL has the potential to lead to lasting damage, elevates the importance of finding ways to minimize the trauma caused by SW exposure. Lowering the SW dose (power and number of SW's) is one obvious approach, but as explained below other strategies have recently been found to be effective as well.

USING SHOCK WAVES TO TRIGGER A RENAL PROTECTIVE RESPONSE

It is hard to define what constitutes a 'typical' SWL treatment protocol. Most centers likely establish a certain regimen and attempt to follow that scheme, but a protocol at one center may differ considerably from that used elsewhere. Whereas some urologists may always deliver a maximum number of SW's all at high power level, others try to minimize SW exposures and start treatment at a low power level, progressively ramping up (on-the-fly) to a plateau setting for the remainder of the case. Such a practice of 'power ramping' may have originated as a means to help acclimate the patient to SW exposure, particularly for treatment under reduced anesthesia [6]. There may be other benefits as well. *In vitro* studies suggest that a gradual increase in pulse intensity results in better stone fragmentation and a recent clinical study reports an improved success rate with a step-wise treatment scheme [12, 13]. The mechanism is unclear but it may be that repetitive stress at low amplitude promotes stone failure by a process of dynamic fatigue, the progressive growth and expansion of fractures [14]. Power ramping may help the stone remain intact longer as opposed to breaking quickly into large pieces, such that once the stone finally breaks up the fragments are smaller in size.

Although power ramping has been credited for over a decade with a low rate of adverse effects (i.e. 0.08% hematoma rate [15]), the role of step-wise treatment in renal injury has only recently been investigated. In a study in which pigs were treated using the Dornier HM3 lithotripter it was observed that animals treated first with a priming dose of 100 SW's at low intensity (12 kV), followed by the remainder of the dose (2000 SW's) at high intensity (24 kV), had a significantly smaller lesion than pigs treated with all SW's at the higher setting [16]. Injury was also reduced when the priming dose at low power was increased to 500 SW's and when the intensity of the priming dose was raised to 18 kV. This suggested that it was not the power level of the priming dose, but something else that was responsible for the reduction in injury seen in these animals.

The precise protocol used in these studies originated with a set of experiments in which opposite poles of the kidney were treated with a full dose of SW's. First the lower pole was treated with 2000 SW's (all SW's at high power) then the upper pole was treated with the same dose. The two treatments were about 3 minutes apart, the time necessary to change the electrode and reposition the focal zone to the upper pole. All subsequent studies related to this original series of experiments incorporated the same 3-minute pause between the first and second doses. That is regardless of the number of SW's or the power level used, the priming dose was followed by a 3-minute break before the main dose was delivered. To test whether this pause in treatment played a role in tissue protection, pigs were treated with a priming dose of 100 SW's at 24 kV followed by a 3-minute break before the main dose (2000 SW's) was delivered, also at 24 kV [17]. The result was consistent with ramping at lower power levels—injury was significantly reduced (0.51±0.14% FRV versus 3.93±1.29% FRV, $p=0.0135$). That is, even when the priming dose was at a high power level renal injury was significantly reduced when the treatment protocol included a 3-minute pause separating the priming dose and the main dose. The precise mechanism for this effect remains to be determined but may involve the transient vasoconstriction observed in the renal vasculature in response to SW treatment [see Handa et al., these Proceedings]. Further work is needed in this area to determine optimal treatment conditions to afford the greatest degree of protection. In addition, these findings raise the possibility that the practice of power ramping without interruption may not be protective after all. This deserves attention since ramping protocols are in increasingly common use. It makes sense that if ramping is beneficial in acclimating the patient to treatment, plus improves stone fragmentation, the effort should be made to determine if a simple modification to the protocol–adding a brief pause in treatment—would improve the safety of treatment as well.

SLOWING THE FIRING RATE TO IMPROVE STONE BREAKAGE AND REDUCE INJURY

Among the parameters of SW delivery that one might expect would have an effect on stone breakage or on adverse effects, the firing rate of the lithotripter stands out as the least likely. Intuitively it makes sense that stone breakage and tissue injury will be affected by the number of SW's and the amplitude of the pulses. It is perhaps more difficult to appreciate that SW rate might matter. Still, several prospective clinical trials have now shown that stone breakage outcomes are significantly better at 60 SW/min compared to the typical rate of 120 SW/min, and animal experiments show reduced injury at slow SW rate (30 SW/min) compared to fast rate (120 SW/min) [8,18-20].

The role of SW rate in stone breakage outcomes has recently been the subject of a critical meta-analysis [21]. That assessment examined all four of the prospective clinical trials that had been published on the topic of SW-rate, including one in which the stone breakage outcome was not improved at the slower rate [22]. The authors were mindful to disclose a number of potential limitations in their assessment. That is, there were only four reports available for analysis, each study used a different type of lithotripter, the treatment protocols and methods of anesthesia were not the same, stone size could not be compared as different methods of measurement were used, patient follow-up was not the same among the studies, different imaging was used to assess outcomes, and treatment success was defined differently. Even with these caveats it was concluded that treatment at 60 SW/min was more effective than at 120 SW/min.

Progress has been made in understanding the acoustics mechanisms at play in the effect of SW rate on stone breakage. *In vitro* studies show that cavitation generated by the negative pressure phase of the SW increases as the rate of SW delivery is increased [23]. This is because micron-size bubbles are spawned during cavitation bubble collapse and persist to seed cavitation generated by the next SW. The faster the SW rate the more micro-bubbles there are to seed cavitation. Increased cavitation acts to reduce the amplitude and duration of the negative pressure phase of SW's [24, 25]. More work must be done to determine precisely how this reduces stone breakage, but studies using high speed imaging show that cavitation bubble dynamics at the surface of model stones is altered at fast SW-rate compared to slow rate [26].

A study in the pig model suggests that slowing the rate of SW delivery reduces renal injury. Pigs were treated at either 120 SW/min or 30 SW/min using a Dornier

HM3 lithotripter operated at 24 kV. The animals treated at the slower rate showed a significantly smaller lesion compared to the pigs treated at faster rate (0.08±0.02% FRV versus 4.6±1.7% FRV, $p<0.005$). This is a fascinating finding as it implies that all that is needed to protect the kidney from SWL trauma is to slow the firing rate of the lithotripter. Studies are currently underway to determine the level of injury that occurs when SW's are fired at 60 SW/min. It may be a difficult decision for some centers to adopt slow SW rate, but the idea that slow rate is both protective and improves the efficiency of stone breakage makes this a particularly attractive option.

SUMMARY AND CONCLUSIONS

The technique of how SW's are delivered in SWL is key to successful outcomes, and recent research suggests several practical strategies to follow that have the potential to reduce adverse effects and improve the efficiency of stone breakage. Besides the well-appreciated relationship between SW dose and tissue injury—with the recognition that it is always best to minimize the number of high amplitude SW's used in treatment—several ideas deserve special emphasis.

- The sequence of SW delivery is important in SWL.
- Power ramping from low to higher amplitude improves stone fragmentation in vitro and increases the success rate in patients, but ramping on-the-fly has yet to be shown to reduce adverse effects.
- A priming dose of SW's followed by a 3-4 minute pause before resuming treatment significantly reduces renal injury in the pig model.
- Multiple prospective clinical trials have demonstrated improved stone breakage outcomes when SW's are delivered at 60 SW/min compared to 120 SW/min.
- Studies in the pig model show that treatment at slow SW-rate (30 SW/min) significantly reduces renal injury compared to treatment at fast SW-rate (120 SW/min). Thus, slowing the firing rate of the lithotripter improves stone breakage and also significantly reduces adverse effects.

ACKNOWLEDGEMENTS

This work was supported by grant DK43881 from the National Institutes of health.

REFERENCES

1. A.P. Evan and J.A. McAteer. Q-Effects of shock wave lithotripsy. In: *Kidney Stones: Medical and Surgical Management*, FL Coe, MJ Favus, CYC Pak, JH Parks, GM Preminger (eds), Lippincott-Raven, Philadelphia, pp. 549-570 (1996).
2. R. Newman, R. Hackett, D. Senior, K. Brock, J. Feldman, J. Sosnowski, and B. Finlayson. Pathological effects of ESWL on canine renal tissue, *Urology* 29, 194-200 (1987).
3. S.J. Karlsen and K.J. Berg. Acute changes in renal function following extracorporeal shock wave lithotripsy in patients with a solitary functioning kidney, *J Urol* 145, 253-256 (1991).

4. A.P. Evan, L.R. Willis, J.E. Lingeman, and J.A. McAteer. Renal trauma and the risk of long-term complications in shock wave lithotripsy, *Nephron* 78,1-8 (1998).
5. J.A. McAteer and A.P. Evan. The acute and long-term adverse effects of shock wave lithotripsy, *Seminars Nephrol* 28, 200-213 (2008).
6. J.E. Lingeman, B. Matlaga, and A.P. Evan. Surgical management of urinary lithiasis. In: Walsh, P.C., Retik, A.B., Vaughan, E.D. Wein, A.J. eds., *Campbell's Urology*, Philadelphia, W.B Saunders Company, Chapter 44, pp: 1431-1507 (2006).
7. L.R. Willis, A.P. A.P. Evan, B.A. Connors, Y. Shao, P.M. Blomgren, J.H. Pratt, N.S. Fineberg, and J.E. Lingeman. Shockwave lithotripsy: dose-related effects on renal structure, hemodynamics, and tubular function, *J Endourol* 19, 90-101 (2005).
8. A.P. Evan, J.A. McAteer, B.A. Connors, P.M. Blomgren and J.E. Lingeman. Renal injury in SWL is significantly reduced by slowing the rate of shock wave delivery, *Brit J Urol Int* 100, 624-627 (2007).
9. A.P. Evan and L.R. Willis. Extracorporeal shock wave lithotripsy: complications. In: *Smith's Textbook on Endourology*. Smith AD, Badlani GH, Bagley DH, Clayman RV, Docimo SG, Jordan GH, Kavoussi LR, Lee BR, Lingeman JE, Preminger GM, Segura JW (eds), Hamilton, Ontario, Canada, BC Decker, Inc, pp: 353-365 (2007).
10. A.E. Krambeck, M.T. Gettman, A.L. Rohlinger, C.M. Lohse, D.E. Patterson and J.W. Segura. Diabetes mellitus and hypertension associated with shock wave lithotripsy of renal and proximal ureteral stones at 19 years of followup, *J Urol* 175, 1742-1747 (2006).
11. J.H. Parks, E.M. Worcester, F.L. Coe, A.P. Evan and J.E. Lingeman. Clinical implications of abundant calcium phosphate in routinely analyzed kidney stones, *Kidney Int* 66, 777-785 (2004).
12. Y. Zhou, F.H. Cocks, G.M. Preminger and P. Zhong. The effect of treatment strategy on stone comminution efficiency in shock wave lithotripsy, *J Urol* 172, 349-354 (2004).
13. D. Demirci, S. Mustafa, E. Yalcin, O. Ekmekcioglu, I. Gulmez and M. Karacagil. Comparison of conventional and step-wise shockwave lithotripsy in management of urinary calculi, *J Endourol* 21,1407-1410 (2007).
14. M. Lokhandwalla and B. Sturtevant. Fracture mechanics model of stone comminution in ESWL and implications for tissue damage, *Physics Med Biol*, 45, 1923-1940 (2000).
15. T.B. Mobley, D.A. Myers, W.B. Grine, J.McK. Jenkins and W.R. Jordan. Low energy lithotripsy with the lithostar: treatment results with 19,962 renal and ureteral calculi, *J Urol* 149,1419-1424 (1993).
16. L.R. Willis, A.P. Evan, B.A. Connors, R.K. Handa, P.M. Blomgren, and J.E. Lingeman. Prevention of lithotripsy-induced renal injury by pretreating kidneys with low-energy shock waves, *J Am Soc Nephrol* 17, 663-673, (2006).
17. B.A. Connors, A.P. Evan, P.M. Blomgren, R.K. Handa, L.R. Willis and S. Gao. Effect of initial shock wave voltage on SWL-induced lesion size during step-wise voltage ramping, *Brit J Urol Int* (Accepted for publication 2008)
18. K.T. Pace, D. Ghiculete, M. Harju, and R.J.D'A. Honey. Shock wave lithotripsy at 60 or 120 shocks per minute: a randomized, double-blind trial, *J Urol* 174, 595-599 (2005).
19. K. Madbouly, A.M. El-Tiraifi, M. Seida, S.R. El-Faqih, R. Atassi, and R.F. Talic. Slow versus fast shock wave lithotripsy rate for urolithiasis: a prospective randomized study, *J Urol* 173, 127-130 (2005).
20. E. Yilmaz, E. Batislam, M. Basar, D. Tuglu, C. Mert and H. Basar. Optimal frequency in extracorporeal shock wave lithotripsy: prospective randomized study, *Urology* 66,1160-1164 (2005).
21. M.J. Semins, B.J. Trock and B.R. Matlaga. The effect of shock wave rate on the outcome of shock wave lithotripsy: a meta-analysis, *J Urol* 179, 194-197 (2008).
22. K. Davenport, A. Minervini, S. Keoghane, J. Parkin, F.X. Keeley, and A.G. Timoney. Does rate matter? The results of a randomized controlled trial of 60 versus 120 shocks per minute for shock wave lithotripsy of renal calculi, *J Urol* 176, 2055-2058 (2006).
23. Y.A. Pishchalnikov, J.A. McAteer and JC Williams Jr. Effect of firing rate on the performance of shock wave lithotriptors. *Brit J Urol Int* (Accepted for publication 2008)
24. Y.A. Pishchalnikov, J.A. McAteer, J.C. Williams Jr,, I. Pishchalnikova, and R.J. VonDerHaar. Why stones break better at slow shock wave rate than at fast rate: In vitro study with a research electrohydraulic lithotripter, *J Endourology* 20, 537-541 (2006).
25. Y.A. Pishchalnikov, O.A. Sapozhnikov, M.R. Bailey, I.V. Pishchalnikova, J.C. Williams Jr,, and J.A. McAteer. Cavitation selectively reduces the negative-pressure phase of lithotripter shock waves, *Acoust Res Let Online* 6, 280-286 (2005).
26. Y.A. Pishchalnikov, M.M. Kaehr, and J.A. McAteer. Influence of pulse repetition rate on cavitation at the surface of an object targeted by lithotripter shock waves. *Proc IMECE2007*-41387, 2007

Effect of Shock Wave Lithotripsy on Renal Hemodynamics

Rajash K. Handa,[a] Lynn R. Willis,[b] Andrew P. Evan [a] and Bret A. Connors [a]

Departments of [a]Anatomy & Cell Biology, and [b]Pharmacology & Toxicology, Indiana University School of Medicine, 635 Barnhill Drive, Medical Sciences Bldg, Indianapolis, IN 46202, USA

Abstract. Extracorporeal shock wave lithotripsy (SWL) can injure tissue and decrease blood flow in the SWL-treated kidney, both tissue and functional effects being largely localized to the region targeted with shock waves (SWs). A novel method of limiting SWL-induced tissue injury is to employ the "protection" protocol, where the kidney is pretreated with low-energy SWs prior to the application of a standard clinical dose of high-energy SWs. Resistive index measurements of renal vascular resistance/impedance to blood flow during SWL treatment protocols revealed that a standard clinical dose of high-energy SWs did not alter RI during SW application. However, there was an interaction between low- and high-energy SWL treatment phases of the "protection" protocol such that an increase in RI (vasoconstriction) was observed during the later half of SW application, a time when tissue damage is occurring during the standard high-energy SWL protocol. We suggest that renal vasoconstriction may be responsible for reducing the degree of tissue damage that normally results from a standard clinical dose of high-energy SWs.

Keywords: Extracorporeal shock wave lithotripsy, PET imaging, sonography, resistive index, "protection" protocol
PACS: 01.30.Cc; 87.19.U-; 87.50.Y-; 87.50.yt

INTRODUCTION

Extracorporeal shock wave lithotripsy (SWL) was introduced in the early 1980's and is widely viewed as an effective noninvasive method of removing kidney stones. However, it is a technology that is not without trauma to the kidney. Early on in the treatment of patients, it was recognized that SWL could damage renal tissue [1] with subcapsular and/or perirenal hematoma rates as high as 32% when MRI or CT methods of detection were employed [1,2], with the incidence of renal hematomas increasing 2-fold for each decade in patient age [3]. Animal studies have revealed that blood vessel rupture with subsequent bleeding is the primary event characterizing the acute renal injury induced by SWL [4]. The hemorrhagic lesion is largely localized to the region of the kidney targeted by the focal zone of the lithotripter, beginning in the renal medulla and spreading into the cortex towards the kidney capsule where a subcapsular hematoma may develop [4]. This vascular injury, together with tubular and interstitial damage, may potentially lead to the permanent loss of functional tissue

CP1049, *Renal Stone Disease 2, 2nd International Urolithiasis Research Symposium,*
edited by A. P. Evan, J. E. Lingeman, J. A. McAteer, and J. C. Williams, Jr.

[4]. Human and animal studies have also shown that another hallmark of SWL is a reduction in renal hemodynamic function in the SWL-treated kidney [5-11], and to a lesser extent in the untreated kidney [7-11]. The acute tissue and functional trauma of SWL will generally resolve over a relatively short period of time without complications, but in some patients may persist and lead to chronic adverse effects [2]. Therefore, there is a continuous effort by investigators to understand how SWs interact with renal tissues in the hope of reducing SWL-induced adverse effects and thus improve the safety of SWL.

EFFECT OF SWL ON RENAL BLOOD FLOW

Acute reductions of RBF and GFR have been observed in the treated kidney within an hour after SWL in dogs [12], pigs [8,9] and humans [2]. The reduction in RBF is transient in most cases, but there are some instances where SWL results in a chronic reduction in renal function that can lead to long-term adverse complications such as hypertension [2].

Pig studies in our laboratory have repeatedly shown that a clinical dose of SWs can result in an acute and transient decrease in RBF of 40-70% in the SWL-treated kidney with a somewhat smaller reduction in RBF in the untreated kidney [8,9]. The mechanism(s) responsible for the reduction in RBF in the SWL-treated kidney has not been identified, but renal sympathetic nerves mediate the vasoconstriction in the unshocked kidney almost entirely [13].

Classic clearance methods have been used to estimate renal hemodynamic function in order to provide a picture of the integrated whole-kidney response to SWL, but this gives no information on the possible regional changes in function. It is likely that regional changes in function do exist based on the fact that tissue injury and blood vessel rupture is localized to the renal pole targeted by the SW [4,9]. Indirect measurements of changes in regional renal blood flow have been gathered from resistive index (RI) measurements taken from blood vessels within, or close to, the SW focal zone and compared to regions remote from this location. The results of these clinical studies suggest that there is a transient increase in RI (implying vasoconstriction) after SWL in the SW-targeted pole of the kidney with less of an increase, or no increase, in RI in remote locations in the same kidney or untreated kidney [7,10,11,14-16]. A localized reduction in intrarenal blood flow after SWL has also been demonstrated by Mostafavi and colleagues who used a more direct approach of Gd-DTPA-enhanced magnetic resonance imaging to demonstrate a reduction in cortical blood flow in the SWL-treated pole of the kidney in 6 of 7 adult patients compared to locations away from the targeted area or the untreated kidney [5].

We have looked at the issue of SWL-induced regional changes in renal blood flow using Positron Emission Tomography (PET) and the radiopharmaceutical tracer, ^{62}Cu-ETS [17]. These studies were done in collaboration with Dr. Mark Green (Department of Industrial and Physical Pharmacy, Purdue University, Indiana), and performed on 6-week-old female Gottingen minipigs that were treated with SWs from a Doli-50 lithotripter (3500 SWs, power setting 6, 120 SWs/min). As shown in Figure 1, renal perfusion appeared constant throughout the kidney before lithotripsy (panel A), with the highest signal in the cortex that has the highest blood flow, whereas 90-min after SWL there was a definite deficit in perfusion in the lower pole of left kidney that was treated with SWs (panel B). There also appears to be a small reduction in the signal from the untreated upper pole of the SW-treated left kidney, but no change in the signal from the untreated, right kidney. Therefore, the PET data indicates that the SWL-induced reduction in renal blood flow is largely localized to the area treated with SWs. Although, visual inspection of the signal intensity would suggest that there was no change in blood flow in the untreated, right kidney after SWL, kinetic models remain to be fitted to the PET data in order to quantify blood flow and determine the degree of reduction in flow in the various poles of the SW-treated and perhaps untreated kidney.

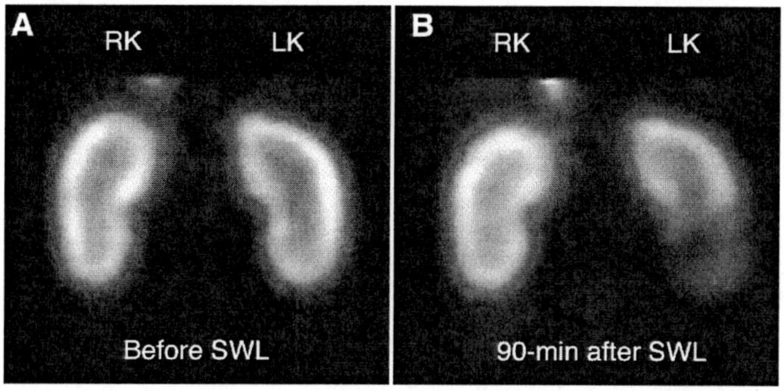

FIGURE 1. PET images of the right (RK) and left (LK) kidney before SWL (panel A) and 90-min after SWL (panel B). The Doli-50 electromagnetic lithotripter delivered 3500 SWs (power level 6, 120 SWs/min) to the lower pole of the left kidney.

LOW-ENERGY SW PRETREATMENT "PROTECTS" THE KIDNEY FROM SW-INDUCED TISSUE DAMAGE

Our discovery of the "protection phenomenon" was serendipitous [18]. Originally, we were attempting to assess whether multiple SWL treatments in a single session to one kidney was a risk factor for renal damage. Treatment of one pole of the kidney with a clinical dose of high-energy SWs (2000 SWs, 24 kV, 120 SWs/min) elicited a hemorrhagic lesion that was ~6% of functional renal volume (FRV), and treatment of the opposite pole of the same kidney with a similar dose of SWs was expected to produce at least the same degree of tissue injury and, thereby, double the amount of injury to the SWL-treated kidney. To our surprise, the second dose of SWs had minimal effect on the tissue, with hemorrhagic lesion that comprised only 0.5% FRV or less. These studies were repeated with the first dose of SWs being of a strength (12 kV) that did not damage renal tissue, and the second dose of high-energy (tissue damaging strength) SWs was still found to have little tissue effects. These results implied that tissue damage was not a pre-requisite for the manifestation of the "protection phenomenon". Additional experiments were performed where low-energy and high-energy SWs were applied to the same area of the kidney and it was found that pretreatment with 500 or even 100 low-energy (12 kV) SWs could protect the kidney from the damaging effects of a clinical dose of high-energy SWs (Figure 2).

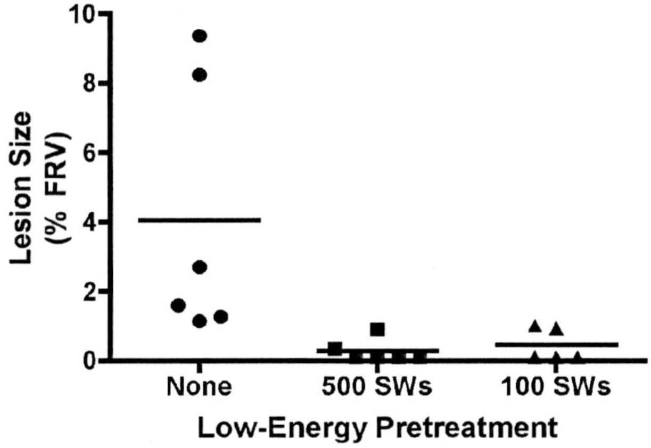

FIGURE 2. The effect of low-energy (12 kV) pretreatment on the hemorrhagic lesion size (% of function renal volume) following a clinical dose of high-energy SWs (2000 SWs, 24 kV, 120 SWs/min). Individual values are shown as well as the mean response (horizontal bar).

The mechanism(s) involved in the "protection phenomenon" is unknown, but we have hypothesized that pretreatment with low-energy SWs will cause renal vasoconstriction, and that this in some way (perhaps impeding factors that can rupture blood vessels, e.g. cavitation activity, and/or reducing blood loss from ruptured vessels) would interfere with the ability of a second dose of high-energy SWs to injure tissue. This hypothesis was based on the observation that SWL treatment with either high-energy or low-energy SWs will evoke comparable renal vasoconstriction measured within 1 hour after SWL [19], our PET imaging data that indicated that SWL-induced renal vasoconstriction was most intense at the site of SW application (see above), and our assumption that renal vasoconstriction is likely initiated during the period of SWL. As a first step in testing that renal vasoconstriction occurs earlier during the "protection" protocol than in the standard protocol, we used resistive index (RI) measurements as a noninvasive method to monitor vascular resistance/impedance to blood flow [20]. This allowed us to track, in real time, the RI of a single intralobar artery located in the lithotripter-targeted pole of the kidney before, during and after SWL protocols that injure the kidney or protect the kidney from injury. These studies were done in collaboration with Dr. Michael Bailey and Marla Paun (Applied Physics Laboratory, University of Washington, Seattle).

Figure 3 shows the change in RI from baseline values for four groups that had similar pre-SWL RI values (~ 0.6). Sham SWL treatment (no SWs) did not alter RI during the entire experimental observation period. Animals treated with a clinical dose of high-energy SWs (2000 SWs, 24 kV, 120 SWs/min) did not show a significant change in RI during SWL, but a rise in RI (vasoconstriction) was observed about 45-min into the post-SWL period (not shown). Animals treated with the SWL "protection" protocol (500 SWs, 12 kV, 120 SWs/min + 3-min pause + 2000 SWs, 24 kV, 120 SWs/min) showed no change in RI after the initial period of low-energy SWL, indicating that pretreatment does not result in renal vasoconstriction as originally hypothesized (see above). However, we did observe an increase in RI during the subsequent application of high-energy SWs that occurred earlier (1000 SWs) and was greater (2-fold) than that observed with standard SWL. The earlier rise in RI was not due to low-energy pretreatment, as pretreatment alone (500 SWs, 12 kV, 120 SWs/min) did not alter RI. Therefore, there appears to be an interaction between the low-energy and high-energy phases of the "protection" protocol that allows the manifestation of renal vasoconstriction at a time that renal injury normally occurs, between 1000 to 2000 high-energy SWs [21]. It would appear that the initial SW stimulus and the interval period between SW applications allows the sensitization of the vasculature and/or a vasoconstrictor system(s) that elicits a robust renal vasoconstriction during high-energy SWL. Our results show only a correlation between the time of renal vasoconstriction and the reduction in renal damage, and do not prove cause and effect. However, our hypothesis that renal vasoconstriction may be responsible for the protection phenomenon is still valid and merits further investigation.

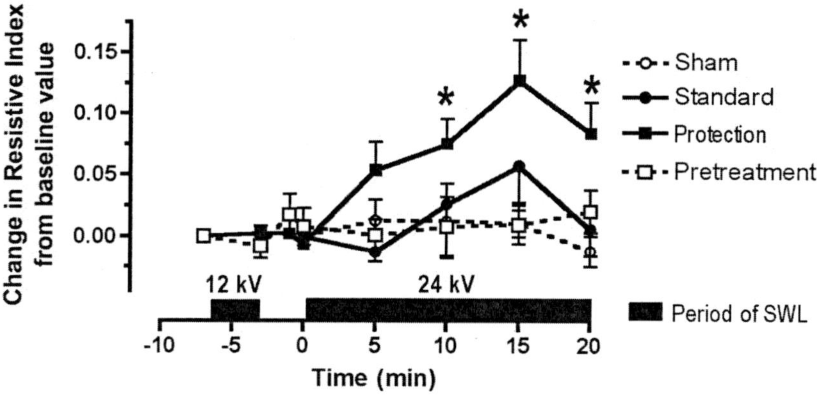

FIGURE 3. The change in resistive index during SWL: Sham protocol (no SWs; n=4), Standard Protocol (2000 SWs, 24 kV, 120 SWs/min; n=7), Protection Protocol (500 SWs, 12 kV, 120 SWs/min + 3-min pause + 2000 SWs, 24 kV, 120 SWs/min; n=8), Pretreatment Protocol alone (500 SWs, 12 kV, 120 SWs/min; n=6). All groups had a similar baseline RI value of ~ 0.6. * = $P < 0.05$ from individual group's baseline (Pre-SW) RI value.

The "protection" protocol is composed of three steps: an initial low-energy SW stimulus, a 3-min interval between SW applications and the clinical dose of high-energy SWs. We have recently reported that the protection phenomenon is independent of the initial SW strength and that reduced tissue injury is apparent whether the initial SW voltage is 12 kV, 18 kV or 24 kV [22]. This would suggest that the interval between SW applications is important in allowing the protection phenomenon to fully develop. Support for this notion has been obtained from two pigs in which the lower pole of the left kidney was pretreated with 500 low-energy (12 kV)

SWs followed by a pause of 10 seconds (minimal amount of time to change the voltage setting on the HM3 lithotripter) and then immediately applying a clinical dose of 2000 high-energy (24 kV) SWs. Under these conditions, subcapsular hematomas were noted on the kidney surface. Surface hematomas were never observed when the "protection" protocol had a 3-min pause between SW treatments. Therefore, our preliminary data from only two experiments suggests that the length of inactivity between the initial and standard SW treatments may be a critical step in manifesting the "protection phenomenon". Clearly, these findings must be shown to be reproducible before we can take this conclusion as a true fact, but the implication is that current clinical SWL protocols that progressively increase SW voltage without a brief pause in treatment may not be invoking the "protection phenomenon" and, therefore, not protecting the kidney from SWL-induced tissue injury.

The long-term consequences of SWL-induced tissue injury are unclear, but some studies have implicated potential adverse effects to include the early onset of hypertension [11,15,23], particularly in older adults [11,15], the development of diabetes [23] and that multiple SWL treatments may alter the type of stone disease [24,25]. Therefore, an anticipated benefit of the "protection" protocol would be not only the reduction in the acute tissue injury resulting from SWL but also preventing some of the potential long-term adverse complications of SWL.

ACKNOWLEDGMENTS

This work was supported by funds from National Institute of Health grants P01-DK43881 and R01-DK67133.

REFERENCES

1. J.V. Kaude, C.M. Williams, M.R. Millner, K.N. Scott and B. Finlayson, *AJR* **145**, 305-313 (1985).
2. J. Lingeman, M. Delius, A. Evan, M Gupta, K. Sarica, W. Strohmaier, J. McAteer and J. Williams, "Bioeffects and Physical Mechanisms of SW Effects in SWL" in *Stone Disease: First International Consultation on Stone Disease*, edited by J. Segura et al., Health Publications, Paris, 2003, pp. 251-286.
3. N.B. Dahr, J. Thornton, M.T. Karafa and S.B. Streem, *J Urol* **172**, 2271-2274 (2004).
4. A.P. Evan and J.A. McAteer, "Q-Effects of Shock-Wave Lithotripsy" in *Kidney Stones: Medical and Surgical Management*, edited by F.L. Coe et al., Lippincott-Raven Publishers, Philadelphia, 1996, pp 549-570.
5. M.R. Mostafavi, D.R. Chavez, J. Cannillo, B. Saltzman and P.V. Prasad, *J Endourol* **12**, 9-12 (1998).
6. A.J. Chan, P.V. Prasad, A. Priatna, M.R. Mostafavai, C. Sunduram and B. Saltzman, *J Endourol* **14**, 117-121 (2000).
7. Y. Aoki, S. Ishitoya, K. Okubo, T. Okada, S. Maekawa, H. Maeda and Y. Arai, *Int J Urol* **6**, 483-492 (1999).
8. L.R.Willis, A.P. Evan, B.A. Connors, G. Reed, N.S. Fineberg and J.E. Lingeman, *J Urol* **156**, 1502-1506 (1996).
9. L.R. Willis, A.P. Evan, B.A. Connors, P. Blomgren, N.S. Fineberg and J.E. Lingeman, *J Am Soc Nephrol* **10**, 1753-1762 (1999).
10. H. Nazaroglu, A.F. Akay, Y. Bükte, H. Sahin, Z. Akkus and A. Bilici, *Scand J Urol Nephrol* **37**, 408-412 (2003).
11. M. Mitterberger, G.M. Pinggera, R. Neururer, R. Peschel, F. Aigner, J. Gradl, G. Bartsch, D. Kendler, F. Karakolcu, F. Frauscher and L. Pallwein, *BJU Int* **101**, 731-735 (2007).
12. S.J. Karlsen, B. Smevik, J. Stenstrøm and K.J. Berg, *J Urol* **143**, 1280-1283 (1990).
13. B.A. Connors, A.P. Evan, L.R. Willis, J.R. Simon, N.S. Fineberg, D.A. Lifshitz, A.L. Shalhav, R.F. Paterson, R.L. Kuo and J.E. Lingeman, *Nephron Physiol* **95**, 67-75 (2003).

14. R. Knapp, F. Frauscher, G. Helweg, D. zur Nedden, H. Strasser, G. Janetschek and G. Bartsch, *J Urol* 154, 955-958 (1995).
15. G. Janetschek, F. Frauscher, R. Knapp, G. Höfle, R. Peschel and G. Bartsch, *J Urol* 158, 346-351 (1997).
16. M.G. Mohseni, M.H. Khazaeli, S.M.K. Aghamir and F. Biniaz, *Urol J* **4**, 217-220 (2007).
17. M.A. Green, C.J. Mathias, L.R. Willis, R.K. Handa, J.L. Lacy, M.A. Miller and G.D. Hutchins, *Nuclear Medicine and Biology* **34**, 247-255 (2007).
18. L.R. Willis, A.P. Evan, B.A. Connors, R.K. Handa, P.M. Blomgren and J.E. Lingeman, *J Am Soc Nephrol* **17**, 663-673 (2006).
19. B.A. Connors, A.P. Evan, L.R. Willis, P.M. Blomgren, J.E. Lingeman and N.S. Fineberg, *J Am Soc Nephrol* **11**, 310-318 (2000).
20. M.E. Tublin, R.O. Bude and J.F. Platt, *AJR* **180**, 885-892 (2003).
21. B.A. Connors, A.P. Evan, P.M. Blomgren, L.R. Willis, R.K. Handa, D.A. Lifshitz, J.E. Lingeman and J. Ying, *J Endourol* **20**, 607-611 (2006).
22. B.A. Connors, A.P. Evan, P.M. Blomgren, R.K. Handa, L.R. Willis and S. Gao, *BJU Int.* In Press (2008).
23. A.E. Krambeck, M.T. Gettman, A.L. Rohlinger, C.M. Lohse, D.E. Patterson and J.W. Segura, *J Urol* **175**, 1742-1747 (2006).
24. J.H. Parks, E.M. Worcester, F.L. Coe, A.P. Evan and J.E. Lingeman, *Kidney Int* **66**, 777-785 (2004).
25. A.P. Evan, J.E. Lingeman, F.L. Coe, Y. Shao, J.H. Parks, S.B. Bledsoe, C.L. Phillips, S. Bonsib, E.M. Worcester, A.J. Sommer, S.C. Kim, W.W. Tinmouth and M. Grynpas, *Kidney Int* **67**, 576-591 (2005).

Clinical Studies of Real-Time Monitoring of Lithotripter Performance Using Passive Acoustic Sensors

T.G. Leighton[a], F. Fedele[b], A.J. Coleman[b], C. McCarthy[b], S. Ryves[c], A. M. Hurrell[d], A. De Stefano[e] and P.R. White[a]

[a]*Institute of Sound and Vibration Research, University of Southampton, Highfield, Southampton SO17 1BJ, UK (Corresponding author: tgl@soton.ac.uk)*
[b]*Medical Physics Department, Guy's and St Thomas' NHS Foundation Trust, Lambeth Palace Road, London SE1 7EH, UK.*
[c]*Stone Unit, Day Surgery Department, Guy's and St Thomas' NHS Foundation Trust, St Thomas Street, London SE1 9RT, UK.*
[d]*Precision Acoustics Ltd., Hampton Farm Business Park, Higher Bockhampton, Dorchester DT2 8QH, Dorset, UK.*
[e]*Radiological Science Group, Medical Physics Department, St Mary's Hospital, Portsmouth PO3 6AD, Hampshire, UK.*

Abstract. This paper describes the development and clinical testing of a passive device which monitors the passive acoustic emissions generated within the patient's body during Extracorporeal Shock Wave Lithotripsy (ESWL). Designed and clinically tested so that it can be operated by a nurse, the device analyses the echoes generated in the body in response to each ESWL shock, and so gives real time shock-by-shock feedback on whether the stone was at the focus of the lithotripter, and if so whether the previous shock contributed to stone fragmentation when that shock reached the focus. A shock is defined as being 'effective' if these two conditions are satisfied. Not only can the device provide real-time feedback to the operator, but the trends in shock 'effectiveness' can inform treatment. In particular, at any time during the treatment (once a statistically significant number of shocks have been delivered), the percentage of shocks which were 'effective' provides a treatment score $TS(t)$ which reflects the effectiveness of the treatment up to that point. The $TS(t)$ figure is automatically delivered by the device without user intervention. Two clinical studies of the device were conducted, the ethics guidelines permitting only use of the value of $TS(t)$ obtained at the end of treatment (this value is termed the treatment score TS_0). The acoustically-derived treatment score was compared with the treatment score CTS_2 given by the consultant urologist at the three-week patient's follow-up appointment. In the first clinical study (phase 1), records could be compared for 30 out of the 118 patients originally recruited, and the results of phase 1 were used to refine the parameter values (the 'rules') with which the acoustic device provides its treatment score. These rules were tested in phase 2, for which records were compared for 49 of the 85 patients recruited. Considering just the phase 2 results (since the phase 1 data were used to draw up the 'rules' under which phase 2 operated), comparison of the opinion of the urologist at follow-up with the acoustically derived judgment identified a good correlation (kappa=0.94), the device demonstrating a sensitivity of 91.7% (in that it correctly predicted 11 of the 12 treatments which the urologist stated had been 'successful' at the 3-week follow-up), and a specificity of 100% (in that it correctly predicted all of the 37 treatments which the urologist stated had been 'unsuccessful' at the 3-week follow-up). The 'gold standard' opinion of the urologist (CTS_2)

CP1049, *Renal Stone Disease 2, 2nd International Urolithiasis Research Symposium,*
edited by A. P. Evan, J. E. Lingeman, J. A. McAteer, and J. C. Williams, Jr.

correlated poorly (kappa=0.38) with the end-of-treatment opinion of the radiographer (CTS_1). This is due to the limited resolution of the lithotripter X-Ray fluoroscopy system. If the results of phase 1 and phase 2 are pooled to form a dataset against which retrospectively to test the rules drawn up in phase 1, when compared with the gold standard CTS_2, over the two clinical trials (79 patients) the device-derived scored (TS_0) correctly predicted the clinical effectiveness of the treatment for 78 for the 79 patients (the error occurred on a difficult patient with a high body mass index). In comparison, using the currently available technology the in-theatre clinician (the radiographer) provided a treatment score CTS_1 which correctly predicted the outcome of only 61 of the 79 therapies. In particular the passive acoustic device correctly predicted 18 of the 19 treatments that were successful (i.e. 94.7 sensitivity), whilst the current technology enabled the in-theatre radiographer to predict only 7 of the 19 successful treatments (i.e. 36.8 sensitivity). The real-time capabilities of the device were used in a preliminary examination of the effect of ventilation.

Keywords: Lithotripsy, Cavitation, Kidney stone fragmentation, ESWL, passive acoustic sensor.
PACS: 43.20.Fn, 43.25.Cb, 43.25.Vt, 43.25.Yw, 43.25.Zx, 43.30.Lz, 43.35.Ei, 43.35.Hl, 43.35.Yb, 43.60.Lq, 43.80.Ev, 43.80.Gx, 43.80.Qf, 43.80.Sh, 43.80.Vj, 87.50.yt.

INTRODUCTION

Background

In the earlier 1990's Leighton and Coleman identified a two-burst structure (Figure 1) present in the time histories of the passive acoustic emissions detected during lithotripsy, and by comparing this structure with the time histories of sonoluminescent emissions, identified the two bursts as relating to cavitational collapses [1-3].

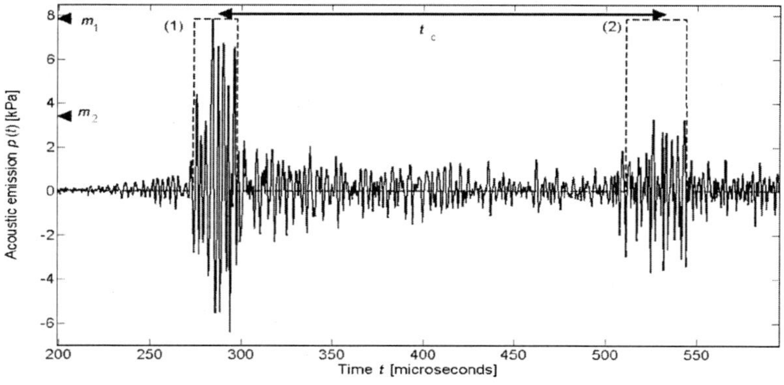

FIGURE 1. Example of the time domain analysis of an *in vivo* signal. The dashed boxes indicate those two portions of the signals that are attributed to the (1) first and (2) second bursts. The two bursts are separated by a collapse time t_c= 246 μs and each of these bursts is then characterised in terms of a maximum amplitude (m_1 = 7.8 kPa and m_2 = 3.3 kPa respectively) [8-12]. The method of calculating these values is discussed in reference [13]. This trace was recorded using one of the clinical prototypes developed in this study (Mark III), and a signal conditioning system that includes a high pass filter at 300 kHz and a preamplifier. The data acquisition system is described in detail by Fedele [11].

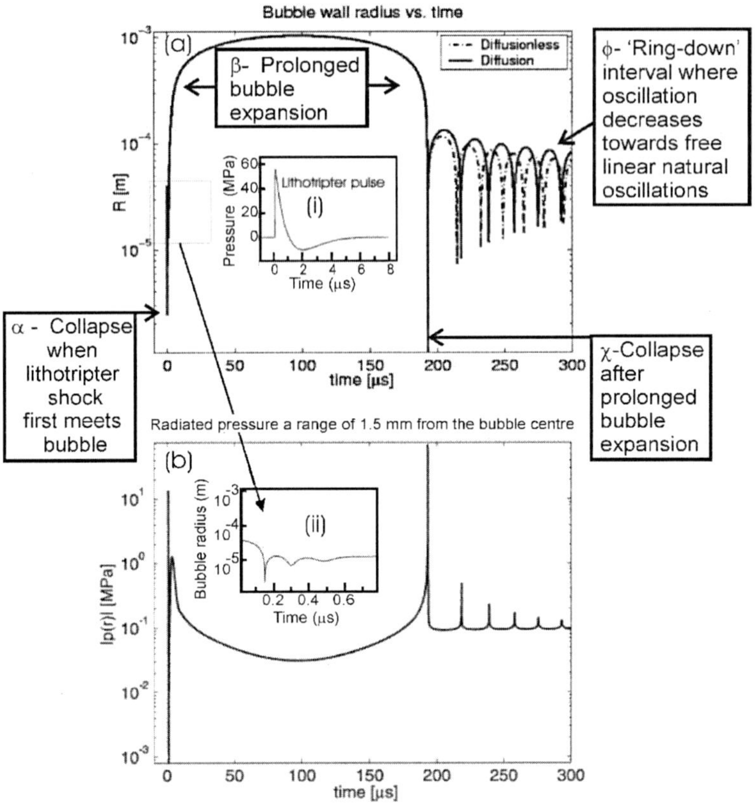

FIGURE 2. An air bubble of initial radius 40 microns in water is subjected in the free field to the lithotripter pulse shown in inset (i) (Peak positive pressure = 56 MPa; Peak negative pressure = -10 MPa). (a) The bubble radius time history, as predicted by the Gilmore model, is shown for conditions with (solid line) and without (dashed line) mass flux across the bubble wall. Note that the inclusion of diffusion makes the final bubble size greater than the initial size, with a consequent slight decrease in the period of the oscillations (i.e. a reduction in the frequency) at the timescales marked ϕ. Inset (ii) shows the micro-rebounds that are visible in the fine detail of the collapse which occurs around t=0. Similar features are seen in the CFD predictions (Turangan *et al.* [7]). (b) On a common time axis with (a) and for the same bubble collapse, the pressure that would be measured 1.5 mm away from the bubble centre is shown. Two main emissions (at $t \approx 0$ μs and at $t \approx 190$ μs) are associated with rebounds in (a), subsequent emissions being smaller. The overall effect of such pairs of emissions from the collapse of a cloud of bubbles was identified as demarcating the interval t_c in the early 1990s [1-3]. Comparison of (a) with (b) suggests that the source of the first peak is the cavitational collapse which results when the lithotripter first meets the bubble (label α). After this collapse, the Gilmore model suggests that the bubble undertakes a prolonged expansion phase (label β), before collapsing again (at which time the second peak in acoustic emission and luminescence is generated; label χ). The bubble must remain spherical and intact in the Gilmore model, so that after this second collapse the bubble oscillates with gradually decreasing amplitude, with a frequency which tends ever more closely to its 'Minnaert' frequency as time proceeds (label ϕ).

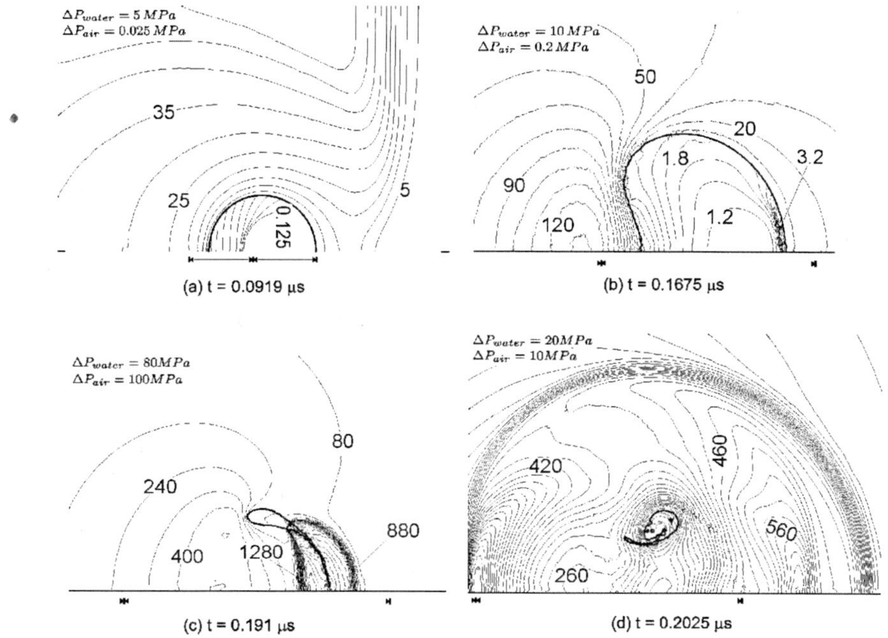

FIGURE 3. An air bubble of initial radius 40 microns in water is subjected in the free field to a lithotripter pulse (propagating from left to right). The axis of rotational symmetry is the horizontal line at the base of each plot. The contour increments in pressure for both air and water are indicated on each plot, the value of selected contours being labelled in MPa. All elapsed times 't' are measured after the lithotripter pulse first meets the upstream bubble wall. (a) The lithotripter pulse has passed over the bubble, travelling further than the slower gas shock within the bubble. An expansion wave is reflected back off the bubble, travelling to the left and upwards in the picture. (b) The bubble involutes as it collapses, to form a liquid jet which will pass through the centre of the bubble. (c) The impact of the jet against the downstream bubble wall generates a blast wave, which propagates outwards in (d). Such liquid impacts and blast waves can generate erosion and biomechanical effects. The high temperatures and pressures attained within the gas can generate chemical effects and luminescence. Movies of this CFD code in operation can be found at the online page associated with the paper [7]: http://journals.cambridge.org/fulltext_content/supplementary/S0022112007009317sup001/index.html Figure reproduced from reference [5].

Furthermore, through use of the Gilmore equation (Figure 2), they identified the time interval between the two bursts (t_c) as corresponding to the period of prolonged expansion between two cavitational collapses: the first collapse occurs when the shock wave from the lithotripter first impacts upon the bubble, and the second collapse occurs over 100 μs later. Using the Gilmore equation, they showed that t_c depended on the initial bubble size and the strength of the lithotripter shock wave, and provided experimental evidence for this [1-4]. Finally, they discussed the possibility that such passive acoustic emissions could be used to monitor the efficacy of lithotripsy treatments in real-time [1-3].

To bring such a concept to fruition required improvements in the simulation capability, since the Gilmore model contains limiting assumptions, most notably that the bubble remains spherical at all times. Alternative methods, which allow for the departure of the bubble wall from sphericity, could not model the blast wave produced when the bubble collapses [5-8]. This blast wave is a vital feature, since the GPa pressures in the diverging blast wave (Figure 3) exceed by two orders of magnitude the compressive pressure in the lithotripter shock wave, and so failure to incorporate them in the model neglects what is potentially a significant contributor both to the far field acoustic emissions and to the stone fragmentation (bearing in mind the differing geometric spreading characteristics of the two waves). Hence a free-Lagrange computational fluid dynamics (CFD) scheme was developed for simulating bubble collapses during ESWL, initially in free field (Figure 3) [5,6] but then incorporating multiple bubbles, bubble cloud effects, the presence of solids in the vicinity of the stone, and the effect of the geometry of that solid on the pressures and stresses induced. The method is outlined in reference [7], with later papers in preparation detailing the multi-bubble stages of the CFD and the far field predictions of the emissions.

In parallel with these CFD studies (and informed by them) a program of *in vitro* tests was conducted in order to progress towards the design of the hardware, software, and rules for the operation of the passive acoustic device for in-theatre real-time monitoring of ESWL [9-12]. These rules were important, since the most challenging component in this study was to condense the myriad of complicated interactions between shock, tissue, stone and bubble into two simple, reliable, and easily observable parameters (m_2/m_1 and t_c; see Figure 1) which could be judged against preset rules in order to assess, in real time, whether each shock delivered to the patient in a given ESWL treatment session was 'effective' [13]. By 'effective', we mean that the shock was (i) on-target, in that the stone was appropriately in the focus of the ESWL device; and (ii) that the shock effectively contributed to the fragmentation of the stone.

Condensing the interpretation of the passive acoustic emissions into two parameters (m_2/m_1 and t_c), despite the myriad sources which can contribute to those interactions, was a considerable task. The simplified explanation for the two-burst structure given above has appealed to idealized descriptions of single-bubble cavitation, and very simplified concepts of scattering from the stone. Since its discovery [1], a range of authors exploited this two-burst structure in ingenious ways [14-17]. One might therefore ask whether the device outlined in this paper relies on cavitation being the major cause of stone fragmentation in order to operate effectively. The answer to this question is no. The cavitational interpretation of the passive acoustic emission was used as a starting point, acting rather as the first 'stepping stone' rather than a 'bridge' between the concept of this device and the implementation of this device in the clinic.

Coleman *et al.* [1] had access to a narrow-band passive acoustic detector, but proposed that use of a wide-band receiver might detect useful resonances. Prior to the clinical trials, the research effort investigated both the information that was available in the time-history of the passive acoustic emissions, and also the information available in the spectral representation (Figure 4), and the time-frequency representation (Figure 5). Data were taken both *in vitro* and *in vivo* [4,9-11,21].

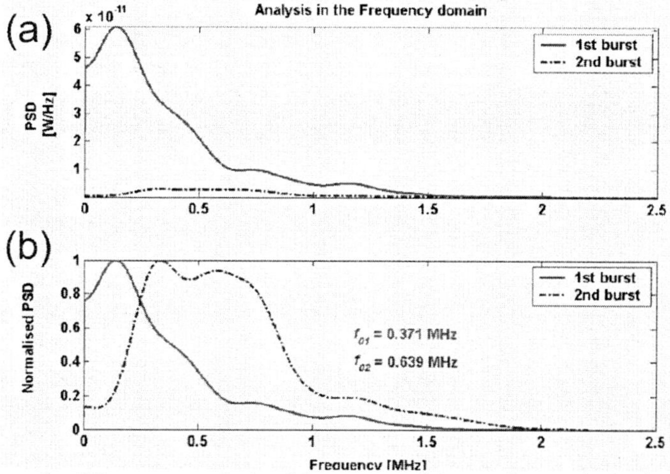

FIGURE 4. Example of frequency analysis of the content of the two bursts obtained *in vitro* from tap water, shown with same absolute reference in (a), but in (b) the same data is shown with the spectrum of each burst normalised to the peak for that burst (effectively increasing the gain for the second burst data). The data were taken prior to the development of the final prototype sensor used in the clinical trials, using a sensor developed at the UK National Physical Laboratory (see [11] for details). With these data the algorithm (Fedele [11]) for detecting the central frequency for the first burst gives an answer of f_{01} =0.371 MHz, and for the central frequency of the second burst it provides f_{02} =0.639 MHz. However such analysis needs to be treated with caution, as the calculated frequencies can be strongly influenced by factors not present in the raw data (see text). Figure reproduced from Fedele *et al.*, 2004 [21]. For further details see Fedele [11].

Although the spectral characteristics of the passive acoustic emissions were investigated as a way of providing a diagnostic of stone fragmentation, and initially provided promising results [9-11,20-21], they proved to be a significantly less reliable method *in vivo* for the device built for this study than was characterization using the time history (see below). It is important to emphasize that this does not imply that a different device, designed specifically for spectral characterisation *in vivo*, might not provide useful information. Owen *et al.* [18] have through careful experimentation exploited the spectral characteristics of such passive acoustic emissions successfully to distinguish *in vitro* between complete and dissected glass spheres at the focus of a lithotripter, and tracked changes in model stone size [19].

The problems encountered with the device of the current study, and which a device designed to exploit spectral characteristics *in vivo* should be designed to counter, are as follows.

Consider Figure 4. Whilst the prototype transducer for use in the clinical trials was being developed, a range of earlier prototypes and other sensors were tested to inform the design process. The data of Figure 4 were taken in tap water using a sensor developed by the UK National Physical Laboratory, which was positioned so as to be primarily sensitive to the region at the lithotripter focus. An algorithm readily provides estimates for the central frequencies of the first and second bursts (f_{01} and f_{02} respectively). However such analysis needs to be treated with caution. To prevent the EM noise from the lithotripter source from dominating the signal, a 200 kHz high-pass filter was used. The peak for the first burst in Figure 4 is below this frequency, so that the central frequency calculated from these data for the first burst will be strongly influenced by the characteristics of the filter.

The spectrum of the second burst appears to show considerable frequency content above the 200 kHz setting of the high pass filter. A weighted average of the energy in this burst provides a sensible estimate for f_{02}. However when such a procedure was attempted *in vivo*, the signal-to-noise ratio above ~500 kHz was significantly reduced, so that the calculated value of f_{02} became heavily dependent upon the upper frequency limit chosen for the averaging [11].

Artificial factors such as these tend to become more problematic (for both the first and second burst) as the signal-to-noise ratio deteriorates, and therefore it was not unsurprising that *in vivo* the spectral characteristics proved to be less useful in discrimination than did the temporal ones for our device. Even *in vitro*, when faced with asymmetric mineral shapes, the initially promising spectral discrimination [11,20] showed less promise than did the time history in being reduced to simple parameters for an automated system to use [9-10,20-21]. For example, the trends in the central frequencies in Figure 6(a) are less significant (when the uncertainties in the error bars are taken into account) than the trends in the time histories for the same data (Figure 6(b)). Therefore the clinical studies were based on parameterization of the time histories rather than the spectral information (recalling however that this does not imply that devices specifically designed to rely on spectral information *in vivo* may not prove to be effective [18,19]).

The remainder of the paper will therefore describe how three automated measurements of the time history were reduced to two parameters to allow automated diagnosis.

Aims and Objectives

To summarise, the goal of this project was to develop a passive 'listening device' (in the form of a single sensor transducer, for simplicity and to minimize cost) which can report, in real-time, the 'effectiveness' of each shock during ESWL, where the 'effectiveness' is judged on two points:

(i) Is the shock on-target (i.e. hitting the stone)?

(ii) Did the shock contribute to stone fragmentation?

Our Ethics permission forbade us from providing operator with any information (in case it altered treatment, or skewed results). Hence the following longer-term objectives could not be included in this study:

- To provide an alternative to using a preset number of shocks;
- To alert operator in real time to the possible need to check targeting;
- To reduce morbidity by reducing exposure to minimum required;
- To reduce retreatment rates (currently at 30-50%).

(a)

(b)

(c)

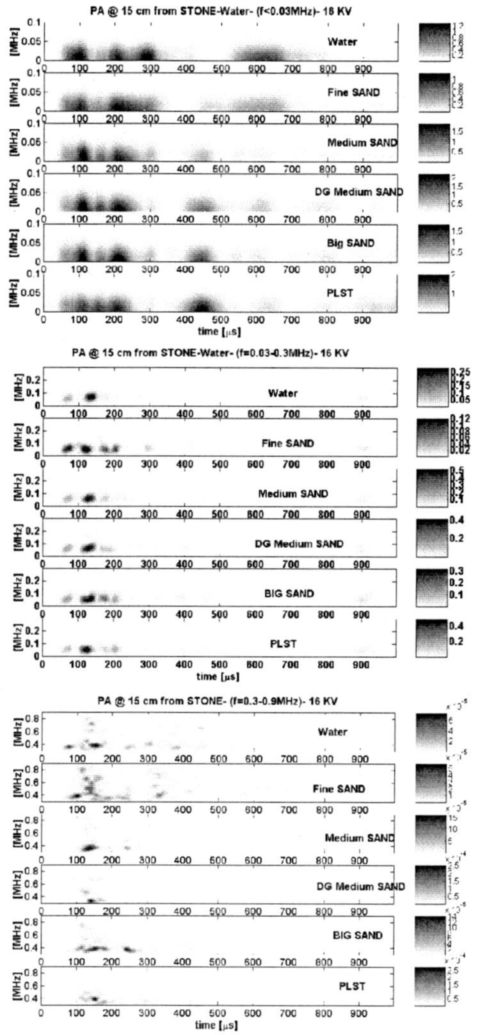

FIGURE 5. Examples of passive signals in time-frequency representation for (a) very low frequency (VLF, <30 kHz); (b) low frequency (LF, 30-300 kHz); and (c) high frequency (HF, 300-900 kHz) bands. Six subplots within (a), (b) and (c) represent *in vitro* scatter from different target materials, using equal volumes of each (33.5 ml), and consisting of (from the bottom upwards, with fragments sizes selected sieves): PLST (Plaster of Paris made using a ratio plaster:water of 2:1 and injected into the target holder in the liquid state by a syringe avoiding air entrainment); Big sand (diameters of 10-30 mm); Medium sand (diameters of 4-10 mm, where DG implies the degassed samples—all other samples are immersed in tap water); Fine sand (diameters of 1- 4 mm). Figure from Leighton *et al.*, 2004 [20]. The data were recorded using one of the prototype clinical sensors developed in this study (Mark I, [11]). The raw data were filtered digitally using Butterworth filters. For further details see Fedele [11].

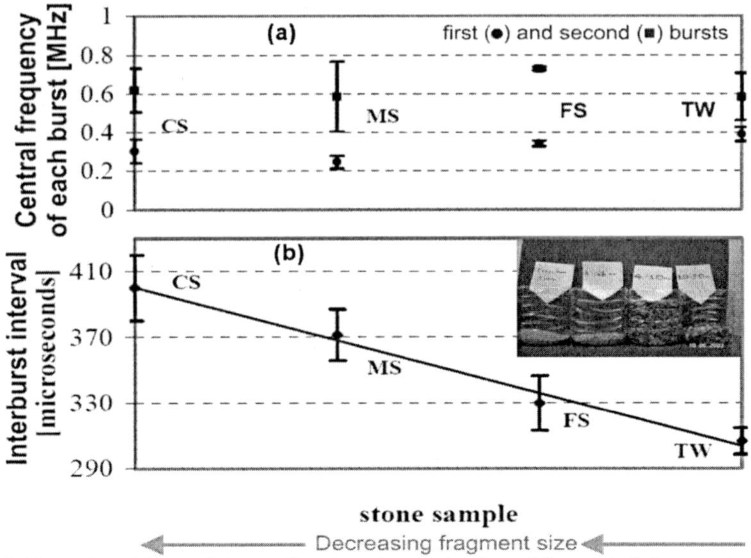

FIGURE 6. Example of the variation with mineral particle size of the central frequencies of the first (f_{01}) and second (f_{02}) bursts, taken with the NPL prototype and a 200 kHz high pass filter (see Fedele [11] for details). A ping-pong ball sample holder contained tap-water (TW), or various samples of stone. Samples of the latter are shown in the inset to part (b) in the following order, from left to right: a very fine sand sample with grain diameter of less than 1 mm is shown on the far left; second from the left is fine sand (FS, grain diameter 1-4 mm); second from the right is medium sand (MS; grain diameter 4-10 mm); on the far right is coarse sand (CS; grain diameter 10-30 mm). Figure reproduced from Fedele *et al.*, 2004 [10,21]. For further details see Fedele *et al.* [9-11].

Given these restrictions, although the device does provide real-time feedback, the ethics permission only allowed us to compare the end-of-treatment score automatically generated by the acoustic system (TS_0) with the treatment score provided by the consultant urologist at the three-week follow-up appointment (CTS_2).

METHODS

Two clinical trials of the device were undertaken (named 'phase 1' and 'phase 2'). [13]. In preparation for these, extensive development stages were conducted. These included the development of the hardware (Figure 7). Informed by input from the CFD simulations [5-7,12], the preparatory stages before the two clinical trials also included the testing of the method *in vitro* and on 51 test subjects *in vivo* [9-12].

The decision as to whether a shock is 'effective' or not, is based on a set of 'rules' (Figure 8). The process by which these rules were derived was detailed elsewhere [9-13]. However a simplified explanation is outlined schematically in Figs. 9 and 10, and will now be described. Bear in mind the comments in the 'Background' section that, whilst this simplified explanation of the rules relies on a cavitational interpretation, this does not mean that for the device to work, cavitation must be the dominant mechanism for stone fragmentation.

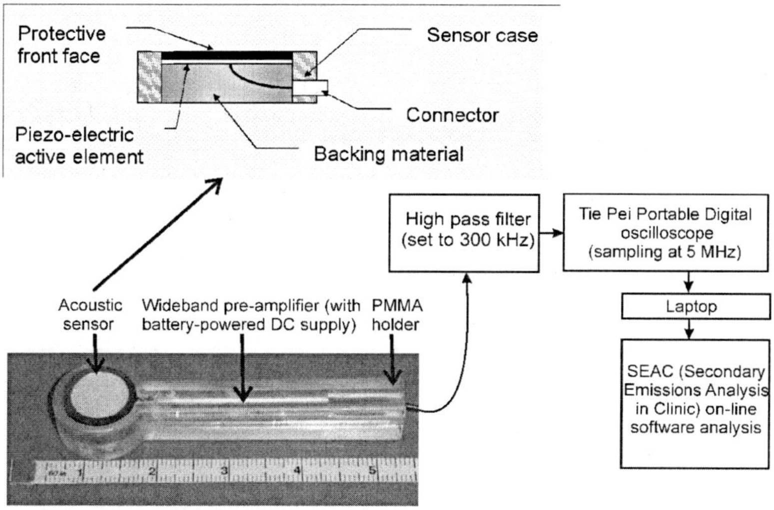

FIGURE 7. Schematic of the apparatus. The signal from the transducer and pre-amplifier (manufactured by Precision Acoustics Ltd.) is high-pass filtered to reduce noise and captured by a portable oscilloscope before being analysed on the laptop using the SEAC (Secondary Emissions Analysis in Clinic) on-line software (see Figure 13). Figure reproduced with permission from [13].

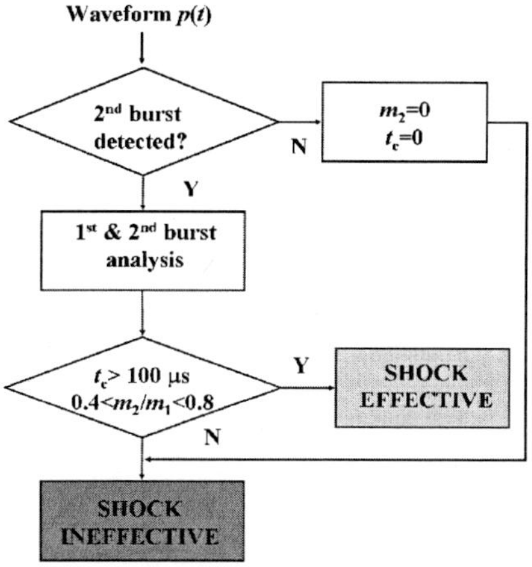

FIGURE 8. A block-diagram of the Secondary Emissions Analysis (SEAC) software. The detected acoustic emission is processed, making use of clinically derived data on the acoustic parameters m_2 / m_1 and t_c, to generate an indication to the operator of the 'effectiveness' of a shock (the 'rules' displayed in the lower diamond correspond to those determined by phase 1 for use in phase 2). Figure reproduced with permission from reference [13].

Figure 9 illustrates a simple interpretation of the two-burst structure outlined in the Introduction. An amplitude m_1 is assigned to the first burst (the temporal peak within the burst is chosen, although a pulse average system could also be used). The interburst period t_c (calculated through a weighted function described in reference [13]) corresponds to the collective prolonged expansion phases of the bubble cloud, after which comes the second burst which has an amplitude m_2. High values of both t_c and m_2 could be taken to indicate strong cavitation, whilst weak cavitation would produce low values of both. The first burst contains components both of the reflection of the incident lithotripter shock wave from the stone, information about the waves which propagate within the stone as a result of ESWL, and cavitation: if, for example the lithotripter shock wave were to miss the stone, a reduction in the reflection component would reduce the value of m_1 (in the same way in which, if a railway worker hits a hammer against the wheel of a locomotive to test for its integrity through its passive emissions, no such emissions are generated if the worker misses the wheel with the hammer - although of course when lithotripter shocks are projected into the body, other scattering sources contribute to m_1 when the stone is not at the focus).

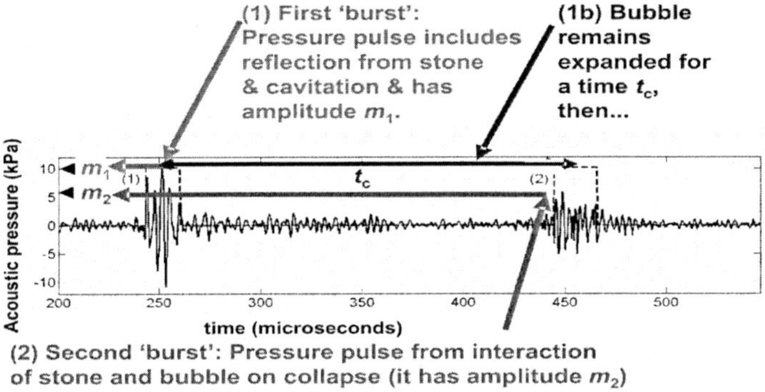

FIGURE 9. Simplified interpretation of a time-history of the detected passive emissions. This emission was recorded *in vivo* using the final clinical prototype (Mark III), and the conditioning system developed in this study. The clinical data acquisition system (that includes the sensor Mark III, a high pass filter at 300 kHz and a preamplifier) is described in reference [11].

Figure 10 shows how the simple interpretation of the time history (Figure 9) can be used to make simplistic predictions about the factors which influence the values of m_1, m_2 and t_c recorded in response to each lithotripter shock wave. To normalize the amplitude results to account for differing sizes of patients, different lithotripter energy levels and coupling efficiencies, the ratio m_2/m_1 is calculated for each shock echo, and this ratio is plotted against t_c. In this way, in real time as each ESWL shock is delivered during a treatment, a point is added to the plot of m_2/m_1 against t_c: if that point falls within a box (the 'strike zone', as shown by the dotted lines on Figure 10), then the shock is taken to have been 'effective'. However if the point falls out of the 'strike zone', the shock is taken to be 'ineffective'.

In this way, the system builds up a real-time picture of how the treatment is progressing. In this idealized scheme, if for example the stone moved out of the focus, the value of m_1 would fall because of the reduction in the reflected component of the incident shock wave. This would cause an increase in m_2/m_1 and the point would fall above the 'strike zone' (as indicated for many of the points in Figure 10). In an alternative scenario, if weak cavitation occurred, both m_2 and t_c would decrease, such that the points would ideally fall below and to the left of the 'strike zone'. If the algorithm fails to detect two distinct bursts in the echo, then both m_2/m_1 and t_c are conventionally equalled to zero, and a point is placed on the origin of the graph shown schematically in Figure 10 (see reference [13] for details).

Having established the principle that an 'effective' shock would result in an echo placed within a 'strike zone' drawn on a graph of m_2/m_1 against t_c, and an 'ineffective' would result in an echo placed outside of this box, the two clinical studies (phase 1 and phase 2) were undertaken.

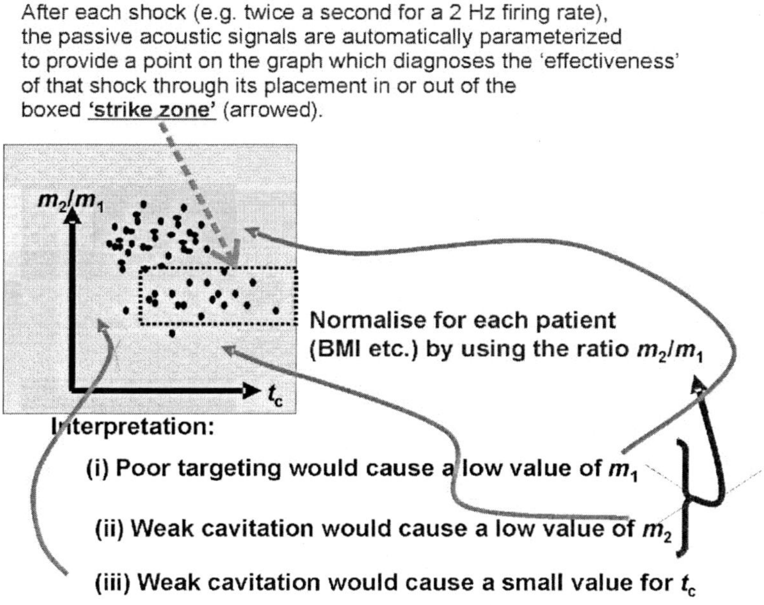

FIGURE 10. Simplified interpretation of how the physical parameters affect the placing of the points (parameterized in terms of m_1, m_2 and t_c) recorded after each ESWL shock (assumed to be acquired two a second for an assumed 2 Hz firing rate). The curved arrows (shown red in the colour version) indicate idealized scenarios (described in the text) through which the points might fall outside of the box (the 'strike zone', shown by dashed lines), indicating that these were 'ineffective' shocks (see text). Readers should note that this is a simplification and are directed to reference [7] for a more rigorous description.

CLINICAL STUDIES

The two clinical studies reported in this paper were carried out by the Medical Physics Department at Guy's & St Thomas' NHS Trust, London on patients treated for stones either in the renal pelvis or the calices on Storz Modulith SLX lithotripter

(Storz Medical AG, Tägerwilen, Switzerland) located in the Stone Unit of the same Trust. The studies received ethics approval and the first study (phase 1) commenced in April 2006 and, together with the phase 2 study, lasted 15 months. The scope of the ethics approval did not allow the ESWL operator to alter the treatments in any way in response to information provided by the output of the passive acoustic device. The study aim was confined, therefore, to examining the correlation between the acoustic data and the clinical outcome. The object of the phase 1 study was to build on the *in vitro* and CFD results to finalise the rules for determining the effectiveness of each shock. In phase 2, these rules were implemented and the system was validated.

A total of 118 patients consented to take part in phase 1. Shock-by-shock sequences of acoustic data from the sensor were retained for the analysis of each treatment. A clinical follow-up three weeks after treatment was obtained for 67 of these subjects in phase 1 (of the remainder, 18 subjects could not tolerate the procedure, for 3 patients the pre-treatment and post-treatment X-Rays were not of adequate quality for reporting, and in 30 further cases the patients failed to return for the follow-up appointment). The acoustic data from these 67 subjects were examined, and a further 37 of these subjects were excluded on the basis that the recorded sequences of the patient in question represented less than 30% of the shocks administered to that patient during the treatment session (phase 1 was used not only to test the 'rules' for the diagnosis, but also to test and enhance the ruggedness of the hardware and software and the procedure by which the nurse recorded ancillary data – such as the lithotripter setting – during the treatment). The remaining 30 subjects constituted the group retained for phase 1 analysis. This high recruitment attrition rate reflected, as explained above, a relatively high incidence of equipment issues early on in the study as well as administrative difficulties in getting X-rays reported. The final group of 30 subjects had an average ($\pm$ 2 standard deviations) of 2473 $\pm$ 1204 shocks administered during treatment using the Storz Modulith. Energy settings from 1 to 6 were used.

A total of 85 patients were recruited to phase 2, of which 49 satisfied the two conditions required for their acoustic data to be included in the trial: firstly, a complete clinical follow-up at three weeks was available; and, secondly, the recorded sequences for each patient represented at least 30% of shocks given to that patient during the treatment session. The attrition rate in phase 2 was considerably better than in phase 1 owing to improved experience with the passive acoustic system. To be specific, treatment was not tolerated by 3 patients, no follow-up was available for 16 patients, and in a further 2 cases the X-rays were of poor quality and could not be interpreted. The equipment was damaged for 15 cases.

The average number of shocks administered in the phase 2 group was similar to that in phase 1, at 2461 $\pm$ 1160. Energy settings from 1 to 6 were used. The operators favoured setting 4 for the majority of treatments in both phase 1 and 2, although some variation occurred in all cases at the start and following realignment of the stone and in some cases higher settings were used.

Leighton *et al.* [13] analyze the results of the two clinical phases separately. This is the appropriate method since the results of phase 1 are used to define the rules, and the results of phase 2 are used to test the rules. For this paper the authors were asked that the data from the two phases be presented in a combined plot, rather than presenting the data from the two phases separately. This is done in Figure 11. However it is noted that Figure 11(a) does include an element of circular argument, since use of the plot to test the effectiveness of the rules would include some of the data that were used to draw up those rules. Readers wishing to see the separate plots are directed to Leighton *et al.* [13].

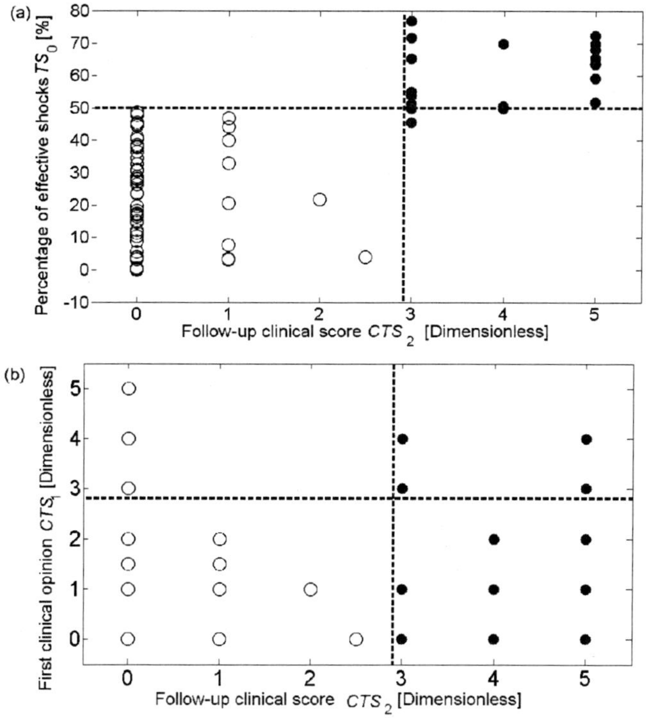

FIGURE 11. The combined results of the phase1 and phase 2 clinical studies. Each point represents a single treatment. The abscissa of both plots (a) and (b) indicates the CTS_2 score, the 'gold standard' provided by the urologist at the three-week follow-up. Using this gold standard, the solid circles indicate 'successful' treatments (i.e. $CTS_2 \geq 3$) and the open circles indicate 'unsuccessful' treatments (i.e. $CTS_2 < 3$), a vertical dashed line showing this demarcation. Both plots contain 79 points, although fewer are visible in (b) because the quantization of the scoring generates overlaps (two patients score CTS_1=3 with CTS_2=5; two patients score CTS_1=3 with CTS_2 =0; three patients score CTS_1=4, CTS_2=5; four patients score CTS_1=2 with CTS_2=0; four patients score CTS_1=1 with CTS_2=1; five patients score CTS_1=1 with CTS_2=3; thirteen patients score CTS_1=1 with CTS_2=0; twenty-nine patients score CTS_1= CTS_2=0). Plot (a) compares the treatment score from the acoustic device (TS_0) with CTS_2. The horizontal dashed line indicates the $TS_0 \geq 50\%$ delineator. Plot (b) does a similar comparison against CTS_2, but this time for the radiographer's initial clinical treatment score, CTS_1. The horizontal line in (b) distinguishes the radiographer's estimate of 'successful' treatments (i.e. $CTS_1 \geq 3$) from the radiographer's assessment of an 'unsuccessful' treatment (i.e. $CTS_1 < 3$). See reference [13] for details of the individual phases which are combined to generate this plot.

Figure 11(a) indicates that the clinical trials showed the acoustic device to be successful. It plots the device-derived score, TS_0 (which is given by the percentage of shocks that lay within the strike zone at the end of treatment) against the gold standard treatment score, CTS_2 (detailed in the following subsection). Compared with the gold standard CTS_2, over the two clinical trials (79 patients) the device-derived score (TS_0) correctly predicted the clinical effectiveness of the treatment for 78 for the 79 patients (the error occurred on a difficult patient with a high body mass index). In comparison, using the current available technology the in-theatre clinician (the radiographer) provided a treatment score CTS_1 which correctly predicted the outcome of only 61 of the 79 therapies (Figure 11(b)). In particular the passive acoustic device correctly predicted 18 of the 19 treatments that were successful (i.e. 94.7 sensitivity), whilst the current technology enabled the in-theatre clinician to predict only 7 of the 19 successful treatments (i.e. 36.8 sensitivity).

Details of the conduct and results of the separate Phase 1 and Phase 2 clinical studies (including details of how CTS_1 and CTS_2 were attained) are provided in the following subsections.

Phase 1 clinical study

In addition to the testing of the hardware, the software and the procedures described above, there were two main goals for the phase 1 study. Both of these goals refer to providing the device with the ability automatically to estimate the success of a treatment (either at the end-of-treatment (TS_0), or during treatment when a significant proportion of shocks have been delivered ($TS(t)$)). They are described below.

The first goal of phase 1 was to define the limits of the strike zone for *in vivo* data. The appropriate limits to define the 'strike zone' for *in vitro* studies had been determined earlier [9,12,13]. However it was important in phase 1 to determine how these limits needed to be adjusted to define the 'strike zone' for *in vivo* measurements.

Specifically, the *in vitro* tests indicated that a possible criterion for determining if a shock had been 'effective' in targeting and fragmenting the stone could be based on the requirement that m_2/m_1>0.4 and t_c~300 μs [9,12,13]. However shorter collapse times could be expected *in vivo* [14]. Therefore phase 1 of the clinical studies examined the validity and application of these 'rules' to the *in vivo* tests. In phase 1, a complete set of acoustic and clinical data was obtained in 30 of the 118 subjects recruited (see above). On the basis of these data it was decided to alter the *in vitro* 'rules' for *in vivo* use such that an 'effective' shock is defined as one in which both $0.40 < m_2/m_1 < 0.8$ and $t_c > 100$ μs. These rules define the limits of the strike zone in Figure 12.

From the preceding discussion, it might be expected that the 'successful' treatments would tend to generate echoes which cluster in this strike zone. To test this hypothesis, a 'gold standard' method (mentioned above) was required for assessing whether a treatment had been successful. This 'gold standard' judgment was arrived at through use of a treatment score, CTS_2, which was provided by the consultant urologist at the 3-weeks patient's follow-up appointment. The CTS_2 score was taken to be the 'gold standard' since the clinical decision on the need for further treatment was based on this. To obtain CTS_2, a form was devised (see Leighton *et al.* [13]) which guided the urologist to base the treatment score for this study on the X-ray images alone. In assessing the need for further treatment, the urologist may in fact take into account other data available at the three-week follow-up (e.g. any reduction in the sensation of pain, comments by the patient on the passing of stone fragments). However, these issues were not used in our study to provide the treatment score CTS_2, as the comparisons involving the latter required an objective and quantitative measure. As a result, the form was designed such that the clinician used only the X-ray image when providing CTS_2.

The judgment of the radiographer immediately at the end of treatment was used to provide the other clinical treatment score CTS_1 - this score was not treated as a 'gold standard' but simply used to compare the judgments of the radiographer at the end of treatment, with the CTS_2 judgment of the urologist at the three-week follow-up. The form for CTS_1 was also designed so that only the X-ray image was used to inform this treatment score.

Details of the forms and the methods used to collect CTS_1 and CTS_2 from the clinicians are given in Leighton *et al.* [13]. Both clinicians used a six point scale of clinical treatment scores (0-5) based on the degree of stone fragmentation (and made without knowledge of the output of the passive acoustic system). They were qualitatively judged by the lithotripter operator, from the X-ray at the end of the treatment (CTS_1), and at the three week follow-up appointment (CTS_2) by a urologist, with '0' indicating no fragmentation, '3' indicating 50% fragmentation and '5' complete fragmentation.

Examination of the data for the two patients shown in Figure 12 reveals that, as expected, the successful treatment (Figure 12(a), judged successful because this treatment was awarded CTS_2=5) indeed shows greater clustering of points within the strike zone than occurs with the unsuccessful treatment (Figure 12(a), for which CTS_2=0). Note also that the process by which the algorithm places particularly 'unsuccessful' points on the origin, detected no such points in the 'successful' treatment of Figure 12(a), but detected 629 such points for the 'unsuccessful' treatment of Figure 12(b).

The second goal of the phase 1 study was to assess what proportion of the shocks in a given treatment need to be 'effective' for the treatment as a whole to be judged as being 'successful' by the acoustic system. The percentage of shocks at the end of a treatment which fell into the strike zone was termed TS_0, and the treatments of Figure 12(a) and 12(b) exhibited TS_0=70% and 20% respectively. In consultation with the clinicians, it was decided that the comparison between the different treatment scores should be based on a bi-modal verdict (in that $CTS_2 \geq 3$ could be termed a successful treatment, and $CTS_2<3$ indicated an unsuccessful treatment). Given this protocol, the critical value for TS_0 to divide between successful and unsuccessful treatments was assessed to be 50%, such that scores of $TS_0 \geq 50\%$ can be usefully classified as 'successful' (see Leighton *et al.* [13] for details of the reasoning). This hypothesis was tested in the Phase 2 clinical study.

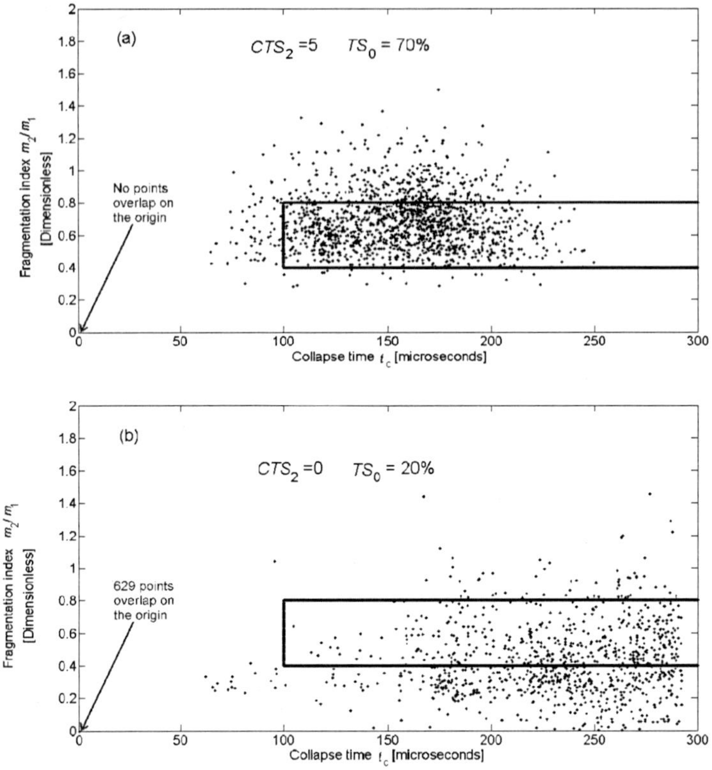

FIGURE 12. Plots from phase 1 of the clinical study giving the values of the acoustic parameters m_2 / m_1 and t_c for each shock from two sample treatments. The first plot (a) is for a 'successful' treatment, as classified by the clinician from the X-rays (CTS_2=5); the second plot (b) is for an 'unsuccessful' treatment as classified by the clinician from the X-rays (CTS_2=0). The area delimited by the solid line ($0.4 < m_2 / m_1 < 0.8$ and $t_c > 100$ μs) represents the semi-empirical rules that appear from the phase 1 study to give the optimum indication of 'effective' and 'ineffective' shocks. It is postulated from the phase 1 study that a large number of 'effective' shocks (i.e. falling within the solid lines) result in a 'successful' treatment. Note that whilst Figure 12(a) contains no points at the origin, Figure 12(b) contains 629 overlapping points at the origin (see the text for explanation; further details can be found in Leighton *et al.* [13]). Figure reproduced with permission from reference [13].

Phase 2 clinical study

Having in phase 1 defined the rules by which the strike zone is delineated ($0.40 < m_2/m_1 < 0.8$ and $t_c > 100$ μs), and the threshold value of TS_0 which will be used to judge whether the acoustic sensor considers the treatment to have been successful (TS_0=50%), the phase 2 clinical study proceeded to test these criteria on 49 of the 85 subjects that were originally recruited. The increased capture rate (59% of the original 85, compared to 25% of the 118 patients who consented to take part in phase 1) reflects a greater robustness of the equipment and a greater familiarity of the nurse with the system. In fact, one reason why only a proportion of shocks in a given treatment were captured arose because, when the operator changed the setting on the lithotripter, the nurse manually had to enter the new setting into the recording software, a task which resulted in some loss of data (and which could be avoided if the device were to be interfaced with the ESWL to detect the setting automatically).

The recording software consisted of a custom-made SEAC (Secondary Emissions Analysis in Clinic) interface. Although the Ethics approval for this clinical work only allowed comparison of the final TS_0 score against the CTS_2 gold standard score given 3 weeks after treatment, the SEAC software provided a real-time display which showed: (i) a cumulative indication of the success of the therapy delivered at any point during a single treatment session (the score $TS(t)$, the proportion of shocks so far in a treatment which were 'effective', and which equals TS_0 at the end of the treatment); and (ii) several features that reflect the ongoing acoustic verdict of the performance of each shock as it is delivered. Several of the latter are featured in Figure 13, which is a screen shot of the SEAC output, with dashed lines added to facilitate the explanation. These dashed lines divide the screen shot into boxes, numbered (1) to (5). A movie of the software running is available at the web site http://www.isvr.soton.ac.uk/fdag/Litho_07/litho_07(main).htm and at the *Ultrasound in Medicine and Biology* website (http://www.umbjournal.org), on the page associated with reference [13].

The SEAC software allows storage of patient identification details (Box 1) and control of the waveform capture via oscilloscope settings (Box 2). Waveform acquisition is triggered from the electromagnetic pickup detected on the generation of each shock, and the 'Analysis start time' slider in Box 2 ensured that there was sufficient delay after triggering to eliminate the electromagnetic signal from the analysis. The lithotripter source power level or setting is manually entered, and displayed in Box 2 along with a virtual red/green 'traffic-light' indicator at the bottom right-hand corner of Box 2. This light is automatically updated after every shock to provide the ESWL operator with real-time feedback as to whether the previous shock has been effective, so that for example a sustained red display in this indicator could prompt the operator to consider re-targeting the stone.

Box 3 in Figure 13 was included to allow additional digital filtering of the data either to improve the signal to noise ratio or to look only at specific frequency components. This option was disabled for the current study. Box 4 records a count of the number of shocks administered and information on software-equipment synchronisation. A *Test On* button (in Box 4) allowed the software to run in test mode (i.e. without saving any data), to check the appropriate settings to use for the specific treatment before starting the acquisition and storage of large quantities of data in the form of voltage waveforms for each shock. The *Start* button began the acquisition of data, and is replaced by a *Stop* button during acquisition.

The end-of-treatment quantitative treatment score (TS_0) is shown in the pop-up window (Box 5). In addition, the graph on the lower left of the screen in Figure 13 shows the waveform captured by the passive acoustic sensor from each shock. It provides a visual clue to the operator as to the ongoing functioning of the acoustic system. The two graphs stacked one-above-another on the lower right of the screen in

Figure 13 plot the single-shock values of m_2/m_1 (upper panel, open circles) and t_c (lower panel, grey crosses) as a visual guide to trends in the effectiveness of a set of shocks. To reiterate a key point, ethics permission would not allow these real time indicators of the effectiveness of the treatment to be communicated to the therapist, and assessments of the equipment performance could only be made by comparing the acoustic score at the end of the treatment (TS_0) with the gold standard delivered three weeks later by the urologist.

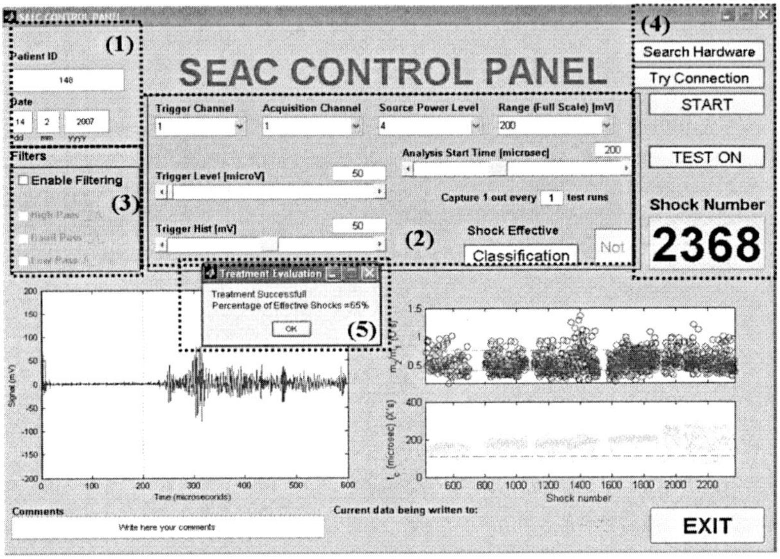

FIGURE 13. A screen shot of the output of the SEAC software interface used by the ESWL operator during phase 2 of the project. The dotted lines demarcating numbered boxes have been added to identify areas in the display (see text for details). Box 5 gives an indication of the percentage of the 2368 shocks given in this treatment which were effective at damaging the stone (TS_0). A score here of 65% indicates a successful treatment. The values of the acoustic parameters (m_2 / m_1 and t_c) for each shock are shown in the graphs on the bottom right hand side of the interface, allowing trends to be noted. The bottom left panel plots the echo time history of the most recent shock, to allow assessment of the extent to which it conforms with the expected structure (noting however from Leighton *et al.* [13] that visual inspection is not as reliable at spotting two-burst structures as plots of the energy time history). In addition to these, there are three other display outputs from SEAC, and these are particularly important. The first of these is the treatment score TS_0 obtained at the end of the treatment (Box 5, described above); the second is the cumulative ratio $TS(t)$ of effective shocks to the total number of shocks given from the start of the treatment to any point during it (which equals TS_0 at the end of treatment); the third indicator is the red/green indicator light which provides feedback on the most recent shock. Trends in these are available (e.g. via the two graphs on the bottom right of the screen). Figure reproduced with permission from reference [13].

This comparison was undertaken in phase 2, using the rules derived in phase 1 (that the strike zone is defined by $0.40 < m_2/m_1 < 0.8$ and $t_c > 100$ μs, and that the acoustic results indicate a successful treatment if $TS_0 \geq 50\%$). The second clinical study (Phase 2) demonstrated almost perfect agreement (kappa=0.94) between the number of 'successful' treatments, defined as greater than 50% fragmentation as determined by X-ray at the follow-up appointment, and the device-derived global treatment score, TS_0. The acoustic system is shown to provide a test of the 'success' of the treatment that has a sensitivity of 91.7% (in that the acoustic device identified $TS_0 \geq 50\%$ for 11 of the 12 treatments for which $CTS_2 \geq 3$) and a specificity of 100% (in that the acoustic device gave $TS_0 < 50\%$ for all of the 37 treatments for which $CTS_2 < 3$). In contrast, the degree of agreement between the two clinical scores CTS_1 and CTS_2 was similar to that found in phase 1. This level of agreement was quantified in this case by kappa=0.38.

Monitoring the effects of respiration

It has previously been suggested [22,23] that the depth of respiration could affect the clinical outcome. The device was used to demonstrate *in vivo* the sensitivity of the passive acoustic sensor to factors that influence targeting. The study is detailed in Leighton *et al.* [13].

Passive acoustic monitoring could possibly be used to provide a real-time check the effectiveness of a system which is designed to use respiration as a trigger for shock production in order to improve targeting, as issue which may be more critical for devices which use small foci rather than wide focus lithotripters [24].

CONCLUSIONS

This paper describes the sequence of studies that led to the first passive acoustic detector for the efficacy of ESWL treatment, which has been proven in clinical trials. The scope of the ethical approval did not allow the output of the sensor to be communicated in theatre to the clinicians. Therefore, we were prevented from testing whether the use of the device affects re-treatment rates. However the study has indicated the clinical usefulness of this technology: in the phase 2 study, the end-of-treatment score (automatically provided in real time by the device) correlated well with the judgment of the consultant urologist given at the patient's 3-week follow-up (kappa=0.94). In particular, this correlation is much better than that between the judgement of the urologist and the end-of-treatment opinion of the radiographer (kappa=0.38 in phase 2). In addition, for the 49 treatments in the second clinical study, the passive acoustic device demonstrated a sensitivity of 91.7% and a specificity of 100%.

The passive acoustic detector provides feedback from acoustic signals *within the patient* as to the interaction between the shock and the tissue. Such passive monitoring offers a range of benefits. At the simplest level, it monitors whether the shock enters the body or whether the shock amplitude reaching the tissue has been degraded, e.g. as a result of poor coupling or loss of coupling (through loss of contact, or bubble formation in the coupling gel). Perturbations on the treatment can be monitored in real time (the example of ventilation has been studied with this device). The current manifestation of the device was designed to be simple and robust: a single unfocused receiver is required, which is robust with respect to use (e.g. placement of the patient), and the operation and the verdict of the device are automatically computed. The data for the clinical studies reported here were obtained by a nurse operating the device. Further discussions of the implications of this technology are given in reference [13].

ACKNOWLEDGMENTS

The Engineering and Physical Sciences Research Council provided a grant from 2000 to 2003 (EPSRC grant, GR/N19243/01, Principle Investigator: TG Leighton; Co-Investigator: AJ Coleman), which was followed by a further grant from 2005 to 2006 (Grant ref: EP/D503310/1; Principle Investigator: TG Leighton; Co-Investigator: AJ Coleman). However over this seventeen-year project, much of the work was undertaken without sponsorship (the average annual income to cover all costs was less than £20k). As such the project relied heavily on the generous donation of equipment and services from a range of munificent sources. From the partner company Precision Acoustics Ltd., T. Gill and D. Bell provided invaluable assistance in developing the passive sensor. R. Tiptaft, J. Glass, D. Phillips and T. Jessop (Urology Department at Guy's and St Thomas' NHS Trust) are gratefully acknowledged for their support during the clinical study. C. McKinnon (Centre for Enterprise and Innovation, University of Southampton) and T. Parlett (Intellectual Property Officer, Guy's & St Thomas' NHS Trust) are thanked for their work in the contractual and commercial aspects of this study. From ISVR, D. Finfer is thanked for assistance in software programming, G. T. Yim is thanked for his advice on computing hardware, and V. Humphrey is thanked for loan of interim replacement transducers and preamplifiers when the apparatus was sent for servicing. NHS Innovations London were kind enough to shortlist the device for their award. All clinical work was approved by the local research ethics committee of Guy's and St Thomas' NHS Foundation Trust.

REFERENCES

1. A. J. Coleman, M. J. Choi, J. E. Saunders and T. G. Leighton, *Ultrasound Med. Biol.* **18**, 267-281 (1992).
2. A. J. Coleman, M. Whitlock, T. G. Leighton, and J. E. Saunders, *Physics in Medicine and Biology* 38, 1545-1560 (1993).
3. T. G. Leighton, *The Acoustic Bubble.* Academic Press, London, 1994, pp. 458-463.
4. K. B. Cunningham, A. J. Coleman, T. G. Leighton, and P. R. White, *Acoustics Bulletin* **26**, 10-16 (2001).
5. T. G. Leighton, *International Journal of Modern Physics B*, **18**, 3267-314 (2004).
6. A. R. Jamaluddin, G. J. Ball, and T. G. Leighton, "Free-Lagrange simulations of shock/bubble interaction in shock wave lithotripsy," in *Proceedings of the Second International Conference on Computational Fluid Dynamics, ICCFD,* Sydney, Australia, 2002, pp. 541-546.
7. C. K. Turangan, A. R. Jamaluddin, G. J. Ball, and T. G. Leighton, *Journal of Fluid Mechanics*. **598**, 1-25 (2008).
8. T. G. Leighton, "From seas to surgeries, from babbling brooks to baby scans: Bubble acoustics at ISVR," in *Proceedings of the Institute of Acoustics*, **26**(1), 357-381 (2004).
9. F. Fedele, A. J. Coleman, T. G. Leighton, P. R. White and A. M. Hurrell, "Development of a new diagnostic sensor for extra-corporeal shock-wave lithotripsy", in *Proceedings of the First Conference in Advanced Metrology for Ultrasound in Medicine, Journal of Physics: Conference Series* **1**, 134-139 (2004).
10. F. Fedele, A. J. Coleman, T. G. Leighton, P. R. White and A. M. Hurrell, "Development of a new diagnostic device for extracorporeal shock-wave lithotripsy", in *Proceedings of the X MediterraneanConference on Medical and Biological Engineering "Health in the Information Society"*, Paper No. 54, 4pp (2004).
11. F. Fedele, "Acoustic sensing of renal stones fragmentation in extracorporeal shockwave lithotripsy", PhD thesis, University of Southampton (2008).

12. T. G. Leighton, F. Fedele, A. Coleman, C. Mccarthy, A. R. Jamaluddin, C. K. Turangan, G. J. Ball, S. Ryves, A. Hurrell, A. De Stefano and P. R. White, "The development of a passive acoustic device for monitoring the effectiveness of shockwave lithotripsy in real time", in *Proceedings of the 7th European Acoustics Association International Symposium on Hydroacoustics*, **11**, 159-180 (2008).
13. T. G. Leighton, F. Fedele, A. J. Coleman, C. McCarthy, S. Ryves, A. M. Hurrell, A. De Stefano, and P. R. White, "A device for monitoring the efficacy of ESWL using passive acoustic emissions," *Ultrasound in Medicine and Biology* (in press), 2008, doi:10.1016/j.ultrasmedbio.2008.03.011.
14. P. Zhong, I. Cioanta, F. H. Cocks and G. M. Preminger, *J. Acoust. Soc. Am.* **101**(1), 2940–2950 (1997).
15. R. O. Cleveland, O. A. Sapozhnikov, M. R. Bailey and L. A. Crum, *J. Acoust. Soc. Am.* **107**(3), 1745-1758 (2000).
16. T. J. Matula, P. R. Hilmo, M. R. Bailey and L. A. Crum, *Ultrasound Med. Biol.* **28**(9), 1199-1207 (2002).
17. M. R. Bailey, Y. A. Pishchalnikov, O. A. Sapozhnikov, R. O. Cleveland, J. A. McAteer, N. A. Miller, I. V. Pishchalnikova, B. A. Connors, L. A. Crum and A. P. Evan, *Ultrasound Med. Biol.* **31**(9), 1245-1256 (2005).
18. N. R. Owen, M. R. Bailey, L. A. Crum, O. A. Sapozhnikov and L. A. Trusov, *J. Acoust. Soc. Am.* **121**, EL41–EL46 (2007).
19. N. R. Owen, O. A. Sapozhnikov, M. R. Bailey, L. A. Trusov and L. A. Crum, "A passive technique to identify stone comminution during shock wave lithotripsy", in *Renal stone disease, Proceedings of the First Annual International Urolithiasis Research Symposium (ed. A. P. Evan, J. E. Lingeman, J. C. Williams Jr. AIP Conference Porccedings)*, pp. 364-367 (2007).
20. T. G. Leighton, A. J. Coleman, F. Fedele and P. R. White, A passive acoustic system for evaluating the in-vivo performance of extracorporeal shockwave lithotripsy, UK Patent Number 0319863.7 (2004).
21. F. Fedele, A. J. Coleman, T. G. Leighton, P. R. White and A. M. Hurrell, *Acoustics Bulletin* **29**, 34-39 (2004).
22. R. O. Cleveland, R. Anglade and R. K. Babayan, *J. Endourol.* **18**(7), 629-633 (2004).
23. M. A. Warner, M. E. Warner, C. F. Buck, J. W. Segura, *J. Urol.* **139**(3), 486-487 (1988).
24. W. Eisenmenger, X. X. Du, C. Tang, S. Zhao, Y. Wang, F. Rong, D. Dai, M. Guan and A. Qi, *Ultrasound Med. Biol.*, **28**(6), 769-774 (2002).

Perspective on Lithotripsy Adverse Effects

Thomas Knoll and Gunnar Wendt-Nordahl

Department of Urology, Mannheim University Hospital, Theodor-Kutzer-Ufer 1-3, 68135 Mannheim, Germany

Abstract. Shock wave lithotripsy (SWL) is an effective and without any doubt the least invasive procedure to treat upper urinary tract calculi. Acute complications are rarely reported and do not require specific treatment in most cases. However, one should be aware that energy levels sufficient for stone breakage are capable of damaging tissue as well, and significant hematoma—not only in the kidney but as well in surrounding organs—has been observed. Furthermore, only little is known about the long-term effects of SWL. Some authors have reported an increased incidence of hypertension and possibly also diabetes mellitus. Such chronic diseases—if indeed related to prior SWL—may be a late result of acute SWL-related trauma but the discussion on the underlying pathogenesis is controversial. Many factors have to be considered, such as the natural history of recurrent stone formers, technical principles of SWL, and differences in treatment protocols. Promising studies are currently underway to optimize stone breakage while limiting potential collateral damage. With this progress, SWL remains a safe treatment option for most urinary calculi.

Keywords: Shock wave lithotripsy, focal zone, hypertension, diabetes mellitus
PACS: 43.80.Sh

INTRODUCTION

Shock wave lithotripsy (SWL), introduced in the early 1980's into clinical practice, has revolutionized active treatment of urinary calculi. Open surgical treatments, routine procedures in those days, were replaced by this non-invasive procedure that allowed for removal of most stones in the ureter or kidney.

After this golden era, today SWL faces more difficult times. Endoscopy, primarily ureteroscopy, has been significantly improved and achieves excellent stone free rates (SFR) with complication rates coming close to those of SWL. At the same time concerns about potential long-term adverse effects of SWL like hypertension and diabetes mellitus have arisen.

This article will review current literature on acute and chronic adverse effects of SWL, potential technical explanations for unwanted energy delivery and possible developments to improve SWL in the future.

Acute Adverse Effects Of Shock Wave Lithotripsy

It is generally accepted that SWL treatment of urinary calculi is a reliable and safe procedure. Recent reports on lithotripsy using third generation devices describe acute

CP1049, *Renal Stone Disease 2, 2nd International Urolithiasis Research Symposium,*
edited by A. P. Evan, J. E. Lingeman, J. A. McAteer, and J. C. Williams, Jr.

complication rates less than 10% [1]. Main reasons for emergency admission are minor events due to pain or infection. Renal or perirenal hemorrhage is only seldom observed. However, there is no doubt that energies that are sufficient for stone breakage potentially have an impact on other structures within the focal zone. Major bleeding complications are rarely reported but can be life threatening if they occur [2].

Numerous studies have investigated the *in vitro* and *in vivo* effects of SWL and it is clear that energy application not only leads to morphological changes like rupture of organ structures, but also induces functional changes like vasoconstriction, alterations of the autonomous neural system or the release of cell mediators and hormones [3-6]. SWL causes acute disturbances of renal perfusion in terms of renal plasma flow and renal resistive index [6]. The underlying mechanisms of these changes are unclear and possibly multi-factorial by means of activation of neural systems, changes in plasma rennin activity or the release of potent vasoconstrictive substances like Big-Endothelin-1 [6,7]. The observations that changes in renal vascular perfusion also take place in the contralateral kidney underline the idea of a systemic response to SWL treatment [7]. Obviously SWL results in a more or less pronounced ischemic situation with consecutive formation of free radicals and lipid peroxidation [5,6]. Keeping in mind that many patients receive multiple recurrent SWL procedures, these effects may accumulate and could contribute to chronic changes.

It is of clinical value to identify patient groups with an increased risk of acute lithotripsy adverse effects. It is generally accepted that SWL is contraindicated in pregnant women and in patients with untreated coagulopathies [9,10]. But there is also some evidence that alterations in renal perfusion are more common in elderly patients [6]. Further studies have to evaluate whether these findings lead to a higher complication rate. However, most reports on SWL agree on favorable results in all subgroups.

Long-term Adverse Effects Of Shock Wave Lithotripsy

Hypertension

Very soon after its clinical introduction several reports suggested an increased rate of hypertension following SWL [3,11-12]. These studies were mostly designed in a retrospective or short-term follow-up fashion and others could not confirm this observation [13-15]. Several aspects may explain such controversial findings: 1. Different lithotripsy machines with different physical principles were used; 2. Follow-up was too short and the study cohort too small; and 3. Only distinct subgroups had a higher risk of developing hypertension. Hypertension is part of the symptoms of the so-called metabolic syndrome (including overweight, dyslipidaemia and diabetes mellitus), which is one of the major problems of industrialized countries. Recent studies strongly suggest that urinary stone disease is a result—if not a substantial part—of this condition [16]. It can therefore be assumed that hypertension is more common in patients with recurrent stone formation and excellent study designs are necessary to discern a substantial dependence of hypertension on prior SWL treatment. However, the observation of Janetschek *et al.* that hypertension is induced only in patients older than 60 yrs. supports the acute findings of Mitterberger *et al.* who reported more sustained alterations in renal perfusion in elderly patients [6,17]. Yokoyama *et al.* reported an increased rate of hypertension with increasing energies leading to the idea of optimizing treatment protocols to reduce SWL adverse effects [12].

Diabetes mellitus

Krambeck *et al.* started a new discussion on SWL safety when they published a 19 year retrospective follow-up study on lithotripsy adverse effects [18]. They reported a significantly higher incidence of hypertension and, for the first time, diabetes mellitus in patients that were treated for proximal ureteral or renal calculi with an unmodified Dornier HM3 in 1985. Although others have not yet confirmed this finding (*e.g.*, Sato *et al.* performed a comparable study that did not detect a higher incidence of hypertension or diabetes mellitus) many studies tried to evaluate possible mechanisms for this finding [19]. While hypertension might result from renal injury, diabetes mellitus was hypothesized to be a consequence of pancreatic collateral damage. The regular reports of acute pancreatitis after SWL demonstrate that such side effects can occur. However, in contrast to these acute effects, diabetes mellitus is a result of an insufficient endocrine system. As SWL is commonly used for the treatment of pancreatic duct stones, prevalence of diabetes mellitus should be significantly increased in such patients if SWL indeed caused endocrine insufficiency. However, the available short-term follow-up literature does not support this idea [20,21]. We performed a prospective evaluation of acute endocrine and exocrine effects of SWL for lower and upper urinary tract calculi and could not demonstrate any significant effect within 24 hours post SWL [22].

Only further prospective long-term studies with regular clinical visits and a detailed data management have the potential to give a definitive answer on such chronic SWL-related complications. Considering the little interest of funding organizations, it is questionable if such studies will ever be performed.

Technical considerations

The ideal focus of SWL is a spherical volume that covers only the region of interest and has no side effects outside this area. However, this ideal cannot be physically achieved with the available lithotripsy devices.

The focal zone, defined as the area of -6dB (50% of maximum energy pressure), differs significantly between the different lithotriptors. The HM3 has a cigar shaped focus of ~100 mm by ~12 mm that covers more than the region of interest, with potential side effects in front and behind the stone, while the focal zone of third generation machines like the Storz Medical SLX are smaller with 25x5 mm (but achieves higher peak energy pressures). In theory, this might lead to minimized side effects and an optimized efficiency. The latter has not been demonstrated so far; in contrast, the HM3 is still considered the golden standard by many urologists. Gerber *et al.* published a comparison of an unmodified HM3 with the Siemens Lithostar and the

Storz Medical SLX [23]. They reported a higher stone free rate and a smaller fragment size after treatment of renal calculi with the HM3. A critical issue of this study, however, is the treatment under general anesthesia with the HM3 and intravenous sedation with the Lithostar and the SLX. There is evidence that SWL success rate can be significantly better with general anesthesia [24].

It is important to realize that lithotripsy machines differ not only in the size of their focal zones, but as well in maximum peak pressures and size or shape of the acoustic reflectors. The electrohydraulic HM3 produces unfocussed shock waves (direct waves) that could have an impact on tissue outside the desired focal zone (in contrast to more recent electromagnetic lithotriptors). Such waves may lead to the formation of cavitation bubbles that are thought to be responsible for side effects like hemorrhage. Matlaga *et al.* recently demonstrated in an experimental *in vivo* setting that SWL after systemic injection of microbubbles leads to severe extrarenal trauma [25].

The impact of maximal peak pressure is often underestimated and the definition of the focal zone as the -6dB area seems questionable. Very recently a new machine has been introduced based on a very large focus, low-pressure principle that achieved excellent results [26]. While increasing peak pressure does not necessarily increase the -6dB zone, the area covered by energies sufficient for stone breakage largely increases. The definition of the focal zone as being limited by the 5 MPa zone seems to better reflect the area of biological effects. The discussion on small versus large focus and low versus high energy will surely continue.

Data from our lab did not support an impact of focal sizes or peak pressure when comparing the small and the large focus of the Storz Medical SLX-F2 [27]. However, we could confirm data that increasing shock wave numbers clearly have a negative impact on renal morphology.

Approaches To Limit Potential Adverse Effects

The mentioned data from our lab underlines that the amount of energy to be applied in SWL should be limited [27]. A further factor that seems to have a significant impact on SWL-related side effects is the rate of shock wave application. It has been demonstrated that a slower rate of 60 shocks/min does not only optimize the stone free rate but also reduces the probability of hemorrhage [28,29]. The underlying mechanism is not well understood but the observations might be related to the accumulation of cavitation bubbles.

A second interesting observation is the reduction of SWL adverse effects after low-energy pre-treatment [30]. The reduced incidence of tissue trauma leads to the hypothesis that low-energy pre-treatment initiates some degree of renal vasoconstriction that protects the kidney from hemorrhage. While being protective against bleeding, such vasoconstriction may lead to renal tissue ischemia and consequently increased free radical activity that itself may cause damage to the kidney. Medical prevention by antioxidative drugs or calcium channel blockers adds another interesting aspect that has to be investigated in further studies [5,8].

SUMMARY

Shock wave lithotripsy remains the safest available treatment modality for urinary calculi. Although shock wave energies may induce tissue damage, acute adverse effects are rare and may depend on individual risk profile but also on lithotripsy principles and different treatment protocols. There is an ongoing controversy on long-term complications of SWL and future studies hopefully will add information on this topic.

The physical properties of the ideal machine have still to be determined, but after a long period with only little success (and probably little efforts) in optimizing shock wave lithotripsy many interesting approaches including improvements of the lithotriptors themselves as well as better treatment protocols are now underway.

REFERENCES

1. H.-G. Tiselius (private communication).
2. J. Beatrice, R. T. Strebel *et al., Eur. Urol.* **52**, 909-911 (2007)
3. J. E. Lingeman, J. R. Woods *et al., JAMA* **263**, 1789-1794 (1990)
4. H. Nazaroglu, A. F. Akay, *et al. , Scan. J. Urol. Nephrol.* **37**, 408-412 (2003)
5. K. A. Al-Awadi, E. O. Kehinde, *et al. , Urol. Res.* **36**, 51-60 (2008)
6. M. Mitterberger, G. M. Pinggera, *et al. , BJU. Int.* **101**, 731-735 (2008)
7. L. R. Willis, A. P. Evan, *et al. , J. Endourol.* **19**, 90-101 (2005)
8. F. Delveccio, B. K. Auge, *et al. , J. Urol.* **169**, 1526-1529 (2003)
9. G. M. Preminger, H.-G. Tiselius, *et al. , Eur. Urol.* **52**, 1610-1631 (2007)
10. H.-G. Tiselius, D. Ackermann, *et al. , Eur. Urol.* **40**, 362-371 (2001)
11. C. M. Williams, J. V. Kaude, *et al. , AJR* **150**, 311-315 (1988)
12. M. Yokoyama, F. Shoji, *et al. , J. Urol.* **147**, 557-558 (1992)
13. C. M. Williams, W. C. Thomas Jr., *et al. , JAMA* **262**, 1952 (1989)
14. J. E. Lingeman, J. Woods, *et al. , J Urol* **141**, 793-797 (1989)
15. A. W. Elves, K. Tilling, *et al. , BJU Int.* **85**, 611-615 (2000)
16. B. West, A. Luke, *et al. Am. J. Kidney Dis.* **51**, 741-747 (2008)
17. G. Jantschek, F. Frauscher, *et al. J. Urol.* **158**, 346-351 (1997)
18. A. E. Krambeck, M. T. Gettman, *et al. , J. Urol.* **175**, 1742-1747 (2006)
19. Y. Sato, H. Tanda, *et al. , Urology* **71**, 586-591 (2008)
20. K. D. Mullen, J. H. Hoofnagle, *et al. , Am. J. Gastroenterol.* **86**, 630-632 (1991)
21. H. E. Adamek, R. Jakobs, *et al. , Gut* **45**, 402-405 (1999)
22. G. Wendt-Nordahl, P. Krombach, *et al. , BJU Int.* **100**, 1339-1343 (2007)
23. R. Gerber, U. E. Studer, *et al. , J. Urol.* **173**, 2013-2016 (2005)
24. L. Eichel, P. Batzold, *et al. , J. Endourol.* **15**, 671-673 (2001)
25. B. R. Matlaga, J. A. McAteer , *et al. , J. Endourol.* **22**, 121-126 (2008)
26. A. P. Evan, J. A. McAteer, *et al. , BJU Int.* **101**, 382-388 (2008)
27. R. Leistner, G. Wendt-Nordahl, *et al. , Urol. Res.* **35**, 165-171 (2007)
28. A. P. Evan, J. A. McAteer, *et al. , BJU Int.* **100**, 624-627 (2007)
29. M. J. Semins, B. J. Trock, *et al. , J. Urol.* **179**, 194-197 (2008)
30. L. R. Willis, A. P. Evan, *et al. , J. Am. Soc. Nephrol.* **17**, 663-673 (2006)

Risk Factors for Stone Recurrence after Percutaneous Nephrolithotomy

Amy E. Krambeck[a], Laureano J. Rangel[b], Andrew J. LeRoy[c], David E. Patterson[a], and Matthew T. Gettman[a]

Departments of Urology[a], Health Sciences Division of Biostatistics[b], and Radiology[c] Mayo Clinic College of Medicine, 200 1st SW, Rochester, Minnesota

Abstract. Recent studies have demonstrated more than 30% of percutaneous nephrolithotomy (PCNL) patients will experience a stone recurrence over a 20 year period. The goal of our study was to identify risk factors for stone recurrence after PCNL. Chart review identified 754 patients treated with PCNL for urolithiasis from March of 1983 to July 1984 at our institution. Of this cohort, 87 patients continued to receive medical care at our clinic and had been evaluated within the last 5 years. Of the 87 patients, 80 had recent radiographic imaging. Average follow-up was 19.2 years and 32 (40.0%) experienced at least 1 stone recurrence. There was no difference in preoperative BMI (p=0.453) or change in BMI (p=0.964) between patients that did and did not have a stone recurrence. Renal stone location (p=0.605) and stone size (p=0.238) were not predictive of recurrence. Patients with calcium oxalate monohydrate stones were less likely to recur (38.7% vs. 41.6%, p=0.004) and those with calcium oxalate dihydrate (COD) were more likely to recur (31.1% vs. 19.6%, p=0.006) compared to other compositions. Diabetes mellitus was not associated with recurrent stones (p=0.810). Those patients with residual stones or fragments <3 mm were more likely to recur and to recur earlier than patients rendered entirely stone free at time of PCNL (p=0.015). Stone recurrences were associated with the late development of renal insufficiency (25% vs. 2.1%, p=0.002). In conclusion, stone composition, as well as the presence of residual fragments was associated with recurrent symptomatic stone events after PCNL. Recurrent stone events were significantly associated with the risk of developing renal insufficiency, further stressing the need for complete stone clearance at time of PCNL.

Keywords: Percutaneous nephrolithotomy; Kidney calculi; Lithotripsy; Diabetes mellitus; Renal insufficiency
PACS: 01.30.Cc

INTRODUCTION

The first percutaneous nephrolithotomy (PCNL) was performed in 1941 by Rupel and Brown in Indianapolis, Indiana through a surgically created tract to the renal collecting system [1]. Despite this early introduction, it was not until specialized techniques for percutaneous access in 1976 [2], functional nephroscopes and specialized instruments in 1980 [3] and tract dilation techniques in 1983 [4] were developed did this treatment method for stone disease become widely utilized. The minimally invasive nature of PCNL has made it an attractive treatment modality for complex upper tract urolithiasis, such that open surgical stone extraction has become

CP1049, *Renal Stone Disease 2, 2nd International Urolithiasis Research Symposium*, edited by A. P. Evan, J. E. Lingeman, J. A. McAteer, and J. C. Williams, Jr.

nearly obsolete [5]. Current indications for PCNL are large stone burdens, lower pole calculi, cystine stone disease, abnormal renal anatomy and stones not amenable to ureteroscopy or shock wave lithotripsy (SWL) [6]. Advantages of PCNL over open nephrolithotomy and SWL have been noted including superior stone clearance, limited convalescence and cost effectiveness [7]. Although major complications are possible, analysis has demonstrated overall safety and effectiveness of PCNL for the therapy of complex calculi [8].

We recently evaluated the long-term anatomic and medical outcomes of PCNL [9]. In a cohort of 87 patients followed for a mean of 19.2 years (range 12.7-23.0) 10.6% developed new onset renal insufficiency, 23.5% diabetes mellitus, and 34.1% hypertension. We compared the development of these adverse medical conditions to a group of 288 patients treated with SWL and a group of 288 patients treated with conservative management for symptomatic stone disease [10]. The PCNL patients were not at increased risk of developing any of these medical conditions compared to SWL or conservative management. Interestingly, 36.8% of the PCNL patients developed a symptomatic stone recurrence. PCNL stone recurrence was significantly less than in the SWL cohort (53.5%). Despite the clear advantage of PCNL over SWL at preventing recurrent stone events, over 1/3 of patients treated with PCNL required subsequent treatment for stone disease. The goal of the current study was to identify potentially, modifiable risk factors for recurrent stone disease after PCNL treatment.

METHODS

Retrospective Chart Review

After Institutional Review board approval, a retrospective chart review of all 754 patients undergoing PCNL for renal or proximal ureteral calculi from March 1983 to July 1984 was performed. This was the first year of extensive PCNL therapy at our clinic using a rapid tract dilation technique. We identified 87 patients who continued to receive care at our clinic and who had returned for a complete physical within the last 5 years. Of this cohort 80 patients had recent radiographic imaging. We specifically focused on the development of recurrent, symptomatic stone disease after PCNL and therefore, all surgical, primary care, urologic and emergency room documents were reviewed for the diagnosis of urolithiasis. Recurrent stone disease was defined as passage of stone material or a symptomatic stone identified on radiographic imaging. Those patients with symptoms concerning for stone recurrence or who took part in regular screening through the stone clinic underwent follow-up radiologic imaging in the form of non-contrast computed tomography scans of the abdomen and pelvis. Hypertension was defined as the diagnosis of hypertension by a physician requiring antihypertensive medications. Diabetes mellitus was defined as the diagnosis of diabetes mellitus by a physician requiring oral hypoglycemic agents or subcutaneous insulin. Renal insufficiency was defined as a serum creatinine >1.4 mg/dL in males or >1.2mg/dL in females. Patients were considered overweight if body mass index (BMI) was >25, but <30, obese if BMI was >/= 30 but <40, and morbidly obese if BMI was >/= 40. Patients were also subcategorized by their major stone composition (greatest percentage component).

Percutaneous Nephrolithotomy Technique

PCNL was performed using standard method previously described [11]. Percutaneous renal access was obtained by Interventional Radiology in the fluoroscopy suite. The patient was then transferred to the operating suite and the access tract dilated to 28 French with fascial dilators. The rigid nephroscope without an access sheath was then used to locate the stone(s). Stone fragmentation and extraction was performed primarily with ultrasonic lithotripsy, but also electrohydraulic lithotripsy and basket extraction. After an intra-operative nephrostogram demonstrated no major injuries or obvious residual stone fragments, a 22 French nephrostomy tube and 6 French percutaneous ureteral catheter were left in place. On postoperative day one the patients underwent an antegrade nephrostogram. If no residual fragments were identified the 6 French ureteral catheter was removed and the nephrostomy tube clamped. If the patient tolerated nephrostomy tube clamping for 24 hours the tube was removed and the patient discharged home on postoperative day 2.

Stone free status was not obtained for all patients in this cohort. If residual fragments were small and thought to be passable, or in a location less likely to result in symptoms (i.e. lower pole) a secondary PCNL was omitted.

Statistical Methods

Associations of PCNL features with various outcomes were evaluated using the chi-square and two-sample t-tests. Time to stone recurrence was analyzed using Kaplan-Meier analysis. Wilcoxon rank sum and chi-square tests were used for comparison of stone composition groups.

RESULTS

Average PCNL follow-up was 19.2 years (range 12.7-23.0). Of the 80 patients 32 (40.0%) experienced at least one stone recurrence. A total of 81 separate symptomatic stone events were noted **Table 1**. Patient demographics and pre-existing medical conditions are listed in **Table 2.** Of those patients with recurrent stone events, 23 (71.9%) had an identified metabolic abnormality: hypercalciuria 8, hypocitraturia 5, hyperuricosuria 3, hyperoxaluria 2, cystinuria 1, hyperoxaluria + hypocitraturia 1, hyperoxaluria + hyperuricosuria 1, medullary sponge kidney 1, and type 1 (distal) renal tubular acidosis 1.

Comparison of stone size, location and laterality between the patients with and without stone recurrence after PCNL is listed in **Table 3**. Stone size, location or laterality at time of initial PCNL was not associated with recurrent stone events. A comparison of major stone compositions between patients with and without stone recurrence after PCNL is listed in **Table 4.** The majority of stones were calcium oxalate monohydrate (COM), calcium oxalate dehydrate (COD), and calcium phosphate (CP) with only 5 uric acid, 2 struvite, and 1 cystine

TABLE 1. Total number of post PCNL recurrent stone events.

	Total (N=80)
Number of Recurrences	
0	47 (58.8%)
1	12 (15%)
2	6 (7.5%)
3	7 (8.8%)
4	2 (2.5%)
5	1 (1.3%)
6	2 (2.5%)
7	1 (1.3%)
12	1 (1.3%)
13	1 (1.3%)

TABLE 2. Comparison of characteristics between patients with and without stone recurrence.

	With Stone Recurrence (N=32)	**Without Stone Recurrence** (N=48)	**p value**
Age at surgery			0.121
N	32	48	
Mean (SD)	53.3 (10.60)	49.0 (11.46)	
Range	(31.3-70.9)	(22.1-71.8)	
Gender			0.842
Female	10 (31.3%)	14 (29.2%)	
Male	22 (68.8%)	34 (70.8%)	
BMI preoperative			0.453
Mean (SD)	29.0 (5.70)	29.8 (6.33)	
Range	(21.0-49.4)	(20.3-59.1)	
BMI current			0.663
Mean (SD)	30.5 (8.98)	29.7 (5.28)	
Range	(18.8-66.2)	(21.3-44.6)	
BMI change			0.964
Mean (SD)	0.1 (0.38)	0.0 (0.20)	
Range	(-0.5-1.8)	(-0.4-0.5)	
1985 DM			0.810
Yes	1 (3.1%)	2(4.2%)	
No	31 (96.9%)	46 (95.8%)	
1985 HTN			0.809
Yes	8 (25.8%)	11 (23.4%)	
No	23 (74.2%)	36 (76.6%)	

Comparison of the main 3 components demonstrated that patients with COM stones at time of PCNL were less likely to have a stone recurrence HR 0.04 (CI 0.01-0.17, $p<0.001$) and patients with COD were more likely to have a stone recurrence HR 0.22 (CI 0.05-0.99, $p=0.04$).

TABLE 3: Comparison of stone location and size between patients with and without stone recurrence after PCNL.

	With Stone Recurrence (N=32)	Without Stone Recurrence (N=48)	p value
Stone side			1.000
Left	20 (62.5%)	30 (62.5%)	
Right	12 (37.5%)	18 (37.5%)	
Location			0.605
Missing	1	1	
Upper	1 (3.2%)	2 (4.3%)	
Mid	1 (3.2%)	2 (4.3%)	
Lower	5 (16.1%)	3 (6.4%)	
Pelvis	14 (45.2%)	29 (61.7%)	
Ureteral	8 (25.8%)	10 (21.3%)	
Lower, Pelvis*	1 (3.2%)	1 (2.1%)	
Pelvis, Ureteral*	1 (3.2%)	0 (0%)	
Stone Size			0.238
N	29	44	
Mean (SD)	1.3 (0.52)	1.2 (0.74)	
Range	(0.5-2.5)	(0.6-4.0)	

*Denotes patients with 2 stones

Stone free status at time of original PCNL was associated with the development of recurrent stone events. Those patients that were rendered stone free were less likely to experience a symptomatic stone recurrence compared to patients with fragments ≤ 3 mm or > 3mm HR 0.40 (CI 0.19-0.83, $p=0.015$). Time to stone recurrence stratified by stone free status at time of PCNL is demonstrated in **Figure 1.**

The development of new onset adverse medical conditions (hypertension, diabetes mellitus, and renal insufficiency) is listed in **Table 5**. More patients with recurrent stone events developed renal insufficiency compared to patients that did not develop a stone recurrence ($p=0.002$).

DISCUSSION

Within one decade, PCNL has evolved from a highly skilled undertaking performed by a few to a routine procedure performed by most urologists, due to major advancements in technique and instruments. PCNL continues to evolve with the introduction of smaller nephrostomy tubes [12] or even tubeless procedures [12, 13] and aggressive treatment of underlying metabolic disorders [14]. Today, PCNL is successful at complete removal of complex stones and is associated with a high stone free rate [15]. Due to the major improvements in this treatment modality it is a widely accepted and readily available treatment option for properly selected urolithiasis patients. In an attempt to improve on already excellent outcomes we identified features of PCNL associated with long-term recurrent stone events.

TABLE 4: Comparison of stone compositions between patients with and without stone recurrences after treatment with PCNL.

	With Stone Recurrence (N=32)	Without Stone Recurrence (N=48)	p value
Calcium Oxalate Monohydrate			0.001
No	19 (61.3%)	11 (23.4%)	
Yes	12 (38.7%)	36 (76.6%)	
Calcium Oxalate Dihydrate			0.008
No	21 (67.7%)	43 (91.5%)	
Yes	10 (32.3%)	4 (8.5%)	
Calcium Phosphate			0.860
No	28 (90.3%)	43 (91.5%)	
Yes	3 (9.7%)	4 (8.5%)	
Uric Acid			0.990
No	29 (93.5%)	44 (93.6%)	
Yes	2 (6.5%)	3 (6.4%)	
Struvite			0.155
No	29 (93.5%)	47 (100%)	
Yes	2 (6.5%)	0 (0%)	
Cystine			0.215
No	30 (96.8%)	47 (100%)	
Yes	1 (3.2%)	0 (0%)	
Mixed stone*			0.215
No	30 (96.8%)	47 (100%)	
Yes	1 (3.2%)	0 (0%)	

*No dominant stone type identified, 40% COM, 20% COD and 40% CP

At long-term follow-up, the rate of stone recurrence after PCNL in this cohort was 40%. Stone recurrence rates of 23-37% after PCNL have been quoted in the literature [9, 16]. When comparing patient, procedure, and stone demographics with recurrent stone events original stone free status, as well as certain stone compositions were associated with recurrent symptomatic stone disease. Data is lacking on the significance of residual fragments after PCNL. The majority of data on residual fragments after stone treatment are from the SWL literature, where the debate has been present for some time. Prior authors have indicated that residual fragments of <4 mm are insignificant and will either pass or result in asymptomatic stone disease [17]. Yet, others have claimed adverse effects associated with residual fragments after SWL [18, 19]. With regards to PCNL, some argue that treatment of the underlying metabolic disorder is paramount. A recent study by Kang et al. found no difference in stone recurrence rates in patients with residual fragments after PCNL treated concurrently with medical management [14]

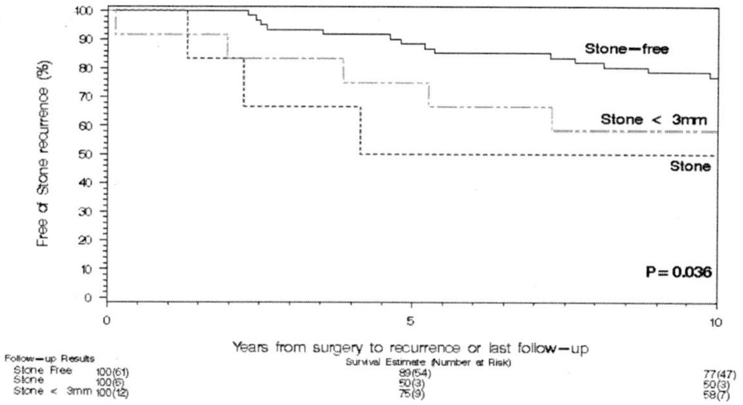

FIGURE 1. Kaplan-Meier curve demonstrating percentage of patients free of stone recurrence each year after PCNL stratified by postoperative stone free status.

TABLE 5: Development of adverse medical conditions between patient with and without recurrent stone events after PCNL treatment at long-term follow-up.

	With Stone Recurrence (N=32)	Without Stone Recurrence (N=48)	p value
New Diabetes Mellitus			0.748
Yes	7 (21.9%)	12 (25%)	
No	25 (78.1%)	36 (75%)	
New Hypertension			0.914
Yes	12 (38.7%)	18 (37.5%)	
No	19 (61.3%)	30 (62.5%)	
New Renal Insufficiency			0.002
Yes	8 (25%)	1 (2.1%)	
No	24 (75%)	46 (97.9%)	

Our data not only demonstrates that residual fragments are significantly associated with recurrent stone events, but also indicates that those patients with residual fragments recur earlier than those patients rendered stone free. At the time of original PCNL for this cohort our treatment philosophy was of the times and similar to the treatment philosophy for SWL. The symptomatic stone was treated and therefore peripheral stones in eccentric calyxes were left undisturbed in patients that did not have struvite or cystine stone disease. Residual fragments smaller than 3mm or in locations less likely to cause symptoms were not treated with a second-look PCNL. Since that time we have learned valuable lessons in urolithiasis treatment. In general, our current PCNL treatment goal is clearance of all stone fragments, thus completely stone-free. All treated patients are then referred to a subspecialized nephrology stone clinic for the initiation of medical management.

We have previously identified a higher rate of stone recurrence in patients treated with SWL compared to those treated with PCNL [9]. Similar findings have been noted by Carr et al. who found at 2 years follow-up the rate of stone recurrence was higher among SWL patients compared to those treated with PCNL [16]. These findings support our current data that residual fragments predispose to stone recurrence. SWL relies on passage of small fragments and may result in one or more residual fragments, whereas PCNL is more likely to remove all fragments at time of treatment.

There were more patients with COM stones without a stone recurrence than patients with stone recurrences. In fact, COM stones were noted to be a negative predictive factor for stone recurrence in univariate analysis. Conversely, COD stone composition was positively associated with stone recurrence, while CP stones were neither positively or negatively associated with stone recurrence. We theorize the majority of patients with COM stones had idiopathic stone disease resulting in the negative predictive factor while the COD stones were associated with underlying metabolic conditions. Prior studies have demonstrated that patients with COD stones form more stones than patients with COM stones [20]. Other investigators have demonstrated that COM stone recurrences are associated with a lack of stone inhibitors, while COD stones are associated with hypercalciuria, high urine pH and decreased urinary citrate [21, 22]. Although all patients in this study were referred to nephrology for metabolic evaluation, we do not know how many patients in either cohort complied with medical stone therapy. Therefore, medical treatment for stone disease could be a significant confounding factor.

Although recurrent stone disease after PCNL was not associated with the development of hypertension or diabetes mellitus, we did see a positive association with the development of new onset renal insufficiency. Stone disease is a known risk factor for the development of end stage renal disease [23]. Recurrent episodes of obstruction, urinary tract infections, and surgical interventions may have contributed to the increased risk of renal insufficiency in the patients with recurrent stone disease. Similarly, concurrent medical conditions (such as morbid obesity or diabetes mellitus) that may have contributed to recurrent stone events could also increase the risk of renal insufficiency. Nonetheless, our presented data supports the concern over recurrent stone disease and should prompt clinicians to minimize factors for stone recurrence. We recommend clearance of all stone fragments and referral for metabolic evaluation should be considered the standard of care.

CONCLUSIONS

At long-term follow-up over 1/3 of PCNL patients experienced a symptomatic recurrent stone event. Location and size of the original PCNL treated stone did not predict stone recurrence. However, stone composition and stone free status were strong predictors of stone recurrence. Time to recurrent stone events was associated with the size of residual stone after PCNL with stone free patients recurring later and patients with stones > 3mm recurring the earliest. Finally, recurrent stone events were associated with the long-term development of new-onset renal insufficiency. Based on these results we recommend complete stone clearance at time of PCNL and referral for metabolic evaluation to prevent long-term morbidity.

ACKNOWLEDGMENTS

We would like to acknowledge Dr. Joseph W. Segura, M.D. This study utilized his original cohort of PCNL patients, enabling us to carry out a unique long-term analysis.

REFERENCES

1. E. Rupel and R. Brown, Nephroscopy with removal of stone following nephrostomy for obstructive calculous anuria. *J Urol* **46,** 177-182 (1941).
1. I. Fernstrom and B. Johansson, Percutaneous pyelolithotomy. A new extraction technique. *Scand J Urol Nephrol* **10,** 257-259 (1976).
2. P. Alken, R. Hutschenreiter, M. Guenther, and M. Marberger, Percutaneous stone manipulation. *J Urol* **125,** 463-466 (1981).
3. J. W. Segura, D. E. Patterson, A. J. LeRoy, G. R. May, and L. H. Smith, Percutaneous lithotripsy. *J Urol* **130,** 1051-1054 (1983).
5. J. W. Segura, Current surgical approaches to nephrolithiasis [review]. *Endocrinol Metab Clin North Am* **19,** 919-935 (1990).
6. D. M. Rudnick and M. L. Stoller, Complications of percutaneous nephrostolithotomy. *Can J Urol* **6,** 872-x (1999).
7. J. W. Segura, G. M. Preminger, D. G. Assimos, S. P. Dretler, R. L. Kahn, J. E. Lingeman, et al, Nephrolithiasis clinical guidelines panel surgery report on the management of staghorn calculi. *J Urol* **151,** 1648-1651 (1994).
8. G. M. Preminger, D. G. Assimos, J. E. Lingeman, S. Y. Nakada, M. S. Pearle, and J. S. Wolf JR., Chapter 1: AUA guideline on management of staghorn calculi: diagnosis and treatment recommendations. *J Urol* **173,** 1991-2000 (2005).
9. A. E. Krambeck, A. J. LeRoy, D. E. Patterson, and M. T. Gettman, Longterm success of percutaneous nephrolithotomy. *J Urol* **179,** 2233-2237 (2008).
10. A. E. Krambeck, M. T. Gettman, A. L. Rohlinger, C. M. Lohse, D. E. Patterson, and J. W. Segura, Diabetes mellitus and hypertension associated with shock wave lithotripsy at 19 years follow-up. *J Urol* **175,** 1742-1747 (2006).
11. J. W. Segura, D. E. Patterson, A. J. LeRoy, H. J. Williams Jr., D. M. Barrett, R. C. Benson Jr., et al, Percutaneous removal of kidney stones: review of 1,000 cases. *J Urol* **134,** 1077-1081 (1985).
12. S. C. Kim, W. W. Tinmouth, R. L. Kuo, R. F. Paterson, and J. E. Lingeman, Using and choosing an nephrostomy tube after percutaneous nephrolithotomy for large or complex stone disease: a treatment strategy. *J Endourol* **19,** 348-352 (2005).
13. M. Goh, J. S. Wolf Jr., Almost totally percutaneous nephrolithotomy: further evolution of the technique. *J Endourol* **13,** 177-180 (1999).
14. D. E. Kang, M. M. Maloney, G. E. Haleblian, W. P. Springhart, E. F. Honeycutt, E. L. Einstein, et al., Effect of medical management on recurrent stone formation following percutaneous nephrolithotomy. *J Urol* **177,** 1785-1789 (2007).
15. P. Downey and D. Tolley, Contemporary management of renal calculus disease. *J R Coll Surg Edinb* **47,** 668-675 (2002).

16. L. K. Carr, J. D'A Honey, M. A. Jewett, D. Ibanex, M. Ryan, C. Bombardier. New stone formation: a comparison of extracorporeal shock wave lithotripsy and percutaneous nephrolithotomy. *J Urol* **155,** 1565-1567 (1996).
17. M.M. Osman, Y. Alfano, S. Kamp, A. Haecker, P. Alken, M. S. Michel, et al., 5-year follow-up of patients with clinically insignificant residual fragments after extracorporeal shock wave lithotripsy. *Eur Urol* **47,** 860-864 (2005).
18. S. B. Streem, A. Yost, and E. Mascha, Clinical implications of clinically insignificant stone fragments after extracorporeal shock wave lithotripsy. *J Urol* **155,** 1186-1190 (1996).
19. A. R. El-Nahas, A. M. El-Assmy, K. Madbouly, and K. Z. Sheir, Predictors of clinical significance of residual fragments after extracorporeal shockwave lithotripsy for renal stones. *J Endourol* **20,** 870-874 (2006).
20. T. Koide, H. Itatani, T. Yoshioka, H. Ito, M. Namiki, E. Nakano, et al., Clinical manifestations of calcium oxalate monohydrate and dihydrate urolithiasis. *J Urol* **127,** 1067-1069 (1982).
21. J. R. Asplin, J. Lingeman, R. Kahnoski, H. Markis, J. H. Parks, F. L. Coe, Metabolic urinary correlates of calcium oxalate dihydrate in renal stones. *J Urol* **159,** 664-668 (1998)
22. A. Costa-Bauza, J. Perello, B. Isern, P. Sanchis, F. Grases, Factors affecting calcium oxalate dihydrate fragmented calculi regrowth. *BMC Urol* **6,** 16 (2006)
23. Junger, D. Joly, F. Barbey, G. Choukroun, M. Daudon, ESRD caused by nephrolithiasis: prevalence, mechanisms, and prevention. *Am J Kidney Dis* **44,** 799-805 (2004).

Urolithiasis and Genitourinary Systems Issues for Spaceflight

Jeffrey A. Jones[a,b,e], Ashot Sargsyan[c], Robert Pietryzk[d], C. Sams[a], Phillip Stepaniak[a], and P. Whitson[a]

[a]*NASA/Johnson Space Center, Houston, TX, USA*
[b]*International Space University, Strasbourg, France*
[c]*Wyle Laboratories, Houston, TX, USA*
[d]*M.S.Enterprise Advisory Services, Inc Houston, TX, USA*
[e]*Baylor College of Medicine, Houston, TX, USA*

Abstract. Genitourinary medical events have shown to be an issue for both short duration and long duration spaceflight, and are anticipated to also be a potential issue for future exploration missions as well. This is based on actual historical pre-, in- and post-flight medical events, as well as assessment of what future flight challenges lay ahead. For this study, retrospective record review, as well as prospective studies of ultrasound and contingency management procedure development, and oral urinary stone prophylaxis were conducted. Results showed that the incidence of prior urinary calculi in- and post-flight was a risk driver for development of on-orbit countermeasures, as well as diagnostic and therapeutic methods for a possible in-flight calculus contingency. Oral potassium citrate and bisphosphonate preparations show promise for prophylaxis in spaceflight risk reduction. We conclude that a properly developed approach of selection, monitoring, and preventive medicine with effective countermeasures, along with early imaging diagnosis and minimally-invasive contingency intervention, should prevent issues such as urinary calculi from having a significant mission impact for exploration-class spaceflight.

Keywords: urinary stones, citrate, risk factors
PACS: 07.87.+v

INTRODUCTION

Spaceflight is associated with numerous environmental hazards as well as numerous physiological changes in adaptation to an altered gravitational field which may affect the health of crewmembers. The longer the duration of the flight, the higher the likelihood that a medical contingency may occur; however, medical symptoms are common even in short duration spaceflight [5].

U.S. spaceflight experience to date from early space vehicles (Mercury, Gemini, Apollo, Apollo-Soyuz) to Space Transportation System (STS-Shuttle) to long duration space platforms (Skylab, NASA-Mir and International Space Station) cumulates to approximately 30,000 crew-days, >80 crew-years. On Shuttle missions from STS-1 to STS-108 (106 Shuttle flights) cumulating 5496 flight days, 588 of 607 (97%) participating crewmembers experienced some medical symptom.

CP1049, *Renal Stone Disease 2, 2nd International Urolithiasis Research Symposium,*
edited by A. P. Evan, J. E. Lingeman, J. A. McAteer, and J. C. Williams, Jr.
2008 American Institute of Physics 978-0-7354-0577-6/08/$23.00

The genitourinary (GU) system is not uncommonly affected during spaceflight [5]. During Shuttle flights to date, approximately 7% (40 discrete on-orbit diagnoses) of participating astronauts have reported GU symptoms during flight. GU health contingencies can secondarily affect other physiological systems, especially in the behavioral health and performance arena. Therefore anticipating the likelihood of GU medical events in space plays a key role in applying the principles of primary, secondary and tertiary preventive aerospace medicine, including having the proper interventional hardware and procedures to avoid adverse effects on the crew and impacts to the mission.

In this manuscript, the incidence of urinary calculi in astronauts and cosmonauts, the risk factors for urinary calculi, possible countermeasures, space flight diagnostic tools and current and future contingency management/ therapeutics will be reviewed.

METHODS

Longitudinal Study of Astronaut Health (LSAH) Database Review

A total of 332 astronauts, active and retired, were evaluated via the LSAH database, from their entry into the astronaut program. The study was reviewed by the NASA/JSC Longitudinal Study for Astronaut Health Executive Committee and approved for release after assuring the non-attributable nature of the data and compliance with the Medical Privacy Act of 1974 and JSC Flight Medicine Clinic policies. All astronauts participating in these clinical data reviews completed a preflight and postflight physical examination as part of the routine medical operations requirements for space flight.

The LSAH control population consists of JSC employees who are matched for age, gender, and body mass index [7]. A total of 927 control patients, comprising 6,475,383 person days of follow-up, were available for review in the LSAH control population database [23].

24h Urine Records from Flight Crew, Pre- and Postflight

Urine samples were collected during 24h periods no earlier than 30 and no later than 10 days before launch (preflight) and beginning immediately after landing (postflight). Additional 24h urine samples were collected for annual medical examinations and in some crew, at the request of the NASA flight surgeons. Diet, activity level, and fluid intake of the astronauts were not directed during the collection periods, i.e., were ad libitum. Prior to return from microgravity, crewmembers consumed the equivalent of approximately 1 liter of physiological saline (as salt tablets swallowed with water, or "Astro-aid"), as part of an established protocol to minimize orthostatic intolerance upon re-exposure to gravity [23].

Urine characteristics associated with renal-stone formation were analyzed by using standard laboratory procedures, as previously described [20, 33-36]. Relative supersaturations of calcium oxalate, brushite, sodium urate, struvite, and uric acid were calculated from biochemical results according to Finlayson's method [3, 22]. Urine samples were collected into containers and stored at approximately 4°C. At the end of each collection period, the container contents were mixed and transferred into a graduated cylinder, total volume and pH were measured, and a 10 mL aliquot was removed for biochemical analyses. A second 10 mL aliquot was acidified with 6 M hydrochloric acid for the analysis of calcium, magnesium, citrate, oxalate and sulfate. For each urine sample, the relative supersaturations were calculated as the activity product in the urine sample to the corresponding mean activity from normal non-stone forming subjects. These unitless ratios indicate the state of urinary supersaturation, a fundamental indicator of the biochemical driving conditions for urinary crystal, and subsequently, stone formation [23].

Potassium Citrate Countermeasure Study Methods

A randomized, prospective, double-blinded placebo controlled study was conducted to evaluate the efficacy of a potassium citrate countermeasure in microgravity during the ISS expeditions 3-6, 8, and 11-14 missions. 24-hour urines were collected pre-, in-, and post-flight, and food, fluid, exercise, and medications monitored before and during the urine collection period [23]. Two 10 mEq potassium citrate (Mission Pharmacal) pills were ingested daily with the last meal of the day from Launch-3 days to Return+14 days. Results were obtained from biochemical analysis of urine samples for urinary factors associated with stone formation and dietary analysis completed to assess environmental influences on the urinary biochemistry.

Diagnosis: Ultrasound Methods

A flight class I, rack-mounted Philips/Advanced Technologies Laboratory model HDI-5000 ultrasound imaging unit (Philips Medical Systems/ATL, Bothell, WA, USA), modified for spaceflight use, is mounted on-board the International Space Station, housed inside one of the Human Research Facility (HRF) racks in the U.S. Destiny Laboratory. For the abdominal, retroperitoneal and pelvic views of the genitourinary system, the C5-2 curved array (convex), broadband probe was utilized.

All imaging protocols were developed by self-scanning, performed by a Crew Medical Officer (CMO), with remote guidance given during the imaging session by voice commands from a ground based team consisting of a radiologist and a urologist, both experienced sonographers.

The CMO was provided approximately 3 hours of total pre-flight instruction time on ultrasound system operation including power-up, check-out, computer interface, and remotely guided image acquisition techniques. A laminated cue card was developed to facilitate the remote guidance activity, by allowing both the on-orbit crewmember and the ground support team to have a common reference point for hardware components and anatomic localization during procedures.

Ultrasound visual data were collected through continuous space to ground video downlink from the ISS video switcher unit, routed through the video base-band signal processor to the Ku-band ISS antenna and from there via the Tracking and Data Relay

Satellite to a receiving antennae at the White Sands Space Harbor and then to the Biomedical Multipurpose Support Room monitor at Mission Control Center, Houston. Secure two-way voice communications between the ISS and the ground team (via the ISS S-band antenna) allowed guidance of probe position and placement, probe movement, and optimal image settings [8].

Treatment: Contingency Methods

The methodology of utilizing flexible endoscopy and ultrasound guidance for stenting the ureter in microgravity or microgravity percutaneous bladder access were developed in a porcine model on the KC-135 parabolic flight aircraft, as previously described [6, 7].

TABLE 1. Sample urinary biochemistry data from stone-forming astronauts after spaceflight (23).

	Normal Range	Sub1	Sub2	Sub3	Sub4	Sub5	Sub6	Sub7	Sub8	Sub9
Calcium (mg/d)	80 - 338	283	102	396	220	403	222	329	353	509
Oxalate (mg/d)	< 45	46.4	49.5	38.7	36.2	23.3	42.5	32.2	50.8	81.0
Uric Acid mg/d)	376 - 1182	968	337	816	616	634	672	394	671	564
Citrate (mg/d)	> 320	653	560	799	583	976	876	524	1709	891
pH	4.70 - 7.80	5.69	6.59	6.08	5.80	5.32	6.86	5.47	5.57	5.37
Total Vol (l/d)	0.8 - 1.8	2.35	1.10	1.97	3.45	1.44	1.91	2.69	3.21	5.42
Sodium (mEq/d)	27 - 287	157	72	244	169	155	147	129	128	114
Sulfate (mmol/d)	0 – 32	25.9	8.5	27.7	20.7	32.8	20.5	31.9	28.1	33.7
Phosphorus (mg/d)	300 - 1300	1078	413	1321	772	1394	879	1324	1316	1778
Magnesium (mg/d)	60 - 158	144	36.3	93	67	92	134	65	128	217
Creatinine (mg/d)	1000 - 2000	2298	884	2044	1812	1843	1673	1927	2687	2385
Potassium (mEq/d)	26 - 123	53	21.3	53	59	53	76	56	75	80
Relative Supersaturation										
Calcium Oxalate	< 2.0	2.28	3.26	2.97	1.97	2.28	1.77	1.64	1.69	2.10
Brushite	< 2.0	0.96	1.47	2.99	0.49	1.14	2.98	0.55	0.40	0.30
Sodium Urate	< 2.0	1.91	2.66	3.83	1.35	1.86	2.26	0.76	0.47	0.11
Struvite	< 75	0.23	10.35	0.60	0.08	0.06	9.72	0.03	0.03	0.01
Uric Acid	< 2.0	3.37	0.45	1.66	3.66	5.04	0.24	2.26	1.80	1.17

N represents the total number of 24 hour urine chemistries performed on each astronaut. Values listed are the means of those analyses. Supersaturation values greater than 2 for calcium oxalate, brushite, sodium urate, and uric acid and greater than 75 for struvite indicate and increased risk for stone formation.

RESULTS

Incidence of Stones

Although astronauts are screened by medical history to select non-stone formers, urinary calculi have been observed on one occasion in-flight and 14 occasions post-flight in space crew [23]. The one in-flight episode occurred in a Russian cosmonaut during a long-duration mission on the Salyut, which nearly resulted in the crewmember being medically evacuated due to inability to control his pain resulting from a stone lodged in the distal ureter. Fortunately, after hours of colicky symptoms resulting from the obstructing calculus, it passed spontaneously, although the stone was not recovered. Eleven U.S. crewmembers have had 14 urinary calculi following their spaceflights, all after missions less than two weeks in duration [23]. The results of urinary biochemistry data from a subset of the astronauts who formed stones post-flight are listed in Table 1. The percent of crew with elevations in urinary stone promoter and inhibitor levels pre- and post- flight are summarized in Table 2.

TABLE 2. Preflight and postflight urinary data of US space shuttle crewmembers (23)

	Preflight		Postflight	
Calcium (mg /dl)	183.0 (5.3)	% Hypercal: 20.8	233.5 (6.5)	% Hypercal: 38.9
Oxalate (mg /dl)	37.8 (0.9)	% Hyperoxal: 22.3	37.0 (0.9)	% Hyperoxal: 15.2
Citrate (mg /dl)	713.7 (16.3)	% Hypocitrat: 6.9	628.8 (17.9)	% Hypocitrat: 14.6
Magnsm (mg/dl)	115.7 (2.5)	% Hypomag: 6.0	99.0 (2.2)	% Hypomag: 15.8
pH	6.05 (0.02)		5.79 (0.03)*	
Total Vol. (L/dl)	2.10 (0.06)		2.00 (0.06)	
		1 L /dl: 13.0%		1 L /dl: 13.1%
		1–2 L/dl: 38.9%		1–2 L /dl: 46.2%
		2 L /dl: 48.2%		2 L /dl: 40.7%
	Relative Supersaturation			
	Preflight		Postflight	
	ratio	% increased risk	ratio	% increased risk
Calcium Oxalate	1.53 (0.06)	25.6%	2.23 (0.07)*	46.2%
Brushite	1.25 (0.06)	19.3%	1.00 (0.06)*	13.1%
Sodium Urate	2.41 (0.11)	44.9%	1.42 (0.07)*	25.8%
Struvite	3.05 (0.83)	0.90%	3.69 (2.21)	0.61%
Uric Acid	1.69 (0.08)	32.8%	2.27 (0.09)*	48.6%

Data represent the mean (SEM) from 24h urine samples collected approximately 10 days before launch (preflight, n=332) and immediately after landing (postflight, n=329). Hypercalciuria >250 mg/dl, hypocitraturia <320 mg/dl, and hypomagnesuria <61 mg/dl

Risk Factors and Quantitating Risk

Space travelers are at risk of urinary calculi due to the mobilization of calcium from the bone when exposed to prolonged microgravity. The principle elements of increased risk during flight are due to 1) increased bone mineral excretion, 2) potential urinary tract infection, 3) urinary retention, 4) perineal hygiene issues.

Micro-g Ca^{++} loss. Due to tight regulation of calcium levels in the blood, the mobilized bone mineral during periods of un-weighting is excreted by the kidney (See Fig. 1), resulting in increased concentration of calcium in the urine, and thereby increased solubility product of calcium salts like calcium oxalate (see Table 1). Based on Skylab data on 59 day flights, calcium loss was not limited to the urine, but also increased in the feces. The losses seem to be associated with increased bone resorption, due to measured increases in bone turnover markers [28-30].

Short duration spaceflight missions are at relatively low risk for in-flight urinary stones, as long as the crewmember is screened to be stone-free pre-flight, because even with increased calcium excretion during the flight, there is not adequate time for a clinical calculus to develop. However, the precursor of a clinical calculus, a nidus of calcium apatite with surrounding calcium oxalate, may form as a "Randall's plaque" on the renal papilla during the short duration mission, and that nidus could provide the seed for later development of a clinical stone event.

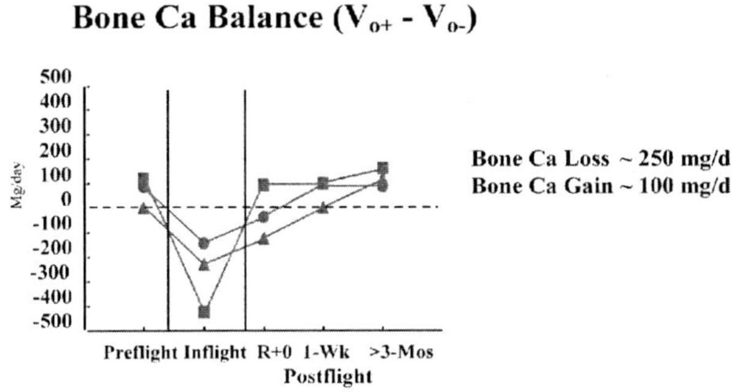

FIGURE 1. Summary of observed in-flight bone calcium balance in mg per day, compared to pre-flight calcium levels, and observed post-spaceflight recovery, from Smith et al [30].

Long- duration spaceflight in LEO (Low Earth Orbit) poses a greater risk for an in-flight stone, as evidenced by the previously discussed actual case. The risk is not theoretical, and is a physiological adaptation consequence of prolonged exposure to micro-gravity. Currently crews onboard the ISS (International Space Station) are staying on- orbit an average of 6 months, long enough for an in-flight stone to from and create a clinical scenario, if countermeasures are not employed to lower the risk. However, program managers are discussing possible ISS missions of up to 12 months in duration with up to 6 crewmembers per expedition, and these missions would obviously expose the crew to longer periods of microgravity, with additional time for an in-flight calculus to form and pass into the ureter, causing renal obstruction. The current human continuous space endurance record is approximately 14 months and was set on the Mir space station.

Summary of bone loss observed in various spaceflight programs to date:

- **Vostok:** Increased fecal and urinary calcium first noticed
- **Gemini:** Loss of approximately 2-4% of bone mass in heel after 4-11 days of spaceflight
- **Apollo:** 3-5% decrease in focal bone mass after 10 days
- **Soyuz:** 8-10% decrease in bone density reported in specific regions

- ♦ **Skylab:** 1-3% per month loss in bone mineral
- ♦ **Mir:** 10% loss of trabecular bone from lumbar spine in one cosmonaut after a 1-year mission
- ♦ **Shuttle-Mir:**
  - With countermeasures: 5.4% decrease in bone density in tibia. Did not return to preflight level in some individuals
  - Without countermeasures: 1.3-1.5% per month decrease in bone density (worst case: 15-22% total in some bones)
- ♦ **ISS:** Preliminary data similar to Shuttle-Mir however trends in later flights with more robust countermeasures towards diminished losses in exercise-targeted regions but significant losses are still being observed and with QCT there are observations of microtrabecular changes that may not be reversible. (11-15, 17)

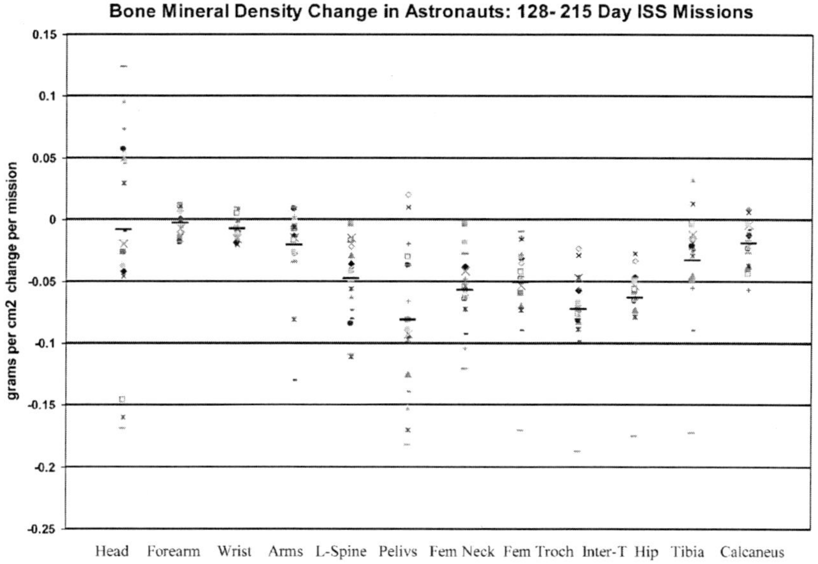

FIGURE 2. Changes in post-flight bone mineral density compared to pre-flight values as measured by DEXA- Dual Energy X-ray Absorpiometry. Fem=Femoral; Troch=Trochanter; Inter-T=Femoral Inter-Trochanteric region.

Urinary tract infections (UTIs) have occurred on multiple occasions during spaceflight with multiple likely causative mechanisms. Certainly individual physical and mental stress, dehydration and hygiene likely played a role during the UTI acquired during Apollo 13. Other hygiene issues such as collection devices and factors such as delayed access to voiding and urinary stasis are thought to also play a role in the UTI cases. One case of prostatitis on the Salyut resulted in sepsis and subsequently a medical evacuation of the patient. Diagnosis of UTI is aided on-orbit by urine chemistry analysis strips (U.S.) and an onboard urine analyzer (Russian). The combination of symptoms plus positive findings of leukocyte esterase or nitrites on the urine strip, make a diagnosis of UTI very likely. The upper tract and proximal ureter could be evaluated with onboard ultrasound. UTIs are easily treated with oral antibiotics flown in the ambulatory medical kit [5].

A question recently under investigation at the NASA/JSC is whether calcifying nanoparticles can play a role in the pathogenesis of human calcific diseases such as urinary and prostatic calculi. Nanobacteria or "nanoparticles" have been found to reproduce more vigorously in bioreactor microgravity simulators, and thus could pose a greater hazard in microgravity than on the ground, if their human pathogenicity is ever proven [1].

Retention- In the history of short-duration flight on the Space Shuttle there have been 5 cases of urinary retention requiring bladder catheterization in the U.S. program. The cause of these cases is again multi-factorial, and includes: pharmacologic side-effects (anticholinergics such as anti-emetics used to treat space motion sickness), delay in voiding (due to schedule and waste control system availability), impaired sensorium, and possibly even microgravity itself (psychological and lack of gravity vector differences in voiding technique) [32]. The added risks associated with long-duration flight for urinary retention are two-fold: 1) possibility of outlet obstruction from prostate or urethral infection/inflammation, and 2) progression or recurrence of a pre-existing condition, e.g. a urethral stricture managed by dilatation, may have time to recur during a long- duration flight. Screening should be performed for pre-flight conditions with potential for recurrence/progression and most likely excluded from long duration flight eligibility.

Hygiene-The onboard waste management system and hygiene of the perineal region can play a contributing role in the development of the above predisposing conditions, as previously described. Collecting fluid and solid waste in microgravity, including the interface with the crewmember's anatomy, has been, and will continue to be, an engineering challenge, especially as we bring requirements for water and carbon recycling systems forward for long duration and planetary missions. Another challenge is during crew suited operations, where currently waste management utilizes Maximal Absorbancy Garments (MAGs) in both Launch and Entry Suits (LES) and Extravehicular Mobility Units (EMU).

Countermeasures for Development of Urinary Calculi

One of the simplest countermeasures to prevent urinary calculi that is applied terrestrially, is increasing the volume of fluid intake. This approach has been applied in short duration Shuttle missions where typically water is plentiful due to it being a by-product of the hydrogen-based fuel cells. Results of increasing fluid intake during these missions have shown reasonable success, as measured by urinary solute concentrations [36]. However, for long duration LEO and future missions to other planetary surfaces and destinations, water may be a limiting consumable. Due to launch mass constraints, prior ISS missions have required restriction of fluid intake to approximately 2 liters/day. So although effective and desirable, oral hydration may not always be optimal for all phases of space missions.

Countermeasures for UTIs include good perineal hygiene, clean urine collection system interface, adequate fluid hydration, and nominal time to void after urge to void sensed (minimal delay in voiding). Occasionally, if the GU system is compromised by an indwelling catheter or intermittent catheterization (ICC-Intermittent Clean Catheterization), then prophylactic antisepsis or antibiotics can be used, e.g. qHS nitrofurantoin while receiving ICC [5].

Longer duration missions will have a longer period of reduced hygiene exposure compared to the terrestrial setting, but current ISS schedules typically provide adequate crew time for personal maintenance relative to the highly packed short-duration flight schedules, and more emphasis on hygiene training and time allocation. Thus far, there has not been a higher rate of UTI in ISS crews relative to prior Shuttle (short-duration) crews.

Countermeasures for urinary retention include avoiding delays in voiding, selection criteria for pre-disposing conditions as mentioned above, plus close monitoring of crew receiving anti-cholinergic medications, to include ICC if required to drain urine from bladder before overdistension injury can occur [32].

Exploration Missions envisioned for the Moon and Mars will vary in mission length from a few weeks, to perhaps 2-3 years. During these missions, the transit phase from LEO to the planetary surface, traversing interplanetary space, will likely expose the crewmember to microgravity for extended periods, ranging from 4-6 days between the Earth and Moon to 4-9 months, depending on the propulsion system and vehicle trajectory. After reaching the planetary surface, the crewmember's musculoskeletal system will be under the influence of reduced or partial gravity. In the case of the Moon, the gravity is approximately 1/6 of that of the Earth, while on Mars approximately 1/3 (0.38g). It is not currently known how well ambulation in partial gravity will maintain the musculoskeletal system on its own, hence the need for both transit phase and planetary surface operational countermeasures.

The possible countermeasures (CMs) for long- duration and exploration-class space missions currently under evaluation at the NASA/JSC, that are antagonistic to the risk of urinary calculi/obstruction, include other approaches to reduce urinary calculus formation during spaceflight aside from hydration mentioned above. They include:

1) Reduce calcium loss via improved musculoskeletal loading (e.g. resistive exercise) [18, 26, 27]

2) Reduce musculoskeletal and neurovestibular dysfunction due to employment of artificial gravity during transit [9, 25, 37]

3) Reduce calcium loss via reduction in bone resorption by employing pharmaceuticals or nutriceuticals/dietary alterations (e.g. vitamin D, bisphosphonates, etc.) [4, 10, 16, 17, 19, 31]

4) Reduce calcium oxalate and uric acid saturation index by supplementing with an orally administered urinary stone inhibitor (e.g. potassium citrate (KCit), potassium magnesium citrate) [38]

Resistive exercise has been the mainstay for counteracting the effects of microgravity on the musculoskeletal system onboard the ISS. Resistive exercise has been used in lesser ways on Skylab and Russian space stations, but a dedicated resistive exercise device was introduced in Node 1 on the ISS, and has been in use for 14+ expeditions of ISS crews. It is thought by applying load to the muscles, tendons, and bones around the joints normally used to weight-bear and ambulate on Earth, that the bone mineral could be preserved [2]. Bedrest studies using resistive exercise support that theory, however the loads and repetitions required to obtain the protective effect seen in bedrest studies, have been difficult to achieve with the interim resistive exercise device (IRED) on ISS [26]. An advanced resistive exercise device (ARED) is under construction for ISS, and perhaps with its operational implementation on the ISS, more protective loading can be achieved.

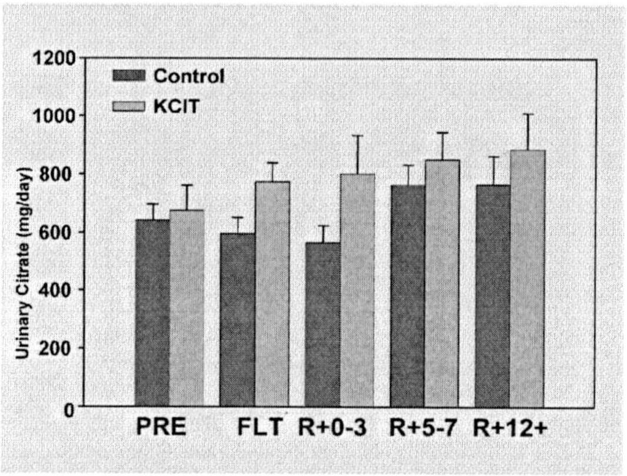

FIGURE 3. Preliminary results of the urinary excretion of citrate in control and KCit supplemented long duration crewmembers [21].

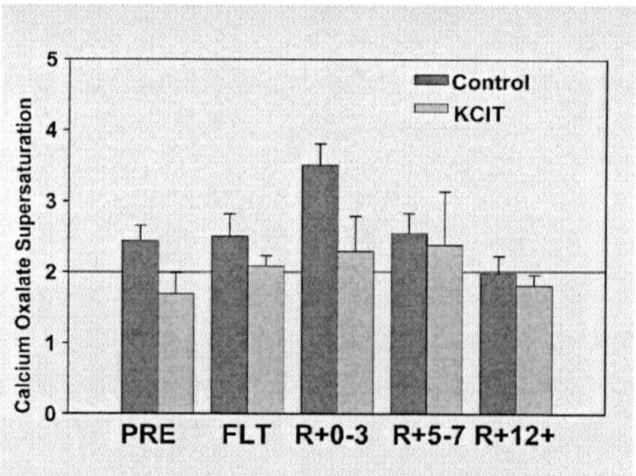

FIGURE 4. Preliminary results from the effect of KCit on calcium oxalate supersaturation in long duration spaceflight [21].

A potential means of mitigating the effects of microgravity while in space is artificial gravity (AG), created by rotating i.e. "spinning" the crewmember. The crewmember could be placed under induced gravity by rotating the entire vehicle or a segment of the vehicle versus spinning the crewmember within a stable vehicle platform, e.g. on a centrifuge. By imparting the load presumably necessary to maintain the bone mineral content, AG provides a means of protecting both the musculoskeletal and genitourinary system from calcium loss associated complications [9]. AG also has the potential to counteract some of the other organ system microgravity adaptive effects, especially in the neurovestibular arena [9]. Research has recently been conducted at the University of Texas Medical Branch (UTMB) in Galveston by a NASA/JSC team to understand the effectiveness of artificial gravity in a controlled bedrest population, as a surrogate to microgravity in space. Still unknown is the magnitude of gravity required to maintain the musculoskeletal system, i.e. do humans require a full 1- gravity level (9.8 m/sec/sec) of force on the system for it to be normally maintained, or will 0.5 or less gravity also preserve the bone mineral levels, or will 2-3 x g be required? Also, what amount of time is gravity loading required to achieve the system conservation objectives? These questions will hopefully be answered by the AG studies at UTMB and other locations.

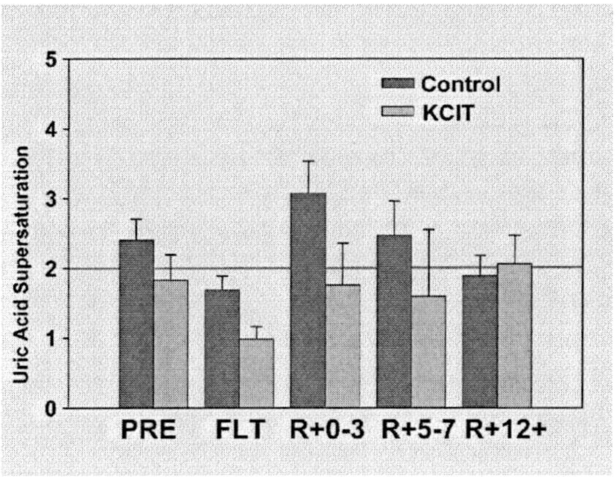

FIGURE 5. Preliminary results from the effect KCit on uric acid supersaturation in long duration spaceflight. (21)

Another potential countermeasure which that has been evaluated in ambulatory bedrest subjects, and extensively in clinical use for osteoporosis patients is the bisphosphonate Aledronate [16, 17]. Bisphosphonates act by inhibiting the action of osteoclasts in mobilizing calcium from bone hydroxyapatite. Bisphosphonates, like AG, have the potential to be protective of both the musculoskeletal and genitourinary systems by reducing the loss of bone mineral calcium. An ISS spaceflight study of the bisphosphonates Aledronate and Zoledronic Acid were recently approved for an in-flight supplemental medical objective (SMO) study on the ISS. It is expected that bisphosphonates could be used synergistically with resistive exercise and perhaps AG if they are operationally approved and employed for exploration missions.

The last countermeasure which may be effective for reducing the risk of urinary calculi in flight is currently under flight study on the Shuttle and ISS, is Potassium Citrate (KCit), in the form of Urocit-K ™ (Mission Pharmacal) [21]. The results from this study are not yet fully evaluated, however prelminary results from the initial 7 expeditionary crewmembers evaluated, comparing to data from historical long duration spaceflight controls, are included in Figures 3-5 [21].

The initial conclusions from the study's preliminary data review are as follows: 1) Urinary citrate levels were maintained with potassium citrate (KCit) supplementation throughout the in-flight and postflight periods; 2) Increased urinary pH levels reduced the risk of uric acid stones, however this pH level may adversely affect brushite stone formation; 3) Crew receiving KCit showed decreased in-flight and early postflight calcium oxalate supersaturation; 4) Urinary volume was still the strongest predictor of renal stone risk, using biochemical methods; 5) The Educational value of this study to crewmembers appears to be evident from the increased urinary volume and decreased risk in both groups compared to Shuttle-Mir.

Diagnosis

Should countermeasures against the effects of microgravity on the bone and subsequently the genitourinary system fail, then early detection of the presence of the calculus is important to prevent development of progressive symptoms and sequelae. For example, should a crewmember develop abdominal pain, then it is also important to discern the etiology of the pain, in order to properly apply therapeutics. If prompt and accurate diagnosis is established, then in the case of LEO or Lunar missions, a medical evacuation may be avoided. For missions to Mars, prompt and accurate diagnosis may be life or mission salvaging, as the crew on the way to Mars or on Mars will not have a short-term medical evacuation option available, and outcome will be totally dependent on the natural history of the disease and the intervention provided. Due to constraints on mass, volume and power available for medical systems, large imaging equipment like Magnetic Resonance Imaging (MRI), and Computed Axial Tomography (CAT) scanners will not be flown to the Moon. Therefore only small, low-power medical imaging devices will be available for exploration. Currently on the ISS, is an HDI-5000 ultrasound device, which NASA/JSC physicians and biomedical engineers have demonstrated to be able to acquire and transport diagnostic-quality from ISS to mission control in Houston. The imaging team at NASA/JSC has been able to remotely guide a non-physician crewmember with one hour of pre-flight training, through a series of ultrasound image acquisition, judged to be of adequate quality to formulate a diagnosis (Figure 6 [8,24]).

Contingency Management/Therapeutics

If a urinary calculus medical contingency develops in-flight, the space medicine system needs to be able to successfully intervene with appropriate secondary and tertiary preventative measures. Currently onboard the Shuttle and ISS include intravenous fluids, parenteral and oral opiate and non-opiate analgesics, and non-steroidal anti-inflammatory agents. Use of this interventional approach has been successful in averting a medical mission termination in a previous spaceflight calculus contingency.

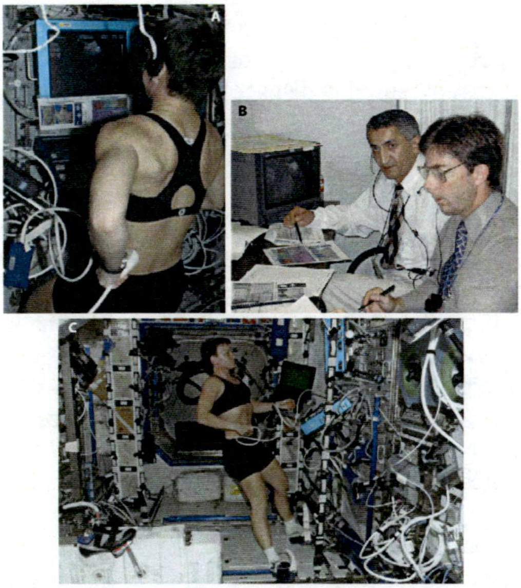

FIGURE 6. A) rear view of ISS Science Officer Peggy Whitson, PhD performing left renal ultrasound using the on-board cue card, with remote guidance from (B) mission control physicians A. Sargsyan and J. Jones employing the same cue card on the ground to guide her in-flight. C) side view of P. Whitson conducting a right upper quadrant ultrasound scan on orbit.

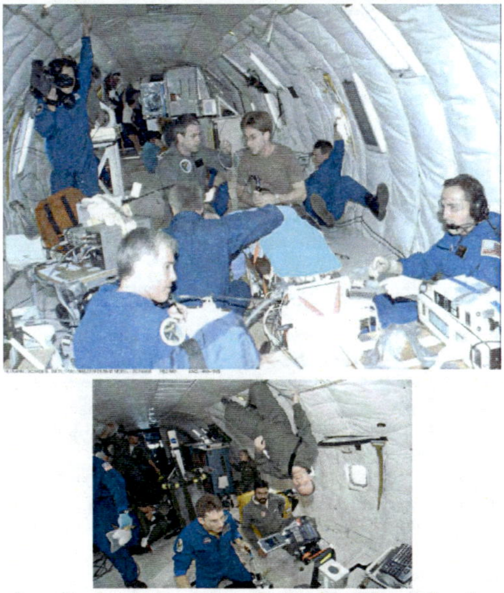

Figure 7. Zero-gravity aircraft simulating spaceflight conditions for (upper) developing ureteral stenting procedure for spaceflight application, (lower) developing laparoscopic techniques for managing a number of transit medical contingencies, e.g. infected obstructing calculus, cholecystititis, appendicitis etc.; from (6)

Also for Mars missions, a contingency management strategy has been developed at NASA/JSC for endoscopic management of a ureteral calculus under ultrasound guidance during microgravity simulated spaceflight conditions (Figure 7) [6].

SUMMARY/CONCLUSIONS

Genitourinary medical events have shown to be an issue for both short duration and long duration spaceflight, and are anticipated to also be a potential issue for future exploration missions as well. This is based on actual historical pre-, in- and post- flight medical events, as well as assessment of what future flight challenges lay ahead. The incidence of prior urinary calculi in- and post-flight drive the need to develop on-orbit countermeasures, diagnostic and therapeutic methods for a possible in-flight stone contingency. A properly developed approach of selection, monitoring, and preventive medicine with effective countermeasures, along with a readily implementable protocol of early imaging diagnosis and minimally-invasive contingency intervention, should prevent GU issues, such as urinary calculi from having a significant mission impact for exploration-class spaceflight.

ACKNOWLEDGEMENTS

We thank Linda Shackelford, Shannon Melton, Mary Wear and Douglas Hamilton at Wyle Laboratories, and Scott Smith at NASA, for their help.

REFERENCES

1. Ciftcioglu, N., R. S. Haddad, D. C. Golden, D. R. Morrison, and D. S. McKay. 2005. A potential cause for kidney stone formation during space flights: enhanced growth of nanobacteria in microgravity. Kidney Int 67:483-91.
2. Convertino, V. A., and H. Sandler. 1995. Exercise countermeasures for spaceflight. Acta Astronaut 35:253-70.
3. Finlayson, B. (ed.). 1977. Calcium stones: some physical and clinical aspects, vol. 337. John Wiley and Sons, NYC, NY.
4. Heer, M. 2002. Nutritional interventions related to bone turnover in European space missions and simulation models. Nutrition 18:853-6.
5. Jones, J. A., R. Jennings, R. Pietryzk, N. Ciftcioglu, and P. Stepaniak. 2005. Genitourinary issues during spaceflight: a review. Int J Impot Res 17 Suppl 1:S64-7.
6. Jones, J. A., S. Johnston, M. Campbell, B. Miles, and R. Billica. 1999. Endoscopic surgery and telemedicine in microgravity: developing contingency procedures for exploratory class spaceflight. Urology 53:892-7.
7. Jones, J. A., A. W. Kirkpatrick, D. R. Hamilton, A. E. Sargsyan, M. Campbell, S. Melton, Y. R. Barr, and S. A. Dulchavsky. 2007. Percutaneous bladder catheterization in microgravity. Can J Urol 14:3493-8.
8. Jones, J. A., Sargsyan, A, Barr, Y, Whitson, P, Melton, S, Hamilton, D. 2008. Diagnostic Ultrasound at MACH 20: Retroperitoneal Imaging in Space. Gold Journal of Urology submitted.
9. Lackner, J. R., and P. DiZio. 2000. Artificial gravity as a countermeasure in long-duration space flight. J Neurosci Res 62:169-76.
10. Lane, H. W., A. D. LeBlanc, L. Putcha, and P. A. Whitson. 1993. Nutrition and human physiological adaptations to space flight. Am J Clin Nutr 58:583-8.
11. Lang, T., A. LeBlanc, H. Evans, Y. Lu, H. Genant, and A. Yu. 2004. Cortical and trabecular bone mineral loss from the spine and hip in long-duration spaceflight. J Bone Miner Res 19:1006-12.
12. Lang, T. F., A. D. Leblanc, H. J. Evans, and Y. Lu. 2006. Adaptation of the proximal femur to skeletal reloading after long-duration spaceflight. J Bone Miner Res 21:1224-30.
13. LeBlanc, A. 1998. Summary of research issues in human studies. Bone 22:117S-118S.

14. LeBlanc, A., C. Lin, L. Shackelford, V. Sinitsyn, H. Evans, O. Belichenko, B. Schenkman, I. Kozlovskaya, V. Oganov, A. Bakulin, T. Hedrick, and D. Feeback. 2000. Muscle volume, MRI relaxation times (T2), and body composition after spaceflight. J Appl Physiol 89:2158-64.
15. LeBlanc, A., V. Schneider, L. Shackelford, S. West, V. Oganov, A. Bakulin, and L. Voronin. 2000. Bone mineral and lean tissue loss after long duration space flight. J Musculoskelet Neuronal Interact 1:157-60.
16. LeBlanc, A. D., T. B. Driscol, L. C. Shackelford, H. J. Evans, N. J. Rianon, S. M. Smith, D. L. Feeback, and D. Lai. 2002. Alendronate as an effective countermeasure to disuse induced bone loss. J Musculoskelet Neuronal Interact 2:335-43.
17. LeBlanc, A. D., E. R. Spector, H. J. Evans, and J. D. Sibonga. 2007. Skeletal responses to space flight and the bed rest analog: a review. J Musculoskelet Neuronal Interact 7:33-47.
18. Monga, M., B. Macias, E. Groppo, M. Kostelec, and A. Hargens. 2006. Renal stone risk in a simulated microgravity environment: impact of treadmill exercise with lower body negative pressure. J Urol 176:127-31.
19. Morey-Holton, E. R., H. K. Schnoes, H. F. DeLuca, M. E. Phelps, R. F. Klein, R. H. Nissenson, and C. D. Arnaud. 1988. Vitamin D metabolites and bioactive parathyroid hormone levels during Spacelab 2. Aviat Space Environ Med 59:1038-41.
20. Pak, C. Y., K. Hill, N. M. Cintron, and C. Huntoon. 1989. Assessing applicants to the NASA flight program for their renal stone-forming potential. Aviat Space Environ Med 60:157-61.
21. Pietrzyk, R., Whitson, P.A., Nelman-Gonzalez, M.A. Jones, J.A. and Sams, C.F. 2005. Renal Stone Risk during Space Flight Assessment and Countermeasure Validation. USRA/DSLS Bioinvestigator's Workshop 2005 Annual Meting Abstract Volume.
22. Pietrzyk, R. A., A. H. Feiveson, and P. A. Whitson. 1999. Mathematical model to estimate risk of calcium-containing renal stones. Miner Electrolyte Metab 25:199-203.
23. Pietrzyk, R. A., J. A. Jones, C. F. Sams, and P. A. Whitson. 2007. Renal stone formation among astronauts. Aviat Space Environ Med 78:A9-13.
24. Sargsyan, A. E., Hamilton, D.R., Jones, JA, Melton, S, Whitson, PA, Kirkpatrick, AW, Martin, D, Dulchavsky, S. 2005. FAST at MACH 20: Clinical Ultrasound aboard the International Space Station. J. of Trauma Injury, Infection and Critical Care 58:35-39.
25. Scott, W. B. 2005. Artificial gravity. Aviat Week Space Technol 162:62-4.
26. Shackelford, L. C., A. D. LeBlanc, T. B. Driscoll, H. J. Evans, N. J. Rianon, S. M. Smith, E. Spector, D. L. Feeback, and D. Lai. 2004. Resistance exercise as a countermeasure to disuse-induced bone loss. J Appl Physiol 97:119-29.
27. Smith, S. M., J. E. Davis-Street, J. V. Fesperman, D. S. Calkins, M. Bawa, B. R. Macias, R. S. Meyer, and A. R. Hargens. 2003. Evaluation of treadmill exercise in a lower body negative pressure chamber as a countermeasure for weightlessness-induced bone loss: a bed rest study with identical twins. J Bone Miner Res 18:2223-30.
28. Smith, S. M., J. M. Krauhs, and C. S. Leach. 1997. Regulation of body fluid volume and electrolyte concentrations in spaceflight. Adv Space Biol Med 6:123-65.
29. Smith, S. M., J. L. Nillen, A. Leblanc, A. Lipton, L. M. Demers, H. W. Lane, and C. S. Leach. 1998. Collagen cross-link excretion during space flight and bed rest. J Clin Endocrinol Metab 83:3584-91.
30. Smith, S. M., M. E. Wastney, B. V. Morukov, I. M. Larina, L. E. Nyquist, S. A. Abrams, E. N. Taran, C. Y. Shih, J. L. Nillen, J. E. Davis-Street, B. L. Rice, and H. W. Lane. 1999. Calcium metabolism before, during, and after a 3-mo spaceflight: kinetic and biochemical changes. Am J Physiol 277:R1-10.
31. Smith, S. M., S. R. Zwart, G. Block, B. L. Rice, and J. E. Davis-Street. 2005. The nutritional status of astronauts is altered after long-term space flight aboard the International Space Station. J Nutr 135:437-43.
32. Stepaniak, P. C., S. R. Ramchandani, and J. A. Jones. 2007. Acute urinary retention among astronauts. Aviat Space Environ Med 78:A5-8.
33. Whitson, P. A., R. A. Pietrzyk, B. V. Morukov, and C. F. Sams. 2001. The risk of renal stone formation during and after long duration space flight. Nephron 89:264-70.
34. Whitson, P. A., R. A. Pietrzyk, and C. Y. Pak. 1997. Renal stone risk assessment during Space Shuttle flights. J Urol 158:2305-10.
35. Whitson, P. A., R. A. Pietrzyk, and C. F. Sams. 1999. Space flight and the risk of renal stones. J Gravit Physiol 6:P87-8.
36. Whitson, P. A., R. A. Pietrzyk, and C. F. Sams. 2001. Urine volume and its effects on renal stone risk in astronauts. Aviat Space Environ Med 72:368-72.
37. Wolfe, J. W., and J. D. Rummel. 1992. Long-term effects of microgravity and possible countermeasures. Adv Space Res 12:281-4.
38. Zerwekh, J. E. 2002. Nutrition and renal stone disease in space. Nutrition 18:857-63.

VI. OTHER TOPICS IN UROLITHIASIS RESEARCH

Frederik Ruysch's Fascination With Urolithiasis

Michael E. Moran[a] and Katherine Ruzhansky[b]

[a]*Renaissance Urology, 4074 SW Gleneagles Circle, Palm City, FL*
[b]*Yale University, New Haven, CT*

Abstract. Frederik Ruysch was born on March 23, 1638, in The Hague, and studied at the University of Leiden, where he graduated in 1664. He married a daughter of a famous architect and became a praelector of the Amsterdam surgeon's guild in 1665. In 1666, his rise continued, as he became elected as the Professor of the Anthenaeum Illustre. In 1668, Ruysch became the chief instructor to the midwives and by 1679 was the forensics advisor to Amsterdam's courts. His anatomical knowledge was second to none, and he gained worldwide notoriety for his discovery of the valves in lymphatics and the vomeronasal organ. Ruysch was keenly interested in dissection and anatomy, and developed his own methods for preservation of specimens. His secret was called liquor balsamicum. Over 300 years ago, Ruysch developed all of his talents to the point of creating a menagerie, of sorts, out of his specimens. The popularity of his rather morbid exhibits attracted such dignitaries as Peter The Great in 1697. Ruysch had several children from his marriage, and his daughter Rachel helped him illustrate many of his collections. Frederik Ruysch became an intriguing historical figure, worthy of some attention at kidney stone meetings, precisely because he chose these concretions to serve as one of the "finishing elements" in several of his collections. The purpose of this presentation is to present to a knowledgeable stone group, the artistic license of one of the first entrepreneurial surgeons and anatomists of the 17th century. Ruysch was a skilled surgeon, obstetrician, and anatomist, keenly interested in the science of anatomy, especially infant and fetal anatomy. In addition, he exhibited his fine collection of urinary stones in a rather unique way, in his "anatomical pieces."

Keywords: urolithiasis, history
PACS: 01.65.+g; 87.19.X-

INTRODUCTION

The history of urolithiasis consists of many eras of varying scientific interest both medically and surgically. Along the pathway to our modern understanding of this disease lie the flotsam and jetsam of some various curious practitioners. People have made names for themselves as specialists in lithotomy in order to promote their fame (and increase their fees). Others have donned religious attire and monikers in order to increase their trustworthiness. One other practice, typified by itinerant lithotomists was to collect stones from patients and carry them about, demonstrate them, in order to show the prowess of the practitioner. Perhaps the most macabre use of human stones was by the famed anatomist and surgeon of 17th century Amsterdam, Frederik Ruysch. This is a historical review of what we know about Ruysch to better understand his utilization of human stones as adornments—decorations if you would prefer—to his elaborate menageries.

CP1049, *Renal Stone Disease 2, 2nd International Urolithiasis Research Symposium,*
edited by A. P. Evan, J. E. Lingeman, J. A. McAteer, and J. C. Williams, Jr.

RUYSCH'S LIFE AND TIMES

Review of published works of Frederik Ruysch included Dutch archival materials of biographical nature and his published catalogues of his anatomical collection [1,2]. In 1691, Ruysch published a catalogue of his collection of anatomical works entitled *Frederici Ruyschii Thesaurus Anatomicus* with illustrations by C.H. Huyberts. This work is now available in an online electronic version for close scrutiny of the anatomical specimens. Of the works most pertinent to this writing, i.e., the human stones, there are no surviving specimens. The illustrations by Huyberts are the only remaining primary source. Descriptions by Ruysch and others suffice for this historical review. Particular attention was given to his illustrations and description utilizing human stones for artistic reality.

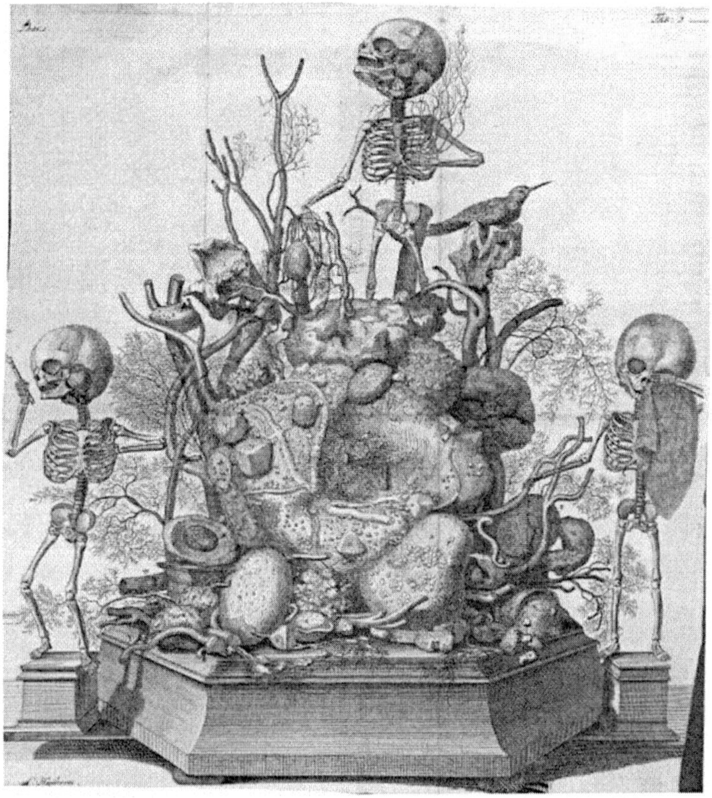

FIGURE 1. This is one of Ruysch's uses of human uroliths [3].

Frederik Ruysch was born on March 23, 1638 in The Hague. His father was a prosperous merchant and Frederik received a tremendous education. He matriculated to the renowned University of Leiden and studied medicine from 1661-1664. He apparently was fascinated by anatomy and anatomical research and probably became very well acquainted with the famed anatomical vanitas, or anatomical demonstrations. Upon his graduation in 1664, Ruysch married the daughter of famed architect in Amsterdam securing an influential circle of friends. In 1665, Ruysch became the praelector of the Amsterdam surgeon's guild following in the luminous pathway of Tulp and others. This appointment, allowed him legal access to dissection of corpses. His skill and renown were enough to secure his being named as the Professor of the Anthenaeum Illustre in 1666. His pathway to success continued with being named the Chief Instructor to Midwives in 1668 and forensic advisor to Amsterdam's courts in 1679.

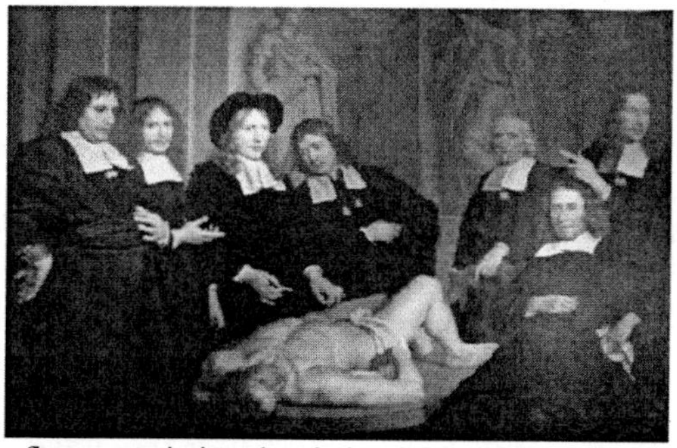

FIGURE 2. This is the first commissioned painting of Ruysch by the Surgeon's Guild in 1670 (Backer), Amsterdam's Historisch Museum.

Ruysch made many significant scientific contributions to anatomy in particular, because of the freedom he was allowed as the praelector. He described the valves in lymphatics and wrote a paper on the vomeronasal organ. He became particularly interested in the preservation of anatomical specimens and developed a secret *liquor balsalmicum* that could keep specially prepared anatomical curiosities life-like, in order to demonstrate the specimens to his students. As praelector of anatomy for the surgical guild, Ruysch utilized his skills in both dissection and preservation of specimens in public demonstrations of anatomy. As a result, his collection of anatomical specimens began to attract increasing attention to his demonstrations. Ruysch began to take a more artistic interest in his specimen presentation, and the collection increased in fame. He was mandated by the guild to perform at least one anatomical dissection annually open to the public. By 1670, Ruysch had achieved such significant renown that the Amsterdam surgeon's guild had famed artist Adriaen Backer paint him in an "Anatomy Lesson" much as Rembrandt had done for Dr. Tulp, another anatomist from the Guild. Ruysch though, would go one better, sitting again in 1683 for a second anatomical portrait, this one by Jan van Neck.

Ruysch's success allowed him to involve his family in his business. His son, Hendrik, became an able anatomic demonstrator and would in turn become a physician. His daughter, Rachel, became an illustrator and collaborator upon the artistic nature of his menagerie and she became a famous painter. Frederik had become Holland's premier anatomist and dissector. He is known to have given at least 31 public dissections, continuing up until his death at age 92. He was also known as a surgeon and obstetrician. His interests are clearly reflected in his anatomical demonstrations. The Anatomical Theater in Amsterdam became Ruysch's own "Rarieiten-kabinetten" or "cabinet of rarities or curiosities." He often worked alone with his son and daughter, improving his secret preservative by minimizing the odor of the dead, improving the water retention of the specimens so that they did not look shriveled, and adding color to make them more spectacular. His published catalogue in 1691, entitled *Frederici Ruyschii Thesaurus Anatomicus*, was lavishly illustrated by the famed artist C.H. Huyberts. Ruysch by this time had begun to add human kidney stones to his animations in order to improve their artistic presentation. Many of the collections animated classical poetry; in all he made more than a dozen tableaux utilizing human kidney and gallstones. Some of his poetic renditions included: *Vita humana lusus* (Man's life is but a game) and *Vita quid est? Fumus fugiens et bulla caduca* (What is life? A transient smoke and a fragile bubble). Frederik Ruysch became an intriguing historical figure, worthy of some attention at kidney stone meetings, precisely because he chose these concretions to serve as one of the "finishing elements" in several of his collections. The purpose of this presentation is to present to a knowledgeable stone group, the artistic license of one of the entrepreneurial surgeons and anatomists of the 17th century.

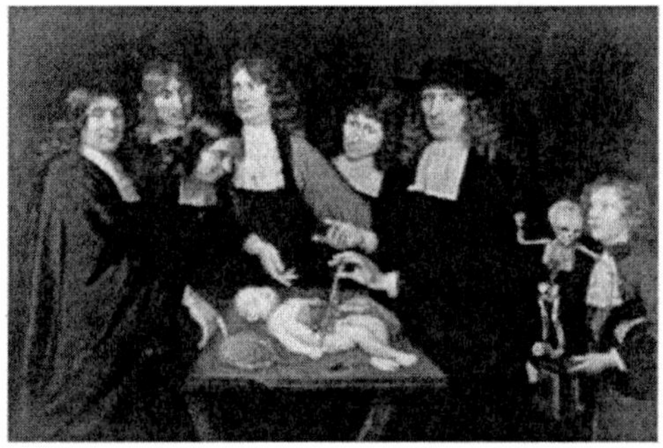

FIGURE 3. This is the second commissioned painting of Ruysch by the Surgeon's Guild in 1683 (van Neck). His son is shown demonstrating a fetal skeleton (also in Amsterdam's Historisch Museum).

RUYSCH'S USE OF KIDNEY STONES: EXHIBITS

Ruysch eventually began to use prosected animal specimens in jars of preservative in even more elaborate displays [4-7]. His most morbidly fascinating exhibits had fetuses dressed in a variety of costumes. Frederik Ruysch combined his skills as a dissector with an obvious natural artistic talent to make some of the most unusual anatomic displays, often utilizing a growing collection of human stone material. He would sift through his collection of calculi in order to obtain particular shapes that added to the scene he had imagined. The haunting character of the C.H. Huyberts drawings are sadly all that remain of these curiosities. Ruysch found a purposeful use for stones extracted from patients in Amsterdam as scenery for his whimsical renderings. By 1697, the fame of his collection had reached Peter the Great who came to visit him and his collection. His "repository of curiosities" included infant and fetal skeletons placed in landscapes accented by human pathology and animal body parts, and human kidney stones were a common decorative item in these displays. In 1717 Ruysch sold his entire ensemble of anatomical displays to Peter the Great for 30,000 guilders. Ruysch eventually developed a relationship with Herman Boerhaave at Leiden and continued to do public anatomical demonstrations. Ruysch in many ways, represents the most extreme showcase for urinary stone disease with his innovative decorative applications within his menagerie. Anatomically, he precedes the current anatomical art of Gunther von Hagens' *Body Worlds* which has been viewed by over 20 million visitors worldwide between 1996-2006.

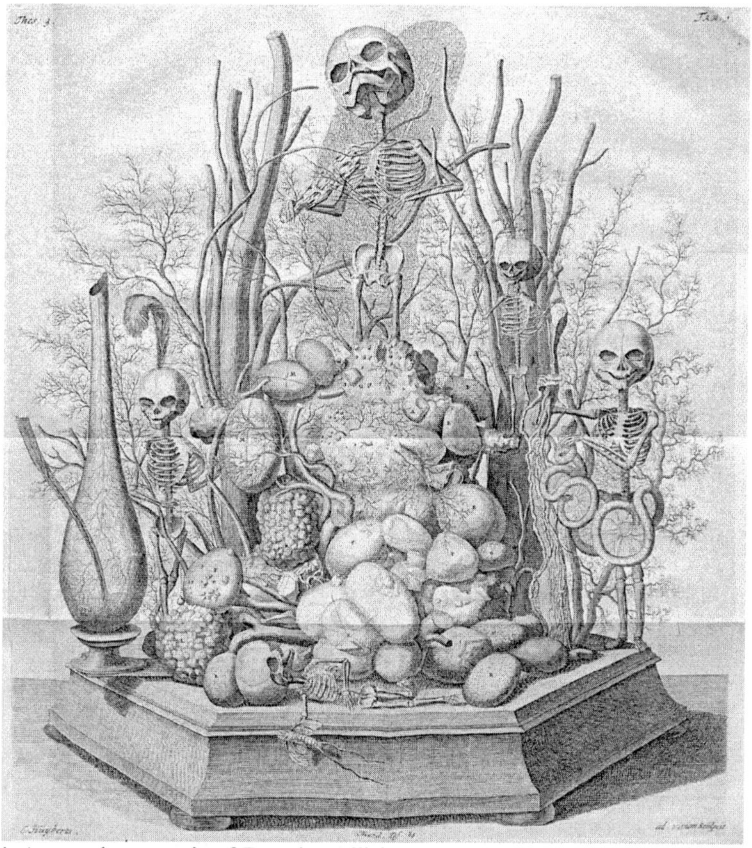

FIGURE 4. A second menagerie of Ruysch's utilizing human kidney stones. The structure to the far left of the "feathered fetus" is a human testicle with tunics [3].

REFERENCES

1. Luyendijk-Elshout,A: Death enlightened: a study of Frederik Ruysch. JAMA 212(1):121-127(1970)
2. Hansen,JV: Resurrecting death: anatomical art in the cabinet of Dr.Frederik Ruysch. Art Bull Dec 1-16 (1996)
3. Ruysch,F: Frederici Ruyschii Thesaurus Anatomicus, Amsterdam 1717.
4. Jones,B, Casey,S: Frederik Ruysch: Vene, vidi et judica nil tuis oculis. (http://laughingbone.blogspot.com/2005/06/frederik-ruysch-vene-vidi-et-judica.html)
5. Ruysch,F: Opera Omnia Anatomica-Medico-Chirugica, 5 vols, Amsterdam 1737.
6. Roach,M: Stiff: The curious lives of human cadavers. WW Norton & Co, NY, 2003.
7. University Anatomical Museum in Leiden and Peter the Great's Kunstkammer in St. Petersburg

Greco-Roman Stone Disease

Michael E. Moran[a] and Katherine Ruzhansky[b]

[a]Renaissance Urology, 4074 SW Gleneagle Circle, Palm City, Fl
[b]Yale University, New Haven, CT

Abstract. Greek and Roman thought had a profound influence upon Western medical practice. From the fall of the Greek civilization to the fall of the Roman, remarkable progress of our understanding of human anatomy and physiology occurred. Here we review the attempts of Greek and Roman thinkers to develop the first understanding of the pathophysiology of urolithiasis, its epidemiology, differential diagnosis of renal versus bladder stones, medications for both colic and prevention, the role of familial syndromes, and dietary management.

Keywords: Urolithiasis, history, Greek, Roman
PACS: 01.65.+g; 87.19.X-

INTRODUCTION

The Greeks and their Roman usurpers have left us a written legacy of intellectual knowledge that transcends all our modern sciences. In medicine, the legacies of such immortal giants as Hippocrates, Diogenes, Heracleitus, Aristotle, Herophilus, and Erasistratus represent the foundations of modern medical ethos and practice. The Roman author Celsus and physician Galen have managed to leave a written legacy that allows historians to recreate medical wisdom from others, less familiar from the literature lost from the pyres of the Library of Alexandria. This represents a review of classic medical writings in order to focus attention upon the "original" Western conceptions of urolithiasis that would ultimately influence the care and management of urolithiasis for more than two centuries.

> *Life is short, art is long, opportunity fugitive, experimenting dangerous, reasoning difficult: it is necessary not only to do oneself what is right, but also to be seconded by the patient, by those who attend him, by external circumstances.*—Hippocrates

The Aphorisms of Hippocrates represent of wealth of information about the ancient knowledge of medicine. Much has been written about the Hippocratic doctrine and specific diseases, such as urolithiasis. Hippocrates lived and wrote during the time of Pericles and rejected superstitious beliefs and attempted to make medicine more philosophical. A review of classic Greek and Roman writings via widely available English translations serve a wealth of information. The Aphorisms of Hippocrates and much of his surviving writings are available in translated form even on the internet. Other sources can be more difficult to trace, but references can be backtracked by a

CP1049, *Renal Stone Disease 2, 2nd International Urolithiasis Research Symposium,*
edited by A. P. Evan, J. E. Lingeman, J. A. McAteer, and J. C. Williams, Jr.

wide variety of medical historical textbooks dedicated to this subject. These were the sources for all of the information about GrecoRoman urolithiasis in this treatise. In addition, any modern authors are also sought to supplement the information that could be culled in this fashion and to insure that no other primary sources were missed.

STONE DISEASE AND GRECO-ROMAN THEORIES

Hippocrates originally describes the shape and location of the kidneys at the back of the loins with concave sides against the large blood vessels. It is attributed to Hippocrates that the paired nature of the kidneys resulted in the notion that disease that affects one, equally affects the other. "The light of the right eye with some disease affected, Is apt to make the left eye similarly infected." Both Aristotle and Plinius believe that the kidney is a lobulated structure (from knowledge of bovine anatomy) and the "portions" of the kidney could be involved with disease while the other portions cope. Galen professes that the kidneys are "hard and firm flesh" because the great looseness of the water that runs through them should not easily effect their flesh. Aristotle believes that the kidneys are given to animals by Nature in order to stiffen and preserve the blood vessels and Galen groups the kidneys with the "glands." Hippocrates also pronounces the difference between renal and bladder stones. Hippocrates, Diocles, Praxagoras, and Galen all believe the kidneys attracted watery fluid by a hidden property and leads to a risk of stone formation, which formed from dietary excess. Aristotle postulates that "all things harden either by heat which dries the dampness, or by cold, which squeezes it out." Two Greek physicians, Ruffus and Aretaeus both suggest that "slimy earthy matter" forms stones when kidneys are too cool, especially in older people with stones.

So stones themselves have a natural hardening tendency that is influenced by heat or cold. Hippocrates goes on to hypothesize that "gravel" does not occur in the kidneys until adulthood. Children who often suffer from bladder stones, supposedly form and grow in the bladder, growing upon a kernel, or nucleus. Galen adds, "the tough slime hardens by the heat of the kidneys and is baked into a stone. That the fire is indeed the cause, but that it does not act by its heat alone, but by drying and hardening the substance and because of other substances which it brings along with the flames…."

Galen professes that children form stones because "they gobble their food and run, leap and play immediately after their meals resulting in the formation of thick water." Hippocrates suggests that a child becomes gravelly if it sucks bad milk and that the milk deteriorates if the nurse eats unwholesome food. Galen continues by suggesting that milk is thick and course by nature and extremely fit to produce stone. And Aristotle questioned "Why none of the animals but Man alone can become gravelly?" Galen proposes to answer this according to the strength or weakness of the organ. According to Galen, this is the reason why grown people and aged persons are more often visited with stone in the bladder, but children more frequently with renal stones.

DISCUSSION

Beginning with Hippocrates, speculations regarding the pathophysiology of stone disease began in the West. Aristotle questions: "Why none of the animals but Man alone can become gravelly?" Stones are mentioned no fewer than in 24 passages of the Hippocratic dogma. Stone formation is discussed in 6 (25%) of these Aphorisms. The Aristotelian perspective is maintained by Hippocrates (heat or cold). Adult vs. pediatric and kidney vs. bladder stones could be attributed to heat, and eventually Galen would reiterate this theme. It is also attributed to Galen for developing the theory of disease transference to a weaker organ…kidney vs. bladder, for instance. Strabo reported a whole town with hot springs that hardened (further evidence of this process)

Through the country of the Cicons
Flows a stream that is most strange;
He who drinks it, pays most dearly,
As it will not spare his life…
Is at once seen stark and stiffening,
Till it is as hard as marble.

The manner of "growing the stone" is explained by Galen when he adds, "the tough slime hardens by the heat of the kidneys and is baked to a stone. But the fire is indeed the cause, but that it does not act by its heat alone, but by drying and hardening the substance." Hippocrates (4th Book of Diseases) adds that stones in young children have their origin in the milk. Red stones arise in the kidney (the color of flesh) all others from the bladder. Galen is noted to not believe this theory of the color origin of stones. Aretaeus states that "the tendency to develop stone of the kidneys is more difficult to prevent than the fecundity of the uterus." Hippocrates talks about the incidence of stones by saying "most between the ages of fourteen and forty-two" and "women do not suffer so frequently of stone as men." Galen astutely notices that "too adipose [patient] can hardly be cured of defects in the kidneys." Plinius [2.5] concludes: "among all greatest pains which a man can suffer in his body, the trickling piss caused by stone has of old been deemed the worst." All ancient Greek and Roman physicians and philosophers had advocated preventative measures. Ovid once penned:

And let the illness not come in,
But check it as it does begin
For once it has obtained firm footing,
It scorns the means for its uprooting.

After the fall of classic Greece and before the rise of the Roman empire, there arose in Alexandria a great medical school. Herophilus of Chalcedon became the first great anatomist, surgeon (~300BC) and named the prostate. Next, came Erasistratus of Chios, also interested in anatomy and physiology (310-250BC). Neither of these great minds left any evidence of an interest in stone disease. The decline of the Alexandrian school followed the deaths of these two great physicians, but their legacy was not entirely lost. Hegetor, Apollonius survived and kept the method alive, but again nothing on urolithiasis is mentioned. Asclepiades of Bynthinia and Schola Medicum taught medicine in the Alexandrian method. Rufus of Ephesus studied at Alexandria in 50 AD and practiced surgery and probably performed lithotomy. Also Marinus of Tyre, Quintus, Numisianus, Satyrus, and Pelops are some further notables, but sadly left no legacy regarding stone disease. Galen of Pergamum (129-199) first studied medicine under Satyrus then left to study with Pelops and then Numisianus until age 28. He then became surgeon to the gladiators and in 161 he went to Rome with Marcus Aurelius as emperor. Much of his philosophy on stones has been presented in this paper, but he also had some surgical experience. Heliodorus, Antyllus, and Oribasius all followed in the footsteps of Galen, but further interest in stone disease follows medicine in general into the Dark Ages. Stone disease essentially did not rise above the hypotheses of Aristotle on the cause and perhaps peaked with Hippocrates on signs, symptoms, causes and therapeutics. Galen certainly added some further insight, but fell short of the experimentalists of Alexandria three centuries before him.

The ancient writers of medicine from Greece and Rome have left a rather significant historical legacy about the topic of urolithiasis. Not only did they document the signs and symptoms caused by bladder and kidney stones, they began to postulate hypotheses about the actual causes of this disease. Hippocrates concludes that between the ages of fourteen and forty-two are the most risky periods of life for stones, thus becoming the first investigator to study incidence as well as pathophysiology. The Hellenistic legacy of these thinkers has persisted to our current era. We no longer follow the admonition to "not cut on those suffering from the stone" but we still seek epistemological truth. The great Greek philosopher Epicurus died from complications of stone disease and it seems fitting to end with his words…

> *I write to you on this happy day which is the last of my life. The obstruction of my bladder, and the internal pains, have reached the extreme point, but there is marshaled against them the delight of my mind in thinking over our talks together. Take care of Metrodorus' children in a way worthy of your lifelong devotion to me and to philosophy.*—Epicurus (341-270 BC)

REFERENCES

1. Saito,H: Descriptions of urinary stone in the Hippocratic Collection. Jap J Urol 96(6):632-639 (2005)
2. Herr,H: 'Cutting for the stone': the ancient art of lithotomy. BJU 2:1464 (2008)
3. Singer,C: A short history of anatomy and physiology from Greeks to Harvey. Dover Publications, NY 1957.
4. http://classics.mit.edu/Browse/browse-Hippocrates.html
5. http://classics.mit.edu/Browse/browse-Galen.html
6. Beagon, Mary (translator). *The elder Pliny on the human animal: Natural History, Book 7.* Oxford University Press, Oxford 2005.
7. Moran,ME: Famous stone patients and their disease. 1st International Urolithiasis Symposium. AI Physics: 412-416 (2007)
8. Eugene O' Connor *The Essential Epicurus*, Prometheus Books, New York 1993.
9. http://www.macalester.edu/~cuffel/herophilus.htm
10. Philip Hardie (ed.), The Cambridge Companion to Ovid. Cambridge: Cambridge University Press, 2002.
11. http://classics.mit.edu/Browse/browse-Strabo.html

Accumulation of Oxalate and Calcium in Organs During a Persistent Oxalate Challenge

Susan Ruth Marengo, Andrea M.P. Romani, and Brian S. Zeise

Department of Physiology and Biophysics, Case Western Reserve University School of Medicine, 10900 Euclid Avenue, Cleveland, Ohio, 44106-4931, USA, srm10@case.edu

Abstract: The body's response to a persistent oxalate challenge is poorly understood. Here we report that calcium (measured by atomic absorbance spectrometry) increases in kidneys in rats exposed to a persistent challenge of 360 µmole/d oxalate for 13D. Time dependent increases in renal concentrations of oxalate and calcium occurred for exposures of 12hr to 13D ($p \leq 0.02$), but these oxalate and calcium concentrations were not intercorrelated ($p=0.8$). Since the calcium concentration was always at least five fold the oxalate concentration, it is unlikely that the entire calcium increase was due to its incorporation into calcium oxalate crystals.

Keywords: oxalate, calcium, rat, minipump, nephrolithiasis, stone disease
PACS: 81.10.Dn

INTRODUCTION

Deposition of interstitial and intraluminal calcium phosphate (CaP) nephroliths in patients with mild idiopathic or persistent hyperoxaluria following bariatric surgery [1] suggests that oxalate affects the physiology of calcium and phosphate. CaP cores and Randall's plaques are common features of calcium oxalate (CaOx) nephroliths in idiopathic hyperoxalurics [2]. In this series of experiments we looked at concentrations of calcium and phosphate in urine and kidneys and compared the accumulation of oxalate and calcium in several organs during a persistent oxalate challenge.

METHODS

Sprague-Dawley rats were implanted with 2 ml, 7d minipumps dispensing PBS or 60 to 360 µmole of potassium oxalate (KOx) for 13 D; procedures were as previously described [3]. 3.3-4.3 µCi/ d of ^{14}C-oxalate (spa. 8 mCi/ mmole) was added to the KOx for determining tissue oxalate concentrations. Urine was collected on D12-13; animals were euthanized and tissues harvested. Urine oxalate concentrations were determined by the oxalate-oxidase colorimetric assay. Urine calcium and phosphate concentrations were determined by University Hospitals of Cleveland Core Laboratories. Tissue oxalate concentrations were determined by scintillation counting. Tissue calcium and phosphate concentrations were determined by atomic absorbance

CP1049, *Renal Stone Disease 2, 2nd International Urolithiasis Research Symposium,*
edited by A. P. Evan, J. E. Lingeman, J. A. McAteer, and J. C. Williams, Jr.

spectrometry in a Perkin Elmer 3100 and by the Fiske-Subbatow colorimetric assay. Statistical analysis was by ANOVA and Fisher's LSD (SPSS) or by linear regression (Prism). Data are expressed as mean ± sem.

RESULTS & DISCUSSION

Calcium excretion was inversely correlated with oxalate excretion in rats treated with PBS or 60-360 μmole KOx/d (Figure 1a, $p \leq 0.02$). The trend for phosphate versus oxalate was similar but not statistically significant (Figure 1b, $p = 0.07$). Plasma concentrations of calcium and phosphate were like those of controls ($p \geq 0.1$).

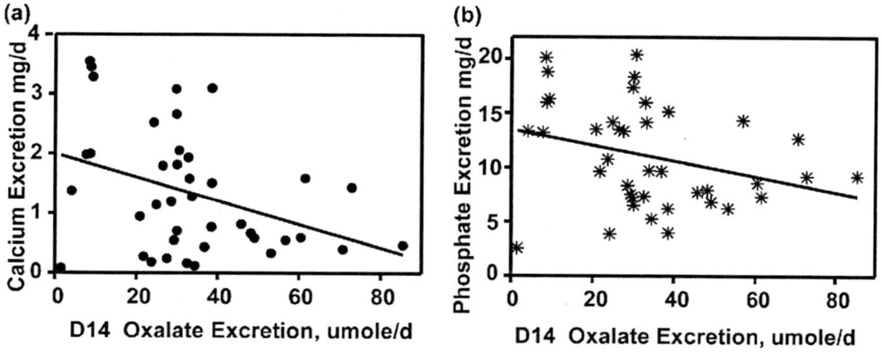

FIGURE 1. Correlation between D 13 urinary excretion of oxalate vs. that of calcium (a: $r^2 = 0.14$, $p \leq 0.02$) or phosphate (b: $r^2 = 0.09$, $p = 0.07$) for rats treated with PBS, 60, 120, 240, 300 or 360 μmole KOx/ d for 13 D (n = 5-7 rats/ dose).

Calcium concentrations were the same in the whole kidney, cortex, medulla, or papilla ($p>0.6$), so these values were pooled for analysis. Although calcium and phosphate concentrations showed similar dose response patterns in all runs, the magnitude of the change varied (1-2 rats/dose/run). Treatment with 360 μmole KOx/d for 13D gave renal calcium concentrations double those in renal tissue from controls ($p \leq 0.001$, Figure 2). Phosphate concentrations doubled in renal tissues from rats treated with 120 μmole KOx/d ($p \leq 0.05$) but not in those treated with 360 μmole KOx (Figure 2). It is not clear if these data manifest a real biphasic response or a statistical artifact, i.e., with more rats the 360 μmole KOx/d treatment might have increased renal phosphate concentrations more proportionately.

To determine the relationship between tissue concentrations of oxalate and calcium, rats were treated with 360 μmole KOx + 3.3-4.3 μCi ^{14}C-oxalate and euthanized after 12 hr to 13 D. Despite the persistent oxalate challenge, several tissues exhibited less than a two-fold increase in oxalate concentration. This was surprising given the large doses of oxalate and the existence of nonrenal oxalate clearance and an exchangeable pool of oxalate beyond the extracellular fluid and plasma [4,5]. Calcium concentrations in these tissues did not change during the oxalate challenge. The overall means for these oxalate and calcium concentrations are shown in Table 1.

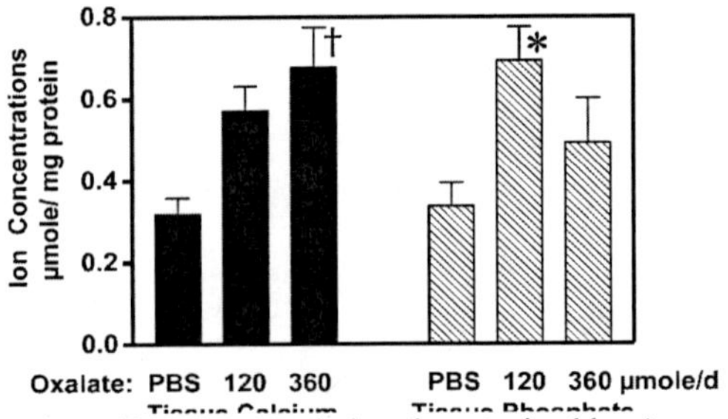

FIGURE 2. Changes in calcium (black bars) and phosphate (striped bars) concentrations in renal tissue. Values for the whole kidneys, cortex, medulla, papilla were not different ($p>0.06$) and tissues were pooled. Rats were treated with PBS, 120 or 360 µmole KOx for 13D (n=9-10 rats/dose). † $p \leq 0.001$ as compared to PBS. * $p \leq 0.05$ as compared to PBS.

TABLE 1. Mean oxalate and calcium concentrations in time course rats for tissues having < 2-fold increase in oxalate and no change in calcium

Tissue	Oxalate µmole/ g wet weight	Calcium µmole/ g wet weight
Spleen	0.052 ± 0.005	16.1 ± 2.4
Lung	0.12 ± 0.013	21.5 ± 1.7
Liver	0.077 ± 0.006	12.3 ± 1.1
Testis	0.026 ± 0.002	13.4 ± 1.1
Skeletal Muscle	0.014 ± 0.004	14.2 ± 2.7

[360 µmole oxalate/d 12hr, 1D, 2D, 7D (n = 4 rats/d), 13D (n = 6 rats/d, mean ± sem)]

In contrast, the kidneys and brain showed larger increases in oxalate concentrations during the time course (Figure 3a,b; $p \leq 0.02$), while the increase in the skin not part of the pump pocket just missed significance (Figure 3c; $p \leq 0.058$). The brain is not usually considered an oxalate reservoir and most neuropathies in hyperoxalurics are associated with the peripheral, not central, nervous system.

Calcium concentrations increased with time of treatment in the whole kidney (Figure 3a; $p \leq 0.001$) but not in the brain or main skin (Figures 3 b & c; $p=0.07$). Calcium concentrations were five (kidney) to >10,000 (brain) times greater than oxalate concentrations in the same tissue, so it is not surprising that most tissues showed no significant increase in calcium concentrations. Since calcium and oxalate crystallize in a one-to-one ratio, we must suspect that at least part of the increase in renal calcium was noncrystalline. Unexpectedly, oxalate and calcium concentrations in the kidney were not correlated ($r^2 = 0.002$, $p=0.8$), while those in the brain were ($r^2 = 0.46$, $p \leq 0.0005$). The correlation between oxalate and calcium concentrations in the skin was not significant ($r^2 = 0.13$, $p=0.1$).

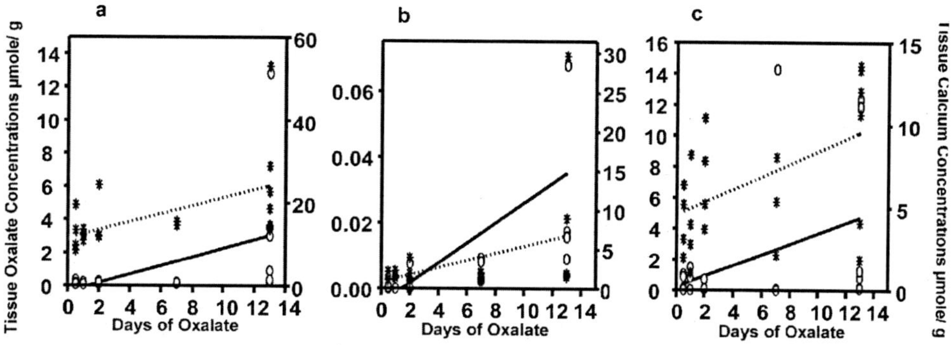

FIGURE 3. Correlation between time vs. oxalate (open circles, solid regression line, µmole/g tissue) or calcium (stars, dashed regression line, µmole/ g tissue) concentrations in whole kidneys (a), brain (b) and skin not part of the pump pocket (c). Rats were treated with 360 µmole oxalate/ d for 12hr, 1D, 2D, 7D (n = 4 rats/ d), or 13D (n = 6 rats/d, mean ± sem)). Correlations between tissue oxalate vs. time are as follows: whole kidney $r^2 = 0.25$, $p \leq 0.02$; brain $r^2 = 0.38$, $p \leq 0.0002$; skin $r^2 = 0.17$, $p \leq 0.058$). Correlations between tissue calcium vs. time are as follows: whole kidney $r^2 = 0.29$, $p \leq 0.001$; brain $r^2 = 0.15$, $p \leq 0.07$; skin $r^2 = 0.15$, $p \leq 0.07$).

Together these data support the hypothesis that calcium concentrations in the kidney do not necessarily correlate with urinary calcium excretion. While increases in renal oxalate concentrations are associated with increases in renal calcium concentrations, other factors are obviously playing significant and probably controlling roles in modulating this increase. Thus oxalate associated increases in renal calcium may be due to secondary effects of oxalate rather than being due to direct effects of oxalate on calcium transport. Because of the difference in magnitude of calcium and oxalate in the kidney, these increases are probably not limited to increases due to the formation of calcium oxalate crystal deposits.

ACKNOWLEDGMENTS

Funding was provided by the AUA Foundation, NIH-DK73730 (SRM), and NIH-HL18708 (AMPR). The technical assistance of Daniel Chen and the editorial assistance of S.E. Brown are gratefully acknowledged.

REFERENCES

1. Evan AP, Lingeman JE, Coe FL, et al. *J Clin Invest* **111**, 607-616 (2003).
2. Randall A. *Int Abs Surg* **71** 209-240 (1940).
3. Marengo SR, Chen DH-C, MacLennan GT, et al. *J Urol* **171**, 1304-1308 (2004)
4. Boer P, Prenen JA, Koomans HA, et al. *Nephron* **41**, 78-81 (1985)
5. Watts RW, Veall N, Purkiss P. *Clin Sci (Lond)* **65**, 627-633 (1983)

Quantitative Analysis of Metabolic Profile and Tamm-Horsfall Protein in Pediatric Stone Patients

M.I. Kogan[a], D.G. Matishov[b], E.F. Shin[b], and V.V. Sizonov[a]

[a]*Rostov State Medical University, Russian Federation, 344034 Rostov-on-Don, 29 Nakhichevansky street*
[b]*Southern Scientific Centre of the Russian Academy of Sciences, Russian Federation, 344006 Rostov-on-Don, 41 Chekhov street*

Abstract. According to some studies, the secretion of urinary glycoprotein Tamm-Horsfall protein (uromodulin) plays a significant part in the suppression of calcium nephrolith formation. The aim of the present study was to detect correlation of Tamm-Horsfall protein with soluble Ca^{2+} in the urine of urolithic patients and compare it with a control group, in order to estimate the degree of the disease progress, as well as the prognosis for the disease. The research included 29 urolithic patients, aged 8,0±0,2 y. The content of soluble Ca^{2+} in fresh urine was estimated by the method of capillary zone electrophoresis. The level of Tamm-Horsfall protein in urine was measured from cryoprecipitate using SDS polyacrylamide electrophoresis and semiquantitative analysis. Urine from the urolithic patients was consistently higher in Ca^{2+} and in Tamm-Horsfall protein concentrations than urine from controls, at all periods of the day.

Keywords: urolithiasis, Tamm-Horsfall protein, uromodulin, soluble calcium, urine
PACS: 87.18.Xr

RESEARCH OF URINE BIOMARKER

At present, the research in the sphere of urogenital pathology is of current importance due to its widespread occurrence, evidence of complications, and increase of disability among the patients. According to published data, urinary glycoprotein Tamm-Horsfall protein secretion (uromodulin) [1] plays a significant role in the suppression of calcium nephrolith formation. Tamm-Horsfall protein is a membrane protein of the epithelium of Henle's loop; it is thought to be involved in binding of soluble Ca^{2+}, removing the latter from the organism and preventing precipitation of insoluble calcium in the form of stones [2]. According to some authors' data, gene mutation of Tamm-Horsfall protein C744G has been detected in patients with medullary cystic renal disease type 2 and familial juvenile hyperuricemic nephropathy, following by the loss of salts—a factor favorable to stone formation [3]. Moreover, in mice lacking Tamm-Horsfall protein, deposition of calcium oxalate in the kidney happens more readily [4]. Since the data on Tamm-Horsfall protein level and soluble Ca^{2+} in urolithic patients' urine are extremely inconsistent, the aim of the present study was to examine these and to compare them with a control group. The obtained results

CP1049, *Renal Stone Disease 2, 2nd International Urolithiasis Research Symposium,*
edited by A. P. Evan, J. E. Lingeman, J. A. McAteer, and J. C. Williams, Jr.

would be significant for the estimation of the degree of development of the disease, prognosis for the disease, and treatment efficacy.

STRATEGY FOR ANALYSIS AND SAMPLE PREPARATION

The study included 29 urolithic patients aged 8,0±1,2 at the average. The control group was composed of 15 conditionally healthy children (aged 8,0±1,0 at the average).

The content of soluble Ca^{2+} in fresh urine was estimated by the method of capillary zone electrophoresis (Kapel' 105, Russia). Normally, the content of Ca^{2+} in the urine is 240 mg/l. Tamm-Horsfall protein extraction in the control group and in urolithic patients was carried out by the method of cryoprecipitation (freezing at -20° for 12 hours, followed by thawing at +4°), worked up by Professor Judah Folkman [5]. The samples were taken before meals into a separate test-tube in the morning, at noon, and in the evening during three days (9 samples from each patient). Mean values of Ca^{2+} and Tamm-Horsfall protein were obtained in the morning, at noon, and in the evening individually in each patient and within the group.

The Tamm-Horsfall protein level dynamics in cryoprecipitate of the urine was estimated by the method of SDS-electrophoresis in polyacrylamide gel (Bio-Rad, USA); the coloring power of protein streaks on the gel, corresponding to Tamm-Horsfall protein, was estimated by a semi-quantitative method. Values of level Tamm-Horsfall protein are expressed in arbitrary intensity units. By means of program Quantity One (Bio-Rad, USA) intensity was defined by signal strength (density in box) within the limits of the allocated area of the image (colored protein spot of Tamm-Horsfall protein). After the procedure of trypsinolysis (Promega) of the protein spots, mass-spectrometric identification (MALDI-TOF-MS Bruker, Germany) of the protein contained in the distinguished streak was carried out.

RESULTS AND DISCUSSION

A decrease of mean values of Ca^{2+} level was seen in the control group at noon ($p<0,05$), and in the evening ($p<0,05$), as compared to morning urines; similarly, an increase of mean values of the Tamm-Horsfall protein level was also seen at noon ($p<0,05$), and in the evening ($p<0,05$), relative to the morning values of the control group. The analysis of protein and electrolyte profile indices in urolithic patients showed higher mean values of soluble Ca^{2+} level in the morning ($p<0,05$), at noon ($p<0,1$), and in the evening ($p<0,05$), as compared to similar indices in the control group. Mean values of the Tamm-Horsfall protein level in patients were also higher in the morning ($p<0,1$), at noon($p<0,1$), in the evening ($p<0,05$), as compared to similar indices in the control group (Table 1).

Thus, it has been shown that both Tamm-Horsfall protein concentration and the concentration of soluble Ca^{2+} in urine were higher in urolithic patients than in controls. But in the urolithic patients, the level of Ca^{2+} was 100-500 % higher than in controls, while the level of Tamm-Horsfall protein was only 180-300 % greater than in controls. On such a small number of patients we cannot establish a correlation between the levels of Ca^{2+} and Tamm-Horsfall protein, however there does seem to be a tendency for these parameters to track together. For this purpose it is necessary to continue research on more representative samples from patients. A lack of correlation between Ca^{2+} and Tamm-Horsfall protein could also be explained by an insufficient quantity of normally functioning Tamm-Horsfall protein secretion or posttranscriptional protein modification (for example, additional glycosylation, phosphorylation) which reduces this protein's ability to bind with Ca^{2+} [2]. Both of these processes could increase the risk of stone formation. To obtain more precise data on the problem, it will be essential to compare the Tamm-Horsfall protein structure in urolithic patients and the control group by the use of mass-spectrometric methods. It will also be necessary to increase the sample sizes of patients and the control group for proper representation in the obtained results.

TABLE 1. Mean values of Ca^2+ and Tamm-Horsfall protein (control group and urolithic patients)

Parametres	Control group (n=15)			Patients (n=29)		
	morning	**noon**	**evening**	**morning**	**noon**	**evening**
Ca^{2+}, mg/l	124,5±8,3	88,3±4,1 1)**	59,4±3,4 1)**	336,6±4,8 2)**	204,8±5,2 2)*	331,5±4,6 2)**
Tamm-Horsfall protein, Intensity x10, conventional units	123,4±4,2	141±3,3 1)**	203,8±4,1 1)**	356,2±5,4 2)*	335,4±3,2 2)*	380±4,4 2)**

Notes: * - p<0,1; ** - p<0,05.

1) probability by Student's t-criterion: morning Ca^{2+}(Tamm-Horsfall protein)/noon Ca^{2+}(Tamm-Horsfall protein), morning Ca^{2+}(Tamm-Horsfall protein)/evening Ca^{2+}(Tamm-Horsfall protein) control group;

2) probability by Student's t-criterion: morning Ca^{2+}(Tamm-Horsfall protein) patient/morning Ca^{2+}(Tamm-Horsfall protein) control group, noon Ca^{2+}(Tamm-Horsfall protein) patient/noon Ca^{2+}(Tamm-Horsfall protein) control group, evening Ca^{2+}(Tamm-Horsfall protein) patient / evening Ca^{2+}(Tamm-Horsfall protein) control group.

ACKNOWLEDGMENTS

The authors gratefully acknowledge the assistance and cooperation of O.N. Darashkevich. We extend special gratitude to Academician RAS G.G. Matishov for expert guidance. We express sincere appreciation to E.I. Goufman for tireless efforts and invaluable advice.

REFERENCES

1. K. Yokomizoi, A. Nakayama, E. Hokazono, A. Ninomiya, R. Miyake, N. Hiratsuka, M. Okuyama, Y. Kato, S. Kobayashi, Y. Ito, K. Shiba, "Analysis of proteins in urinary tract stones and urine of urolithic patients", *Rinsho Byori.*, 2005 Dec, 53(12), pp. 1109-1115.
2. M. Jaggi, Y. Nakagawa, L. Zipperle, B. Hess, "Tamm-Horsfall protein in recurrent calcium kidney stone formers with positive family history: abnormalities in urinary excretion, molecular structure and function", *Urol Res.*, 2007 Apr, 35(2), pp. 55-62.

3. M.T. Wolf, B.B. Beck, F. Zaucke, A. Kunze, J. Misselwitz, J. Ruley, T. Ronda, A. Fischer, F. Eifinger, C. Licht, E. Otto, B. Hoppe, F. Hildebrandt, "The Uromodulin C744G mutation causes MCKD2 and FJHN in children and adults and may be due to a possible founder effect", *Kidney Int.*, 2007 Mar, 71(6), pp. 574-81, Epub 2007 Jan 24.
4. L. Mo, L. Liaw, A.P. Evan, A.J. Sommer, J.C. Lieske and X.-R. Wu. Renal calcinosis and stone formation in mice lacking osteopontin, Tamm-Horsfall protein, or both. *AJP - Renal Physiology* 293(6):F1935-1943 (2007).
5. J.J. Marler, S.J. Fishman, S.M. Kilroy, J. Fang, J. Upton, J.B. Mulliken, P.E. Burrows, D. Zurakowski, J. Folkman, M.A. Moses, "Increased expression of urinary matrix metalloproteinases parallels the extent and activity of vascular anomalies", *Pediatrics*, 2005 Jul, 116(1), pp. 38-45.

Is It Worth Upgrading Your Flexible Ureterorenoscope? A Clinical Analysis

Gunnar Wendt-Nordahl[a], Tuna Mut[b], Peter Alken[a], Thomas Knoll[a]

[a]*Department of Urology, University Hospital Mannheim, Germany.*
[b]*Istanbul Faculty of Medicine, Department of Urology, Istanbul, Turkey*

Abstract. The new generation semiflexible ureterorenoscopes (URS) offer an improved deflection of 270° in both directions and a stiffer sheath. It is postulated that stone access and removal are facilitated compared to the conventional devices. In our study, we aimed to determine the difference in efficacy of stone treatment comparing the new and the conventional flexible URS. A total of 90 patients with upper urinary tract stones were included into a retrospective study. 29 cases were treated with the last generation flexible URS (11274 AA, Karl Storz Endoscopy, Germany) between 01/2000 and 07/2003 and 61 cases were treated with the new flexible URS (Flex-X, Karl Storz Endoscopy, Germany) between 12/2005 and 05/2007. The patients underwent standard clinical and radiological workup before the procedure. Patients' and stone characteristics, stone free rate and complications were compared between the two groups. Treatment success was defined as complete stone removal or insignificant residual fragments <4mm requiring no further intervention. Stone access was possible in 97% and 100% for the conventional and new URS group. Immediate treatment success was 38% for the conventional versus 70% for the new flexible scope ($p=0.0032$). For the subgroup of lower pole stones mean stone size was 6.6 mm (conventional scope, 16 patients) versus 5.3 mm (new scope, 51 patients). Stone access was possible in 94% versus 100% and treatment success was 31% versus 69% ($p=0.0004$) for the old compared to the new scope. No major complications were observed. Minor complications were comparable in both groups. Our study suggests an advantage of the new flexible ureterorenoscopes compared to their predecessors. They offer an increased stone free rate especially in the treatment of lower pole stones.

Keywords: Flexible ureterorenoscopy; stone free rate; lower pole stones
PACS: 01.30.Cc

INTRODUCTION

The introduction of flexible ureterorenoscopy (URS) has lead to a new dimension in diagnosis and treatment of upper urinary tract diseases, especially for urinary tract calculi and tumors. Constant progress in miniaturization has led to the development of flexible scopes with tip diameter less than 9F, active tip deflection in both directions and incorporated working and irrigation channels.

However, due to the miniaturization, the scopes, especially the deflection system, became more fragile requiring high maintenance costs [1]. Another problem is the loss of maximal tip deflection when tools are inserted into the working channel. Furthermore, the insertion of working tools leads to a reduction in irrigation, impairing the vision during surgery [2].

CP1049, *Renal Stone Disease 2, 2nd International Urolithiasis Research Symposium,*
edited by A. P. Evan, J. E. Lingeman, J. A. McAteer, and J. C. Williams, Jr.

To overcome these problems, a new generation of flexible ureterorenoscopes has been introduced in recent years. They offer a stiffer sheath allowing a bare ureter passage in most cases, are more durable and lead to reduced maintenance costs [3-5]. Furthermore, they offer an exaggerated maximal tip deflection of >270° which is maintained when working tools are inserted into the working channel [3,6]. The higher maximal tip deflection of the new generation scopes is postulated to offer an easier stone access compared to the conventional flexible URS, especially for lower pole stones. Our study was undertaken to determine if the new scopes offer a higher stone free rate compared to their predecessors.

MATERIAL & METHODS

90 patients with upper urinary tract stones treated with flexible URS in the University Hospital Mannheim, Germany, were included in this retrospective analysis. 29 of these patients (conventional URS group) were treated with the last generation flexible URS (11274 AA, Karl Storz Endoscopy, Germany) between January 2000 and July 2003. 61 patients (Flex-X group) were treated with a newer generation flexible URS (Flex-X, Karl Storz Endoscopy, Germany) between December 2005 and May 2007. Patients' demography and stone characteristics, intraoperative data as well as treatment success and associated complications were recorded from the patients' charts and compared between the two groups. Treatment success was defined as complete removal of all stones or insignificant residual fragments, smaller than 4mm, requiring no further intervention.

Prior to the procedure, all patients underwent a standard clinical and radiological workup. Under general anesthesia, the procedure started with a cystoscopy and a hydrophilic guidewire was passed up the ureter into the kidney. Afterwards, the flexible URS was passed over the guidewire into the kidney. In case of anticipated multiple ureter passages, an access sheath was placed in the ureter. In none of the patients was a further intramural dilation process required. A thorough inspection of the complete collecting system followed before stone removal was initiated. Whenever necessary, the stones were fragmented before extraction. A double-J catheter was placed in case of multiple ureter passages or residual calculi.

RESULTS

Patients' demography and stone characteristics are listed in Table 1. Patients' age, gender and treated side were comparable in both groups. Size, number and location of the treated stones were also comparable in both groups, although the proportion of lower pole stones was higher in the group treated with the new flexible URS (84% versus 55%).

Intraoperative data and complications are shown in Table 2. Operation time was comparable for both groups; an access sheath was used in 20% and 30% in the conventional and Flex-X group, respectively. Lithotripsy was performed using a holmium laser in the majority of cases in both groups and stone removal was accomplished using nitinol baskets or graspers.

TABLE 1: Patients' demography and stone characteristics

	Conventional	Newer
Number of patients	29	61
Mean age (years)	59±14	52±15
Gender (male:female)	15:14	36:25
Side (left:right)	14:15	32:29
Stone size (mm)	8.8±3.0	8.5±3.3
Number of stones		
Single	18 (62%)	37 (61%)
Multiple	11 (38%)	24 (39%)
Stone localization		
Renal pelvis	3 (10%)	8 (13%)
Upper calyx	4 (14%)	7 (11%)
Middle calyx	11 (38%)	10 (16%)
Lower calyx	16 (55%)	51 (84%)
Pretreatment with Double-J	23 (79%)	30 (49%)

TABLE 2: Intraoperative data and complications

	Conventional	Newer
Operation time (min)	103±40	99±48
Access sheath	6 (21%)	19 (31%)
Lithotripsy		
Laser	11 (38%)	41 (67%)
Ballistic	3 (10%)	0
Stone removing tool		
Nitinol basket	13 (45%)	45 (74%)
Grasper	9 (31%)	2 (3%)
both	5 (17%)	7 (11%)
Complications		
Perforation	1 (3%)	1 (2%)
Abortion for bleeding	2 (7%)	4 (7%)
Fever	2 (7%)	3 (5%)

Stone access was possible in 97% and 100% for the conventional and new URS group, respectively (see Figure 1). Immediate treatment success was significantly improved in the new flexible URS group (38% versus 70%; p=0032).

For the subgroup of lower pole stones stone access was also comparable in both groups (94% versus 100% for the conventional and new scope, respectively; see Figure 2). With 31% versus 69% treatment success was significantly higher in the new flexible URS group (p=0.0004).

No major complications were observed. Minor complications, including perforation (3% versus 2%), abortion because of bleeding or impaired visibility (7% versus 7%) and transient postoperative fever (7% versus 5%) were comparable in both groups (see Table 2).

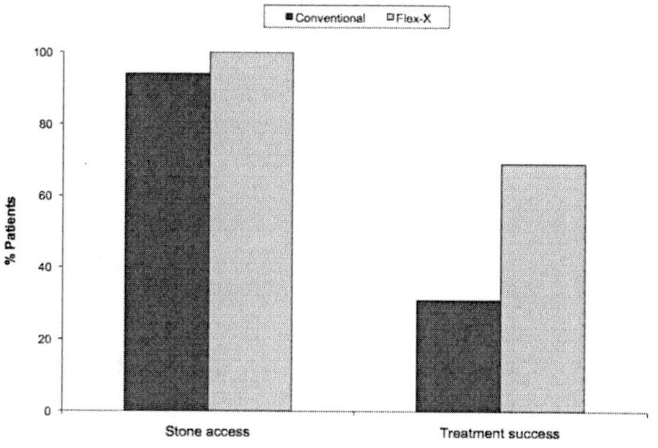

FIGURE 1. All stones: Stone access and treatment success. The newer ureterorenoscope offered an improved treatment success (p=0.0032).

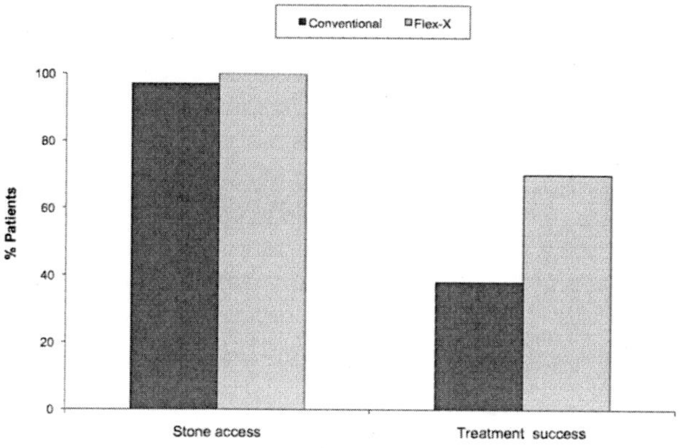

Figure 2. Lower pole stones: Stone access and treatment success. The newer ureterorenoscope offered an improved treatment success (p=0.0004).

DISCUSSION

Flexible URS is widely used as minimal invasive treatment option in upper urinary tract stone therapy. Conventional flexible scopes offer a maximal active deflection of 150° and insertion of working tools such as nitinol baskets or laser probes lead to a further loss of active deflection [3;6]. Furthermore, the vulnerability of conventional flexible ureterorenoscopes leads to a high repair frequency and high associated maintenance costs [1]. To overcome these problems, a new generation of flexible URS has been introduced in recent years. They offer a higher maximal active deflection of >270° in both directions and a stiffer sheath allowing for a bare ureter passage in many cases. Furthermore, the scopes are more durable leading to a reduction in maintenance costs[5]. It was demonstrated in a large series that the higher active deflection of the new generation flexible scopes offers greater access to the lower pole compared to the conventional devices indicating advantages for intrarenal stone treatment [4]. In our study, we found stone access feasible in 97% of all cases and 94% of lower pole stones when the conventional flexible URS was used. However, despite the feasible access, treatment success (defined as complete stone removal or residual fragments <4mm requiring no further intervention) was only 38% for all stones and was further reduced to 31% in the subgroup of lower pole stones. An explanation is the loss of maximal active deflection when working tools are inserted either impairing or completely preventing the access to the lower pole.

In contrast to that, the new generation flexible URS offered stone access in all patients regardless of the localization. With a treatment success of 70% for all cases, the new generation device offered a success rate almost twice as high as that achieved with the conventional scope. This advantage in treatment efficacy was even more pronounced in the subgroup of lower pole stones, where a success rate of 69% was reached with the new generation flexible URS.

It should be noted that the retrospective nature of our study means that uncontrolled factors could have affected the results. For example, it is probable that increasing surgical experience improved the results in the newer instrument. Similarly, the quality of intracorporeal grasping devices has also improved over time, and our study did not take that into account any effect of changes in auxiliary equipment. Nevertheless, the results of the study are in accordance with our subjective assessment of the newer ureterorenoscopes, that they offer improved utility over older models.

In conclusion, our study demonstrates that flexible URS is a safe and efficient treatment modality for upper urinary tract stones. As the new generation flexible ureterorenoscopes provide an improved treatment efficacy, it seems advisable to switch to these devices despite the high acquisition costs.

REFERENCES

1. Afane,J.S., Olweny,E.O., Bercowsky,E., Sundaram,C.P., Dunn,M.D., Shalhav,A.L., McDougall,E.M., and Clayman,R.V. (2000) Flexible ureteroscopes: a single center evaluation of the durability and function of the new endoscopes smaller than 9Fr. 164, 1164-1168.
2. Michel,M.S., Knoll,T., Ptaschnyk,T., Kohrmann,K.U., and Alken,P. (2002) Flexible ureterorenoscopy for the treatment of lower pole calyx stones: influence of different lithotripsy probes and stone extraction tools on scope deflection and irrigation flow. 41, 312-316.
3. Wendt-Nordahl,G., Trojan,L., Alken,P., Michel,M.S., and Knoll,T. (2007) Ureteroscopy for stone treatment using new 270 degrees semiflexible endoscope: in vitro, ex vivo, and clinical application. 21, 1439-1444.
4. Johnson,G.B., Portela,D., and Grasso,M. (2006) Advanced ureteroscopy: wireless and sheathless. 20, 552-555.
5. Traxer,O., Dubosq,F., Jamali,K., Gattegno,B., and Thibault,P. (2006) New-generation flexible ureterorenoscopes are more durable than previous ones. 68, 276-279.
6. Pasqui,F., Dubosq,F., Tchala,K., Tligui,M., Gattegno,B., Thibault,P., and Traxer,O. (2004) Impact on active scope deflection and irrigation flow of all endoscopic working tools during flexible ureteroscopy. 45, 58-64.

Morphology of Major Stone Types, As Shown by Micro Computed Tomography (micro CT)

Molly E. Jackson, Christian A. Beuschel, James A. McAteer, and James C. Williams, Jr.

Department of Anatomy and Cell Biology, Indiana University School of Medicine, Indianapolis, IN 46202, USA

Abstract. Micro CT offers the possibility of providing a non-destructive method of stone analysis that allows visualization of 100% of the stone's volume. For the present study, micro CT analysis was completed on stones of known composition with isotropic voxel sizes of either 7 or 9.1 µm. Each mineral type was distinctive, either by x-ray attenuation values or by morphology. Minor components, such as the presence of apatite in oxalate stones, were easily seen. The analysis of stones by micro CT opens up the possibility of exploring the stone as an encapsulated history of the patient's disease, showing changes in mineral deposition with time.

Keywords: Urinary Calculi, micro computed tomography
PACS: 81.70.Tx

INTRODUCTION

Clinically, Fourier-transform infrared spectroscopy (FT-IR) or x-ray diffraction are used for stone analysis [1], but these methods require hand dissection, a skill that probably varies from lab to lab [2], and can easily miss minor stone components. We have previously described the use of micro CT for analyzing stones [3]. The present study utilizes the state-of-the-art SkyScan 1172 micro CT system to assess internal structure of kidney stones and to visualize minor stone components.

METHODS

Relatively pure stones, each containing at least 90% of one mineral, were used, including stones of calcium oxalate monohydrate (COM), calcium oxalate dihydrate (COD), brushite, apatite, uric acid, and cystine. Each stone was scanned using the Skyscan 1172 Micro CT System (Kontich, Belgium) with isotropic voxel sizes of either 7 or 9.1 µm, depending on the stone size, yielding final image stacks of between 200-600 MB. Scans required 45-60 min, including computer reconstruction time.

CP1049, *Renal Stone Disease 2, 2nd International Urolithiasis Research Symposium,* edited by A. P. Evan, J. E. Lingeman, J. A. McAteer, and J. C. Williams, Jr.

RESULTS

Each mineral type was distinctive, either by its x-ray attenuation values (as for apatite, the highest, and uric acid, the lowest) or by its morphological characteristics. Minor mineral components, such as the presence of calcium oxalate in uric acid and cystine stones, were easily seen. Most COM stones exhibited low absorbing areas (voids) and various forms of concentric ring layering between different concentrations of the mineral. Two examples of COM stones are shown in Figure 1.

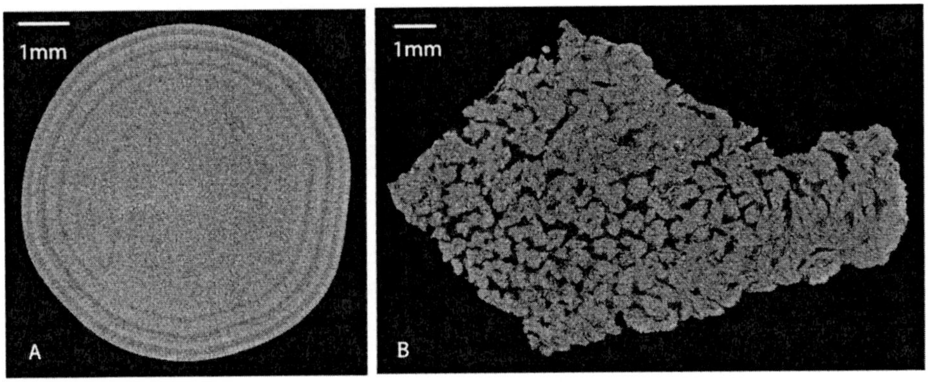

FIGURE 1. A) Cross section of typical COM stone showing regions of lower concentration of mineral and concentric layering. B) Cross section of COM stone showing voids throughout stone and large crystals making up the bulk of the stone. The polygonal shapes of the crystals are seen easily when scrolling through the image stack. The morphology of polygonal crystals suggests that this stone began as COD, and then was transformed to the more stable COM through the process crystalline conversion [4]. Although the mineral is now COM, the original conditions that caused the stone to grow to this size were those that favored the growth of COD crystals [5,6].

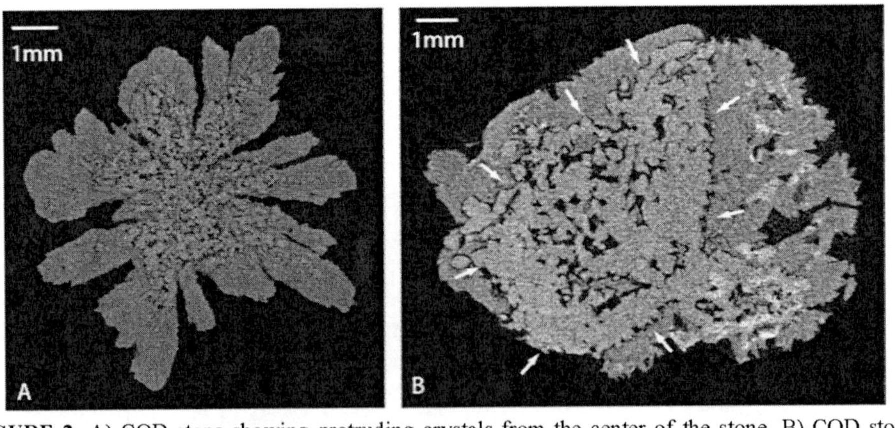

FIGURE 2. A) COD stone showing protruding crystals from the center of the stone. B) COD stone showing a large region with higher X-ray absorbing mineral (shown within arrows), indicating conversion of mineral to COM.

COD stones generally showed the morphology expected of this mineral that forms as bi-pyramidal crystals (Figure 2). The micro CT images of COD stones also frequently showed slightly brighter (more x-ray-dense) regions, which probably represent areas of the stone that have undergone conversion of COD to COM. Such conversion is to be expected for any stone that resides in the urinary tract for extended time, as described above.

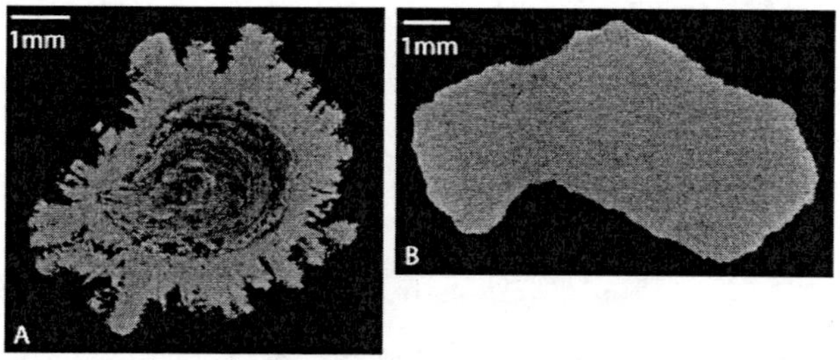

FIGURE 3. A) Cross section of a brushite stone having a shell of radiating crystals and a core suggesting the layering of apatite mineral. B) Cross section of brushite stone not containing voids or different minerals, apparently having very tightly packed crystals.

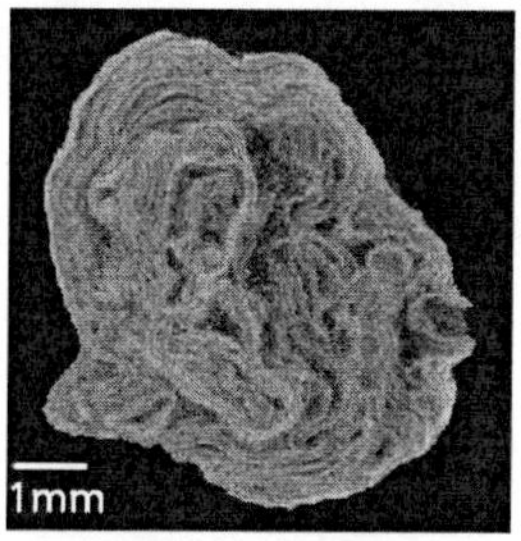

FIGURE 4. Apatite, showing multiple x-ray-dense layers.

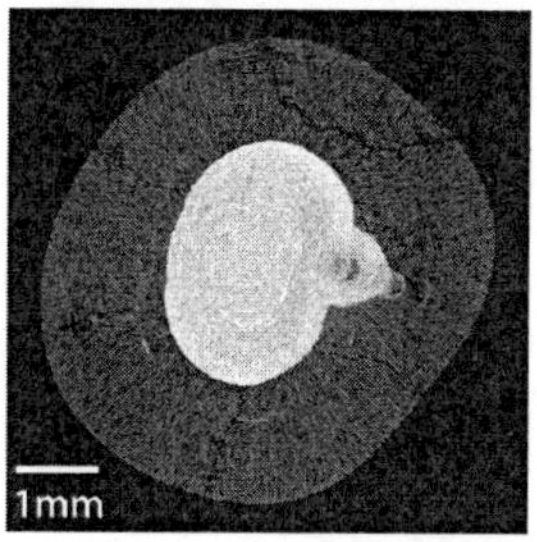

FIGURE 5. Cross section of uric acid stone containing a core of COM.

Brushite displayed highly X-ray absorbing mineral. Many brushite stones showed radial crystals protruding out toward the surface of the stone, with void regions throughout the stone and a rough outer edge (Figure 3A). Others displayed an evenness of micro CT appearance (Figure 3B), apparently due to tight packing of the brushite crystals, which are long and easily seen by stereomicroscope.

Apatite stones showed highly absorbing mineral often forming multiple bright layers separated by less x-ray dense layers (Figure 4). Some apatite stones also showed large internal void regions, perhaps representing areas dominated by protein.

Uric acid stones showed the lowest x-ray densities (Figure 5), with the layers of uric acid often visible, separated by narrow dark regions. The example shown in Figure 5 turned out to be a mixed stone, with a core of COM that was surrounded by a thick layer of uric acid. This morphology strongly suggests that the calculus began as a COM stone, and implies a significant alteration in the physicochemical properties of the patient's urine over time.

Cystine mineral was intermediate in x-ray density, though rough cystine stones tended to display more spots of higher X-ray absorbing mineral and also more voids (Figure 6), as has been described previously [7].

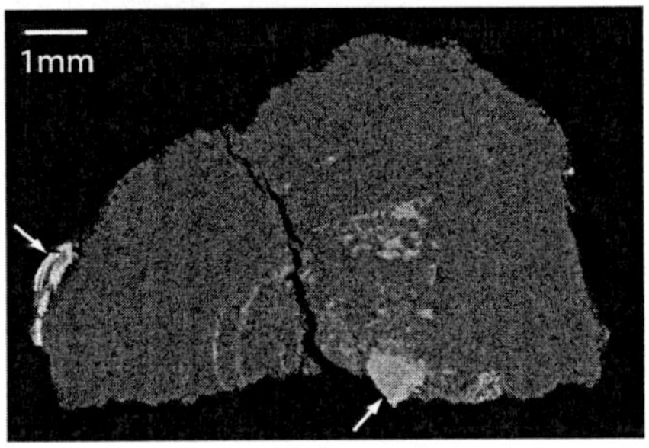

FIGURE 6. Cross section of a cystine stone with internal structure containing voids (dark spots) and highly absorbing mineral (calcium salts, shown with arrows).

CONCLUSIONS

Micro CT, allows complete visualization of stone components in three dimensions. In the present study, minor mineral components were easily seen in four of the five stone types, and layering between different densities of mineral was seen in all of the stone types used in this study. These alterations in the deposition of mineral almost certainly are a consequence of changes in the patient's urine properties over time. Thus, the stone becomes a record of the urine supersaturations. Micro CT allows the determination of minerals making up this record. With further study, it may be possible to relate the records of these layers directly to disease processes, inferring the patient's history from the stone.

ACKNOWLEDGMENTS

Funded by NIH R01DK59933 and S10RR023710. Special thanks to Dr. J.E. Lingeman and Beck Analytical for providing stone specimens.

REFERENCES

1. G. Schubert. Stone analysis. Urol Res 34 (2):146-150 (2006).
2. G.P. Kasidas, C.T. Samuell and T.B. Weir. Renal stone analysis: why and how? *Ann Clin Biochem* 41:91-97 (2004).
3. C.A. Zarse, J.A. McAteer, A.J. Sommer, S.C. Kim, E.K. Hatt, J.E. Lingeman, A.P. Evan and J.C. Williams, Jr. Nondestructive analysis of urinary calculi using micro computed tomography. *BMC Urology* 4:15 (2004).
4. M. Daudon, C.A. Bader and P. Jungers. Urinary calculi: review of classification methods and correlations with etiology. *Scanning Microsc* 7(3):1081-1106 (1993).
5. M. Daudon and R.J. Reveillaud. Typage morphologique des calculs oxalocalciques et données étiopathogéniques *Annales d'Urologie* 19(5):299-308 (1985).
6. B.B. Tomazic and G.H. Nancollas, Calcium oxalate hydrates. Dissolution, transformation and crystallization studies, in *Urolithiasis. Clinical and Basic Research,* edited by L. H. Smith, W. G. Robertson and B. Finlayson (Plenum Press, New York, 1981), pp. 453-457.
7. S.C. Kim, E.K. Hatt, J.E. Lingeman, R.B. Nadler, J.A. McAteer and J.C. Williams, Jr. Cystine: helical computerized tomography characterization of rough and smooth calculi in vitro. *J Urol* 174:1468-1471 (2005).

Gender Distribution of Pediatric Stone Formers

Thomas E. Novak, Bruce J. Trock, Yegappan Lakshmanan,
John P. Gearhart, and Brian R. Matlaga

*James Buchanan Brady Urological Institute, Johns Hopkins Medical Institutions,
600 N. Wolfe St., Baltimore, MD, 21287*

Abstract. Recent epidemiologic evidence suggests that the gender prevalence among adult stone-formers is changing, with an increasing incidence of stone disease among women. No similar data have ever been reported for the pediatric stone-forming population. We performed a study to define the gender distribution among pediatric stone-formers using a large-scale national pediatric database. Our findings suggest that gender distribution among stone formers varies by age with male predominance in the first decade of life shifting to female predominance in the second decade. In contrast to adults, females in the pediatric population are more commonly affected by stones than are males. The incidence of pediatric stone disease appears to be increasing at a great rate in both sexes. Further studies should build on this hypothesis-generating work and define the effects of metabolic and environmental risk factors that may influence stone risk in the pediatric patient population

Keywords: nephrolithiasis, pediatrics, epidemiology
PACS: 87.19.X-

INTRODUCTION

Recent epidemiologic evidence suggests that the prevalence of stone disease in the United States may be increasing [1]. Furthermore, the gender distribution among stone formers, which has been classically reported to be a three-to-one male predominance, has now been reported to be moving closer to parity [2]. The epidemiology of kidney stone disease in the pediatric population has not been as well defined as it has been for the adult population. In particular, our understanding of the gender-specific prevalence among pediatric stone formers is limited, due in great part to the fact that the published literature on this subject consists of small, single-institution series, which are not easily applied to population-wide estimations. There has never been a nationally representative analysis to define the gender distribution within this unique population.

In the United States, the Kids' Inpatient Database (KID) is the only large-scale, national dataset that captures children's use of hospital services. As such, it is an ideal instrument with which to assess illness within the pediatric population. Therefore, we performed a study to define the gender distribution among pediatric stone formers using this large-scale national pediatric database.

CP1049, *Renal Stone Disease 2, 2nd International Urolithiasis Research Symposium,*
edited by A. P. Evan, J. E. Lingeman, J. A. McAteer, and J. C. Williams, Jr.

METHODOLOGY

The KID is a part of the Healthcare Cost and Utilization Project (HCUP), which is sponsored by the Agency for Healthcare Research and Quality (AHRQ). This is the only dataset on children's use of hospital services in the United States, and is a sample of discharges from all community, non-rehabilitation hospitals in states participating in the HCUP. The KID contains information on all patients, regardless of payer, including persons covered by private insurance, Medicaid, Medicare, and the uninsured. The KID includes a core set of patient data found in a typical discharge abstract, such as demographics (e.g., age, gender), diagnostic codes, procedure codes, payer and financial data, and discharge disposition. The KID does not contain physiologic or laboratory patient data.

KID data are collected and compiled in a uniform manner from all participating states. There are three iterations of the KID: 1997, 2000, and 2003. In the present study, we analyzed all three of the datasets. The 1997 version contains 1,905,797 total discharges from 22 states, the 2000 version contains 2,516,833 total discharges from 27 states, and the 2003 version contains 2,984,129 total discharges from 36 states. Hospitalizations for stone disease were identified using the International Classification of Disease 9 Clinical Modification (ICD-9-CM) codes 592.0 (renal calculus) and 592.1 (ureteral calculus).

RESULTS

Stone prevalence, stratified by age quartile and gender, are presented as Table 1. In the first decade of life, stone disease is more prevalent among males than among females. However, in the second decade of life, females are more commonly affected than are males. Within a single sex, the distribution by age group changed from 1997 to 2000, but has remained constant in the 2000 and 2003 datasets. Of note, there was a dramatic increase in treated stone disease across both genders. The rate of increase was greater among the female gender, 365%, than among the male gender, 274%.

TABLE 1. Age and gender distribution among pediatric stone formers.

Age Quartile (years)	1997		2000		2003	
	Male n (%)	Female n (%)	Male n (%)	Female n (%)	Male n (%)	Female n (%)
0-5	98 (13.1)	66 (5.1)	111 (6.9)	95 (2.9)	169 (8.2)	111 (2.4)
6-10	136 (18.2)	101 (7.8)	208 (13.0)	186 (5.6)	269 (13.2)	256 (5.4)
11-15	213 (28.6)	275 (21.3)	327 (20.4)	410 (12.1)	452 (22.1)	589 (12.5)
15-20	299 (40.1)	852 (65.8)	954 (59.6)	2645 (79.5)	1153 (56.5)	3766 (79.8)
Total	746	1294	1600	3327	2042	4722
p-value	<0.0001		<0.0001		<0.0001	

DISCUSSION

The gender distribution of pediatric stone disease differs from adults and appears to change during childhood. While boys are affected more commonly in the first decade, girls predominate in the second. Because of the lack of prior studies such as our present work, it is not known whether this change represents a shift or the natural pattern with adolescence (and puberty) ushering in either physiologic or sex-specific environmental changes that are responsible. In a study of first-degree relatives of stone formers, Bergsland *et al.* reported that age and gender had a profound influence on calcium oxalate parameters in urine [3]. Among non-stone-forming relatives, younger patients and males demonstrated higher levels of calcium oxalate supersaturation and crystal growth inhibition. The difference in growth inhibition was lost, however, in stone forming patients. These authors hypothesized that the loss of this inhibition might play a role in the rising incidence of nephrolithiasis in young males starting in the third decade [3]. The present data would suggest that this pattern of male inhibition might be even more pronounced during the second decade of life. It is interesting to note that the magnitude of increased risk of stone development in obese patients appears to be greater in adult women versus men [4].

Puberty marks a time of great growth and hormonal changes, which can plausibly affect stone pathogenesis. Heller *et al.* have investigated hormonal effects on calcium oxalate stone formation, comparing the urine chemistries of post-menopausal women with and without estrogen replacement. These authors noted that estrogen treatment resulted in a lowering of urinary calcium excretion and calcium oxalate saturation [5]. Unfortunately, similar studies on the role of pubertal hormonal changes on stone development have been lacking. The predominance of female stone formers in the second decade of life could represent a lithogenic effect of estrogen in females or a protective effect of testosterone in males. It is also possible that the primary effect of the hormones on stone formation is not directly on urine chemistry, but on body habitus and such an effect on stone pathogenesis may be secondary. For example, under the influence of androgens, the growth of lean body mass is greater in boys following puberty, while females sustain a relative increase in adiposity. While bone growth is ongoing from infancy to adolescence, puberty marks the start of a period of rapid sex steroid dependent bone growth and mineralization. The acquisition of early bone mineralization appears to be preferentially driven by estrogen and is greater in females at this age [6,7]. The impact of estrogen stimulated adiposity and enhanced bone mineralization in young females after puberty on urine chemistry and stone formation is not known, but is an area of open research.

Our analysis of the KID databases suggests that the prevalence of stone disease appears to be increasing in the pediatric population. VanDervoort *et al.* originally proposed such a rise in the pediatric patient population when they reported a 4.6-fold increased in outpatient pediatric stone encounters at a single institution between two time points (1994-1996 and 2003-2005) [8]. The present report lends support to this claim, as we report a statistically robust analysis of the pediatric population. In fact, our data may even underestimate the true prevalence of pediatric stone disease, as the

KID database captures only inpatient visits. The Urologic Diseases in America project noted a significant shift toward outpatient treatment of adult nephrolithiasis over the preceding decade with refinements in medical management and minimally invasive surgery [9]. Although the pediatric population is a unique cohort of patients, and there may be a bias towards admitting patients with stones that is greater than in an adult population, this trend may still be present. Should such a shift towards outpatient treatment be true in children, the actual prevalence of stone disease may be significantly higher than what we have presented.

The question of why pediatric stone disease may be increasing is a complicated one that will require prospective hypothesis testing trials to answer. The coincident rise in obesity during this same time period may have a causative role. The prevalence in adult obesity doubled between 1980 and 2002; however, in children aged 6-19 years, it nearly tripled in the same time period. The most recent NHANES survey, too, noted ongoing significant increases in obesity among children between 1999-2004 [10]. In a prospective, epidemiologic study of 3 large cohorts, Taylor *et al.* noted an increased risk of nephrolithiasis in adult patients who were overweight or obese [4]. A cross-sectional analysis of adults over the age of 20 from NHANES III reported that metabolic syndrome traits are associated with a self-reported history of kidney stones [11]. Obesity is associated with a number of lithogenic derangements, which makes this an attractive hypothetical target [12].

CONCLUSIONS

The gender distribution among pediatric stone formers varies by age; in the first decade of life, males predominate, whereas in the second decade of life, females predominate. Overall, though, females in the pediatric population have an increased incidence of treated stone disease than do males. Furthermore, the incidence of treated stone disease appears to be increasing at a great rate in the pediatric population. Further studies should build on this hypothesis-generating work and define the effects of metabolic and environmental risk factors that may influence stone risk in the pediatric patient population.

REFERENCES

1. K. K. Stamatelou, M. E. Francis, C. A. Jones et al., *Kidney Int* 63, 1817-1823 (2003).
2. C. D. Scales, Jr., L. H. Curtis, R. D. Norris et al., *J Urol* 177, 979-982 (2007).
3. K. J. Bergsland, J. M. Kinder, J. R. Asplin et al., *J Urol* 167, 2372-2376 (2002).
4. E. N. Taylor, M. J. Stampfer, and G. C. Curhan, *JAMA* 293, 455-462 (2005).
5. H. J. Heller, K. Sakhaee, O. W. Moe et al., *J Urol* 168, 1923-1927 (2002).
6. A. Arabi, M. Nabulsi, J. Maalouf et al., *Bone* 35, 1169-1179 (2004).
7. D. Yilmaz, B. Ersoy, E. Bilgin et al., *J Bone Miner Metab* 23, 476-482 (2005).
8. K. VanDervoort, J. Wiesen, R. Frank et al., *J Urol* 177, 2300-2305 (2007).
9. M. S. Pearle, E. A. Calhoun, and G. C. Curhan, *J Urol* 173, 848-857 (2005).
10. C. L. Ogden, M. D. Carroll, L. R. Curtin et al., *JAMA* 295, 1549-1555 (2006).
11. B. West, A. Luke, R. A. Durazo-Arvizu et al., *Am J Kidney Dis* 51, 741-747 (2008).
12. B. G. Duffey, R. N. Pedro, C. Kriedberg et al., *J Urol* 179, 1401-1406 (2008).

Effect of the Test Basket on Lithotripter Shock Waves, Cavitation Field, and Stone Breakage

Yuri A. Pishchalnikov, James A. McAteer, Anthony J. Zancanaro, Joshua S. Neucks, Irina V. Pishchalnikova, and James C. Williams, Jr.

Department of Anatomy and Cell Biology, Indiana University School of Medicine, 635 Barnhill Drive, Indianapolis, IN 46202, USA

Abstract. The performance of shock wave (SW) lithotripters is often assessed by measuring the breakage efficiency of model stones. Such in vitro tests are usually performed by positioning the stones in plastic mesh baskets. We asked if the plastic mesh affects the properties of SWs, and whether this alteration influences cavitation fields and stone breakage efficiency. Experiments were conducted using a research electrohydraulic lithotripter patterned after the Dornier HM3 (HM3-clone), and a clinical electromagnetic lithotripter (XX-ES). Shock waves were measured at the geometric focus (F2) of the HM3-clone lithotripter using a fiber-optic probe hydrophone (FOPH-500). A 2.5×4mm extruded polypropylene mesh was positioned ~8mm or ~40mm prefocally. Cavitation bubbles were recorded using a multiframe high-speed camera (Imacon 468). Breakage of gypsum cement stones was assessed using the XX-ES lithotripter. SWs generated by this lithotripter propagate downward, so that when stones were positioned in an open-top basket, SWs could reach the stone without passing through the mesh that held the stone. This was compared to a mesh basket in the form of a cylinder, with which SWs had to pass through the mesh to reach the stone. Acoustic measurements showed that the mesh had little effect on the leading positive-pressure phase of the SW, but attenuated to some degree the tensile component of the pulse. Proximity of the mesh to F2 affected the waveforms such that the mesh positioned at 40mm prefocally was almost acoustically transparent, but the effect was much more pronounced when the mesh was within several millimeters of F2. High-speed camera images showed that cavitation was reduced beyond the mesh. Stone breakage was less efficient when SWs had to pass through the mesh to reach the stone. When SWs had to pass through the mesh, the number of SWs to break stones was 634±125 SWs, which was greater ($P<0.002$) than the 448±44 SWs needed to break stones in the open-top basket. These findings show that mesh material—generally considered to be acoustically "invisible"—may have a measureable effect on lithotripter SWs, cavitation fields, and stone breakage efficiency. These factors should be kept in mind when interpreting in vitro test results, particularly in studies assessing the performance of SW lithotripters or in studies on the mechanisms of SW action.

Keywords: shock wave lithotripsy, stone basket, cavitation bubbles, stone breakage efficiency.
PACS: 43.80.Vj, 43.80.Gx, 43.25.Yw, 43.35.Ei.

INTRODUCTION

The performance of shock wave lithotripters is often assessed by measuring the breakage efficiency of model stones. Such in vitro tests are usually performed by positioning the stones in plastic mesh baskets. We asked if the plastic mesh affects the properties of shock waves (SWs), and whether this alteration influences cavitation fields and stone breakage efficiency.

CP1049, *Renal Stone Disease 2, 2nd International Urolithiasis Research Symposium,*
edited by A. P. Evan, J. E. Lingeman, J. A. McAteer, and J. C. Williams, Jr.

MATERIALS AND METHODS

Experiments were conducted using a research electrohydraulic lithotripter patterned after the Dornier HM3 (HM3-clone lithotripter) [1], and a clinical electromagnetic lithotripter (XX-ES; Xi Xin Medical Instruments Co. Ltd., Suzhou, PRC) [2, 3].

A test mesh made of extruded polypropylene (XN 1678, Industrial Netting Inc., Minneapolis, MN, USA) was used in this study. The mesh had a hole size of about 2.5×4mm, the center-to-center distance 3.6mm across and 5.1mm along rows, a thickness of ~0.9mm, and a 60% nominal open percentage (Fig. 1).

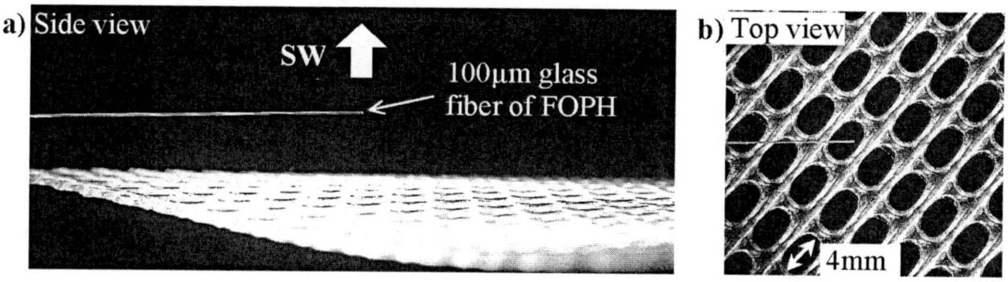

FIGURE 1. Experimental setup for measurements with the fiber-optic probe hydrophone (FOPH).

For acoustic measurements a flat sheet of the mesh was positioned ~8mm or ~40mm prefocal to the focal point (F2) of the HM3-clone lithotripter (Fig. 1). Shock waves were measured at F2 using a fiber-optic probe hydrophone (FOPH-500, RP Acoustics, Leutenbach, Germany). Waveforms were recorded in alternating sets of 30 SWs with and without the mesh. Average temporal profiles were calculated by realigning individual SWs at the half amplitude of their shock fronts [4, 5].

Visual observations to assess the effect of mesh on the cavitation field were performed in the test tank of the HM3-clone lithotripter. For these experiments a flat sheet of the mesh was positioned at the focal plane of the lithotripter (i.e., at F2, perpendicular to the acoustic axis, which was at 14° to the vertical). Cavitation bubbles were recorded using a multiframe high-speed camera (HS-camera, Imacon 468, DRS Hadland, Inc., Cupertino, CA), as previously described [6].

The effect of mesh on stone breakage was tested using the XX-ES lithotripter. Shock waves generated by this lithotripter propagate downward (the shock head sits above the treatment table) so that when stones are held in an open-top basket, SWs impact the stone directly without first passing through the mesh. Two mesh baskets were constructed (Fig. 2). Both baskets had a cylindrical shape but one of the baskets had an open top to allow SWs to reach the stone before passing through the mesh (Fig. 2a). The other basket (Fig. 2b) was a complete cylinder (~12mm diameter), and SWs had to pass through the mesh before reaching the stone. The open-top basket was larger (radius of curvature 15mm) than the closed basket to prevent particles from leaving the basket over the open top. Gypsum cement cylinders (6.5mm diameter by 7.5mm length) were used as stone phantoms [7]. The distance from the top edge of the mesh basket (Fig. 2b) to the center of the stone was ~8mm, so that SWs traveled ~8mm from the mesh to the center of the stone. Shock waves were fired at 9.3kV, 60 SW/min and the number of SWs needed to break stones to completion was counted.

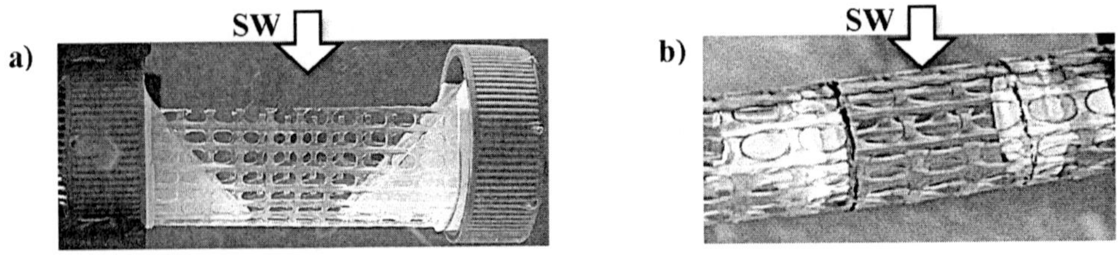

FIGURE 2. Two stone baskets made of the 2.5×4mm mesh: an open-top basket **(a)**, and a basket in the form of a cylinder **(b)**. The open-top basket **(a)** allowed the SWs generated by the XX-ES lithotripter (SWs propagate downward, arrow) to reach the stone without passing through the mesh.

RESULTS AND DISCUSSION

The mesh had little effect on the leading positive-pressure phase of the SW, but attenuated the tensile component of the wave (Fig. 3a). The mesh positioned ~8mm prefocal to the focal point of the HM3-clone lithotripter caused 40% reduction in both the momentum flux (time integral of pressure) and energy density (time integral of squared pressure) of the negative-pressure phase of the SW (Fig. 3a).

As the negative-pressure phase provides the energy for the growth of cavitation bubbles, we hypothesized that reduction in the tensile component of the SWs should be associated with reduced cavitation [8]. High-speed camera images appear to support this hypothesis. Figure 4 shows a high-speed camera sequence showing growth and collapse of cavitation bubbles along the axis of the HM3-clone lithotripter with the mesh positioned at the focal plane of the lithotripter. Proximal to the mesh, the cavitation bubble cloud appeared to be denser (frames 280-480μs) and lived longer (frames 480-580μs) than cavitation bubbles located distal to the mesh.

Figure 4 also provides a slight hint that cavitation was increased in the proximal vicinity of the mesh (frames 280-480μs). This increased cavitation may be, in part, due to the partial reflection by the mesh. In addition, the mesh could provide extra nucleation sites for cavitation. Zooming up the HS-camera lens on the mesh showed that cavitation bubbles were consistently formed at both the proximal and distal surfaces of the mesh. A high-speed camera sequence showing the formation of cavitation bubbles at the distal surface of the mesh is shown in Fig. 5.

Previous studies have shown that cavitation reduces the negative-pressure of the SW [4, 9, 10, 11]. Thus, it seems reasonable to suggest that additional cavitation bubbles formed in association with the mesh (Figs. 4-5) could be responsible for the observed reduction in negative-pressure phase of the SW distal to the mesh.

As cavitation fields could vary dramatically from shot-to-shot [10], a strict study would require a statistical analysis of cavitation fields. This was not attempted in this work. With this caveat, Fig. 4 shows that the cavitation bubble cloud extended up to ~4cm prefocally, which means that at that distance cavitation was not as strong as in the focal area of the lithotripter. When the mesh was positioned at that distance (40mm prefocally), the momentum flux and energy density of the negative-pressure phase of the SWs were reduced only by ~16% (Fig. 3b). This suggests that when cavitation was diminished, the mesh had little-to-no effect on SWs.

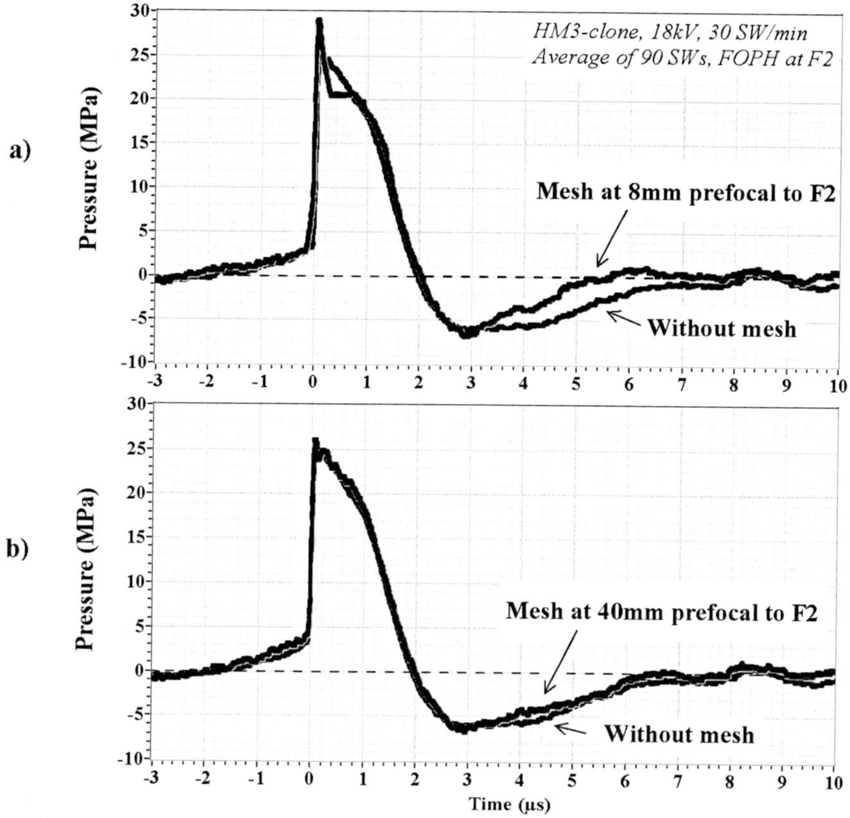

FIGURE 3. The mesh had little effect on the leading positive pressure phase of the SWs, but attenuated the tensile component of the pulse. The mesh at 8mm **(a)** reduced the momentum and the energy density of the negative-pressure phase by 40% (20.5 versus 12.3 μs×MPa, and 95 versus 57 μs×(MPa)^2, respectively). This effect was negligible when the mesh was positioned at 40mm prefocal to F2 **(b)**.

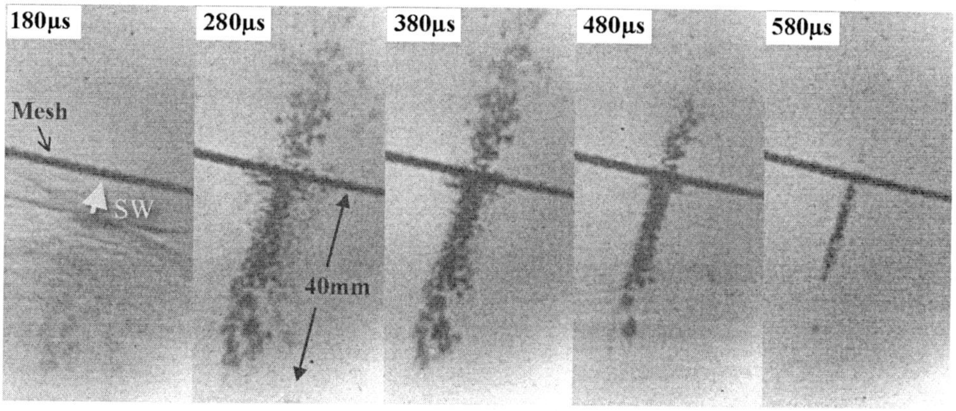

FIGURE 4. Shadowgraph photography of cavitation bubbles proximal to and distal to the mesh. Shadow of the shock front is seen at 180μs. Subsequent frames (280-580μs) show growth and collapse of cavitation bubbles (bubbles are visible as dark spots). Cavitation was reduced beyond the mesh.

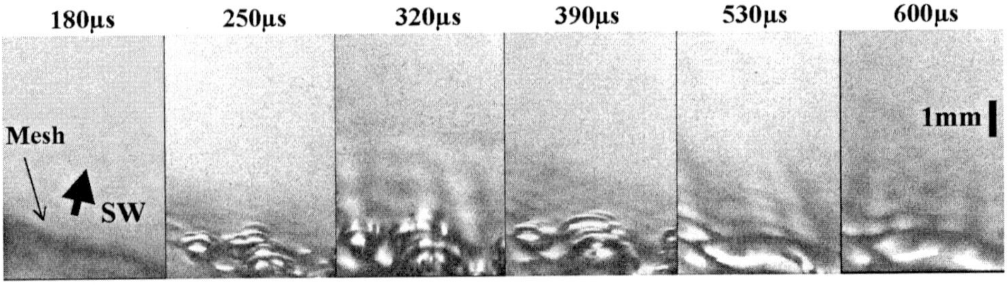

FIGURE 5. Cavitation bubbles on the distal surface of the mesh. The first frame (180μs) was recorded immediately prior of the arrival of the shock front to the mesh (see the first frame in Fig. 4). No bubbles were observed prior to or during the passage of the leading positive-pressure phase of the SW. The negative-pressure phase of the SW gave rise to the growth of cavitation bubbles. While bubbles were consistently observed at the distal surface of the mesh, few bubbles were typically seen beyond the mesh with this field of view of the camera.

These and other [4,6,9,11] high-speed camera observations show that, after the passage of the lithotripter pulse, cavitation bubbles continue their inertial growth for several hundred microseconds and then start to collapse. This lifespan of cavitation bubbles is very short in comparison to the 0.5-2 second interval between SWs. As the incoming SWs did not encounter large cavitation bubbles, the leading positive-pressure phase of the pulse was unaffected by cavitation bubbles [4,9,11]. Small pressure oscillations (seen immediately beyond the shock front in Fig. 3a) were most likely caused by diffraction of the SW on the polypropylene filaments of the mesh. However, no reduction of the positive-pressure phase of the SWs was detected.

Stone breakage was less efficient when SWs had to pass through the mesh to reach the stone (Fig. 6). When SWs had to pass through the mesh, the number of SWs to break stones was 634±125 SWs, which was greater ($P<0.002$) than the 448±44 SWs needed to break stones in the open-top basket (baskets are shown in Fig. 2).

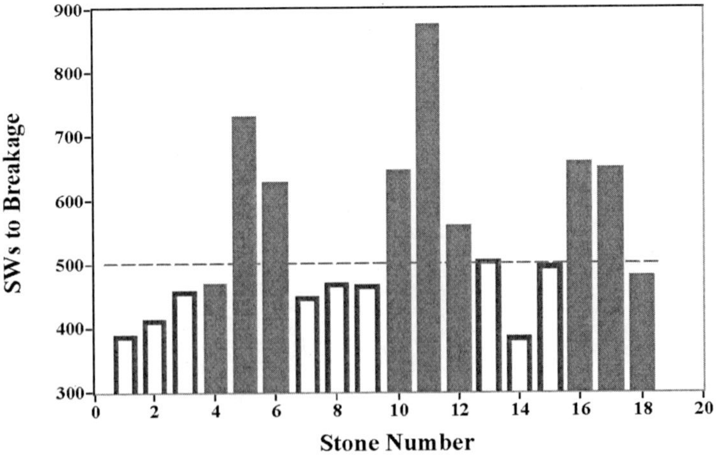

FIGURE 6. Stone breakage using the open-top basket (empty bars) and the closed cylindrical basket (filled bars). Significantly more SWs were needed when SWs had to pass through the mesh (filled bars).

These findings show that meshes used to hold model stones for assessment of lithotripter performance or for studies of the mechanisms of SW action have an effect on waveforms, cavitation, and stone breakage. The positive-pressure phase of the SW was not much affected, but the negative-pressure component was attenuated (Fig. 3a).

Since this effect involves cavitation, it is likely threshold dependent and nonlinear. This means that the mesh can be acoustically transparent for small-amplitude waves, but starts to affect pressure waves when their amplitude exceeds the cavitation threshold. The reduction of the negative-pressure phase was negligible when the mesh was positioned 40mm prefocally (Fig. 3b). However, when the mesh was positioned in the strong acoustic field—in the vicinity of the focus of the lithotripter—it consistently reduced the negative-pressure phase of the SWs (Fig. 3a). This attenuation of the negative-pressure phase of the SWs caused a reduction in cavitation beyond the mesh (Fig. 4). Since cavitation is understood to play a prominent role in stone comminution, it seems reasonable to suggest that mesh stone holders—even materials generally considered to be acoustically "invisible"—may have a measureable effect on stone breakage. The present results for stone breakage (Fig. 6) support this hypothesis. These factors should be kept in mind when interpreting in vitro test results, particularly in studies on the mechanisms of SW action in stone breakage.

ACKNOWLEDGMENTS

Supported by a grant from the National Institutes of Health (DK-43881).

REFERENCES

1. R. O. Cleveland, M. R. Bailey, N. S. Fineberg, B. Hartenbaum, M. Lokhandwalla, J. A. McAteer and B. Sturtevant, *Review of Scientific Instruments* **71 (6)**, 2514-2525 (2000).
2. W. Eisenmenger, X. X. Du, C. Tang, S. Zhao, Y. Wang, F. Rong, D. Dai, M. Guan and A. Qi, *Ultrasound Med Biol* **28 (6)**, 769-774 (2002).
3. A. P. Evan, J. A. McAteer, B. A. Connors, Y. A. Pishchalnikov, R. K. Handa, P. Blomgren, L. R. Willis, J. C. Williams, Jr., J. E. Lingeman and S. Gao, *BJU Int* **101 (3)**, 382-388 (2008).
4. Y. A. Pishchalnikov, O. A. Sapozhnikov, M. R. Bailey, I. V. Pishchalnikova, J. C. Williams, Jr. and J. A. McAteer, *Acoust Res Letters Online* **6 (4)**, 280-286 (2005).
5. Y. A. Pishchalnikov, J. A. McAteer, R. J. Vonderhaar, I. V. Pishchalnikova, J. C. Williams, Jr. and A. P. Evan, *J Urol* **176 (5)**, 2294-2298 (2006).
6. Y. A. Pishchalnikov, O. A. Sapozhnikov, M. R. Bailey, J. C. Williams, Jr., R. O. Cleveland, T. Colonius, L. A. Crum, A. P. Evan and J. A. McAteer, *J Endourol* **17 (7)**, 435-446 (2003).
7. J. A. McAteer, J. C. Williams, Jr., R. O. Cleveland, J. Van Cauwelaert, M. R. Bailey, D. A. Lifshitz and A. P. Evan, *Urol Res* **33 (6)**, 429-434 (2005).
8. Y. A. Pishchalnikov, M. M. Kaehr and J. A. McAteer, in *2007 ASME International Mechanical Engineering Congress and Exposition* (Seattle, WA, November 11-15, 2007, 2007), The American Society of Mechanical Engineers, New York, paper IMECE2007-41387, pp. 1-10.
9. Y. A. Pishchalnikov, J. A. McAteer, J. C. Williams, Jr., I. V. Pishchalnikova and R. J. Vonderhaar, *J Endourol* **20 (8)**, 537-541 (2006).
10. Y. A. Pishchalnikov, Kreider W., J. A. McAteer, J. C. Williams, Jr., , I. V. Pishchalnikova and M. R. Bailey, in *Acoustics for the 21st Century*, (Proceedings of the 19th International Congress on Acoustics, Madrid, Spain, 2-7 September 2007), paper NLA-02-005-IP, pp. 1-6.
11. Y. A. Pishchalnikov, J. A. McAteer and J. C. Williams, Jr., *BJU Int*, in print (2008).

A Prototype Ultrasound Instrument To Size Stone Fragments During Ureteroscopy

Mathew D. Sorensen[a], Joel M. H. Teichman[b] and Michael R. Bailey[c]

[a]*Department of Urology, University of Washington School of Medicine 1959 NE Pacific Street, Box 356510, Seattle, WA 98195*
[b]*Division of Urology, Providence Healthcare and Department of Urologic Sciences, University of British Columbia, 2775 Laurel Street, Vancouver, BC V5Z1M9*
[c]*Center for Industrial and Medical Ultrasound, Applied Physics Laboratory, University of Washington 1013 NE 40th Street, Seattle, WA 98105*

Abstract. An intraoperative tool to measure the size of kidney stones or stone fragments during ureteroscopy would help urologists assess if a fragment is small enough to be removed through the ureter or ureteral access sheath. The goal of this study was to determine the accuracy and precision of a prototype ultrasound device used to measure *in vitro* stone fragments compared to caliper measurements. A 10-MHz, 10-french ultrasound transducer probe was used to send an ultrasound pulse and receive ultrasound reflections from the stone using two methods. In Method 1 the instrument was aligned over the stone and the ultrasound pulse traveled through the stone. The time between reflections from the proximal and the distal surface of the stone were used along with the sound speed to calculate the stone size. Although the sound speed varied between stones, it was unlikely to be known during surgery and thus was estimated at 3000 m/s for calculations. In Method 2 the instrument was aligned partially over the stone and the ultrasound pulse traveled through water with a sound speed of 1481 m/s. Time was determined between the reflection from the proximal stone surface and the reflection from the tissue phantom on which the stone rested. Methods 1 and 2 were compared by linear regression to caliper measurements of the size of 19 human stones of 3 different stone types. Accuracy was measured by the difference of the mean ultrasound and mean caliper measurement and precision was measured as the standard deviation in the ultrasound measurements. For Method 1, the correlation between caliper-determined stone size and ultrasound-determined stone size was $r^2=0.71$ ($p<0.0001$). In all but two stones accuracy and precision were less than 1 mm. For Method 2, the correlation was $r^2=0.99$ ($p<0.0001$) and measurements were accurate and precise to within 0.25 mm. We conclude that the prototype device and either method measure stone size with good accuracy.

Keywords: ultrasound, ureteroscopy, stone fragment size
PACS: 43.80.Vj

BACKGROUND

Ureteroscopy often requires extraction of stone fragments by grasping them in a basket and pulling them along the ureteral tract. Fragments may be too large to pass easily but must be small enough to fit through the ureter [1]. Basket removal of fragments may be faster than continued intracorporeal lithotripsy, provided delays are not incurred from attempting to extract fragments too large to remove through narrow

CP1049, *Renal Stone Disease 2, 2nd International Urolithiasis Research Symposium,* edited by A. P. Evan, J. E. Lingeman, J. A. McAteer, and J. C. Williams, Jr.

portions of the ureter or the ureteral access sheath. Attempted extraction of large fragments may result in injury to the ureter or time lost repositioning the stone into the collecting system, disassembling the basket apparatus, or breaking the stone within the basket [2]. Currently, estimating stone size during ureteroscopy is subjective. This report describes a prototype ultrasound technology to size stones or stone fragments that may be adapted for digital ureteroscopy.

METHODS

Single stones from 19 separate patients were obtained from a stone reference laboratory (Figure 1). All stones were > 95% pure composition. Three different types of stones (7 calcium oxalate monohydrate, 6 cystine, 6 calcium hydrogen phosphate dihydrate), of a variety of shapes were rehydrated for 24 hours in deionized water. Each stone was placed on a solid planar surface and its height from the surface measured using manual calipers; mean and standard deviation were recorded (Figure 2). The stone was then placed in the same orientation on a planar kidney tissue phantom (Sylgard silicone elastomer, Dow Corning Corporation, Midland, MI; plastic microspheres, The PQ Corporation Valley Forge PA; and nickel powder, Alfa Aesar, Ward Hill MA) and submerged in 20°C water.

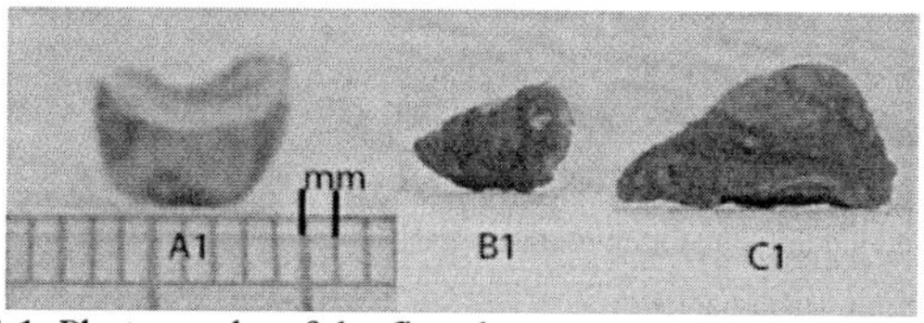

FIGURE 1. Photographs of the first three stones measured in this study.

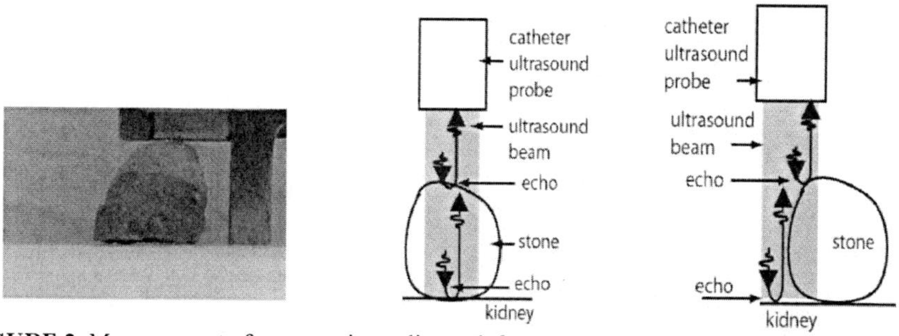

FIGURE 2. Measurement of stones using calipers (left), Method 1 (center) and Method 2 (right).

A 10 MHz, 1/8" diameter (10 french) transducer probe (model M112, Panametrics NDT [now Olympus NDT] Waltham MA) sent and received ultrasound pulses through a pulse receiver (Model 5072PR, Olympus NDT) at 100 Hz. The received signals were displayed in real time on a digital oscilloscope. Ultrasound measurements were then obtained using two different methods (Figure 2). In Method 1, the wave traveled through the stone returning echoes from structure throughout the full thickness of the stone. In Method 2, ultrasound beam was placed so that some of the pulse reflected from the stone's proximal surface and some from the kidney tissue phantom on which the stone rested.

In Method 1, there is continuous signal from the internal structure of the stone. The time of interest was determined from the duration of the signal (Figure 3). In Method 2, the time of interest was determined from the start of each signal. There was negligible detected echo between the two signals because of few scattering objects in the water. Stone thickness was calculated by

$$D = ct/2 \qquad (1)$$

where D = thickness of the stone; c = speed of sound; t = time. The "2" is included because the pulse passes through the stone once, reflects from the distal side and passes back through the stone a second time. The accuracy of Method 1 could be improved if the exact sound speed for each stone were known and used, but since this is unlikely to be known intraoperatively, we used 3000 m/s in all cases [3]. In Method 2, the sound speed of water (or urine in practice) is predictable within a few percent and for 20°C water the sound speed is 1481 m/s. Measurements were all repeated three times and mean and standard deviations are reported.

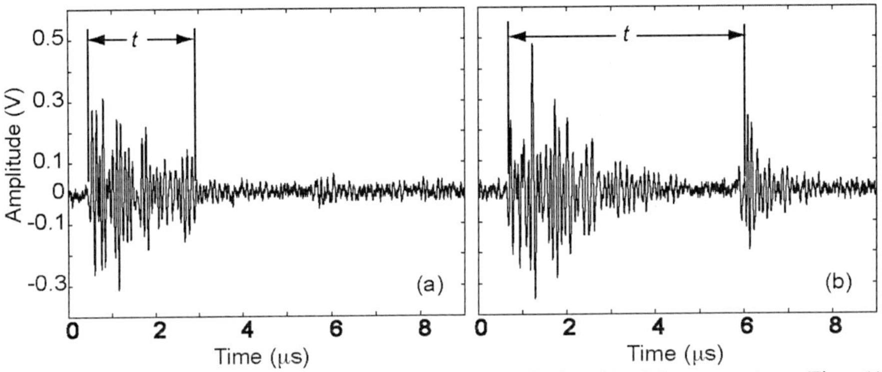

FIGURE 3. Representative signal for Method 1 (a) and Method 2 (b) of the same stone. Time (t) of interest was measured for the duration of Method 1 spike and the difference between the two spikes for Method 2. Note the t measured with Method 1 is roughly half that measured with Method 2 because the sound speed in stone (Method 1) is roughly twice that of the sound speed in water (Method 2).

The operator aligned the transducer by hand and recorded three signals for each of the two methods. The operator aligned the transducer probe visually but made final decisions by watching the oscilloscope and aligning to capture a clear signal. The signals were then analyzed by a blinded investigator to determine the time of interest used to calculate stone size. Regression analyses were performed to evaluate the correlation between mean caliper measurements and ultrasound based measurements.

RESULTS

Both Method 1 and Method 2 yielded a measurement for each stone (Figure 4). Caliper measurements and the two ultrasound measurements were all very similar with error bars smaller than the mean values. Both ultrasound methods slightly overestimated the size of some stones and underestimated the size of other stones, but with no observed differential effect of stone type. In all cases, the precision indicated by the standard deviation was less than 1 mm in Method 1 and 0.2 mm in Method 2. Compared to caliper measurement, accuracy was excellent for all stones using Method 2 while Method 1 differed from caliper measurements by more than 1mm for three stones. Correlation between the caliper measurements and Method 1 measurements was r^2=0.71 ($p<0.0001$). Correlation between the caliper measurements and Method 2 was r^2=0.99 ($p<0.0001$).

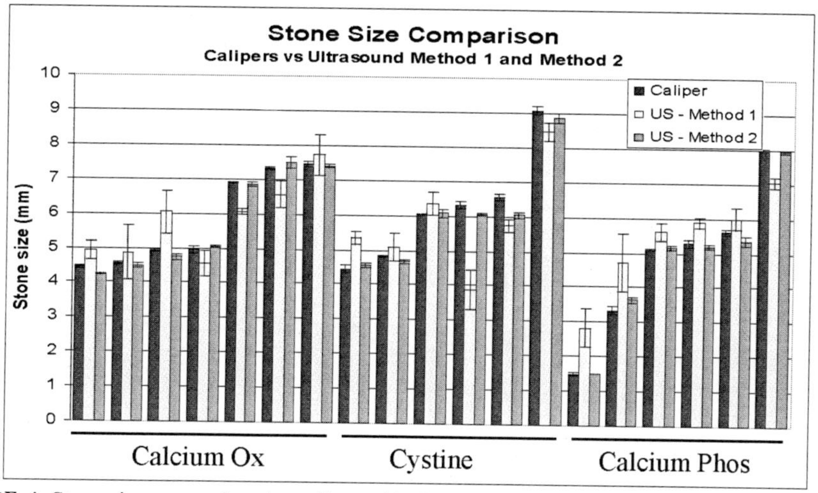

FIGURE 4. Stone size comparison by calipers (black), Method 1 (white) and Method 2 (gray). Mean and standard deviation of three measurements are shown.

CONCLUSIONS

Instrument-based ultrasound accurately and precisely measured stone fragment size by two methods. The methods rely on obtaining reflections from the stone and, for Method 2, the surface upon which the stone rests. Measurements were made using a hand-held transducer as would be done in surgery. Flat, hard surfaces give the strongest reflections; however, even irregularly shaped stones and a soft tissue kidney phantom produced reflections that registered nearly one-half volt on the oscilloscope. Both methods by this measure were sensitive and could survive the drop in sensitivity likely to occur when a smaller transducer is trialed for clinical use. This technology offers promise for real-time fragmentation size measurements during ureteroscopy.

ACKNOWLEDGMENTS

This work was supported by grants NIH DK43881 and NSBRI SMS00402.

REFERENCES

1. J.M.H. Teichman, G.J. Vassar, J.T. Bishoff, G.C. Bellman, *J Urology* Jan;**159(1)**:17-23 (1998).
2. J.M.H. Teichman, A.D. Kamerer, *Journal of Urology* Nov;**164(5)**:1602-3 (2000).
3. C.J. Chuong, P. Zhong, G.M. Preminger, *Journal of Endourology* Dec;**7(6)**:437-44 (1993).

Author Index